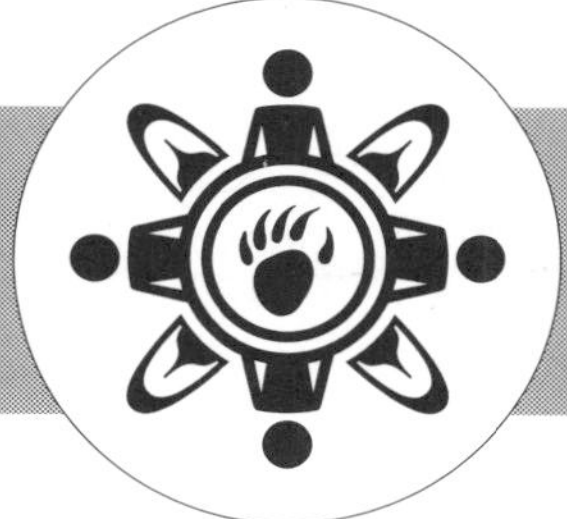

The Path to Healing

Report of the National Round Table on Aboriginal Health and Social Issues

Royal Commission on Aboriginal Peoples

Available in Canada through
your local bookseller
or by mail from
Canada Communication Group – Publishing
Ottawa, Canada K1A 0S9

Canadian Cataloguing in Publication Data
National Round Table on Aboriginal Health and Social Issues
(1993: Vancouver, B.C.)
The path to healing: report of the
National Round Table on Aboriginal Health and Social Issues

Cat. no. Z1-1991/1-11-4E
ISBN 0-660-15173-1

1. Native peoples – Canada – Health aspects.
2. Native peoples – Canada – Social conditions.
I. Canada. Royal Commission on Aboriginal Peoples.
II. Title. III. Title: Report of the National Round Table on
Aboriginal Health and Social Issues.

E78.C2N37 1993 971'.00497 C93-099614-3

Issued also in French under the title:
Sur le chemin de la guérison.

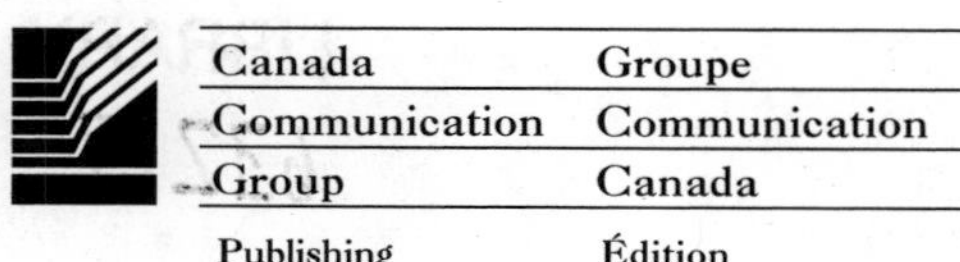

Contents

Members of the Royal Commission on Aboriginal Peoples

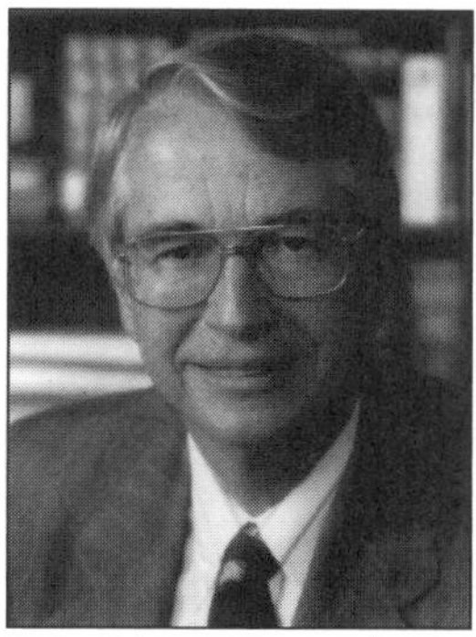

René Dussault, j.c.a.
Co-Chair

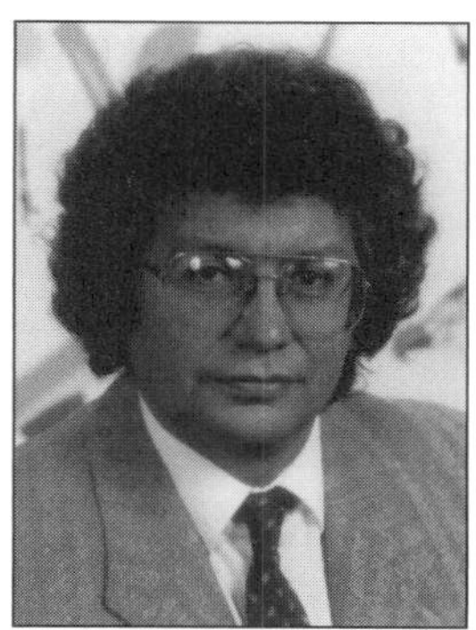

Georges Erasmus
Co-Chair

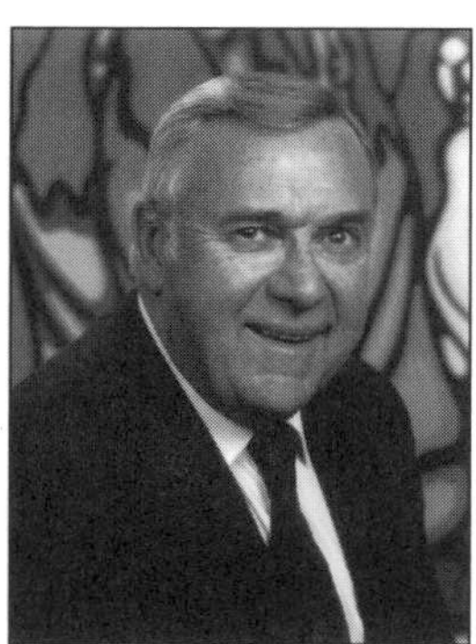

Allan Blakeney
Commissioner

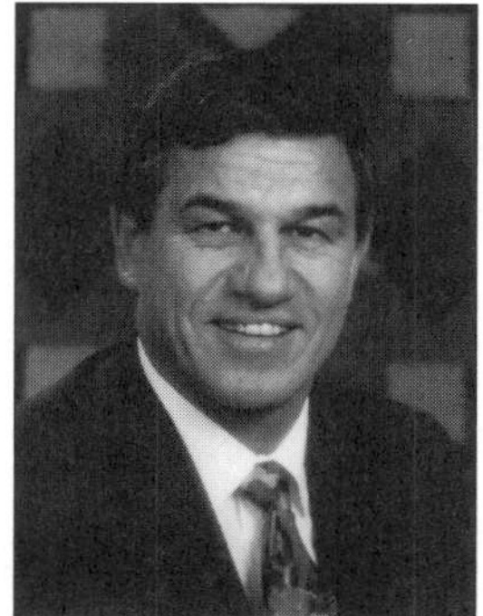

Paul Chartrand
Commissioner

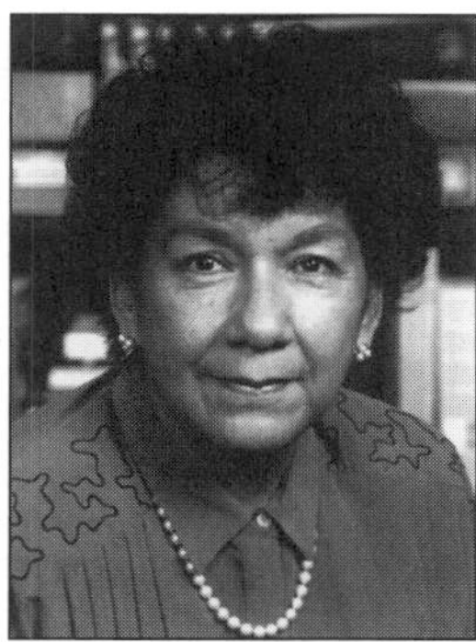

Viola Marie Robinson
Commissioner

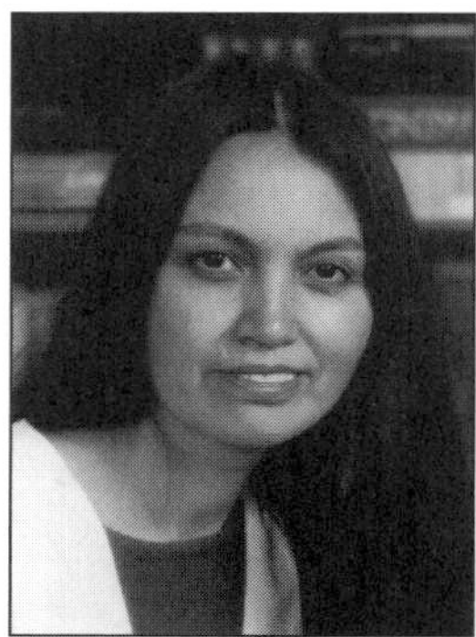

Mary Sillett
Commissioner

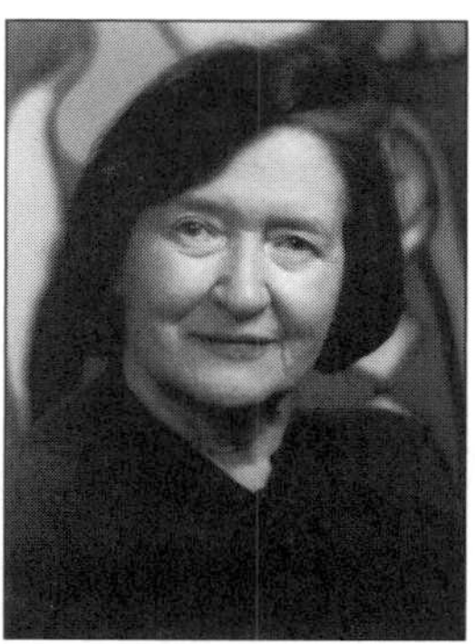

Bertha Wilson
Commissioner

Preface

The Royal Commission on Aboriginal Peoples has undertaken to host a series of National Round Tables on selected themes. The Round Tables bring together academics, practitioners, political leaders and community leaders with knowledge and expertise on the selected themes in order to assist the Commission in the preparation of recommendations for the final report.

The National Round Tables all have a similar format. We invite certain experts or leading-edge thinkers to produce papers on a series of questions that we intend to ask participants to consider. In the course of panel presentations, round table discussions and plenary sessions, participants have the opportunity to put forward their views and recommendations as they relate to the questions. A rapporteur is asked to write a report based on the proceedings of the round table setting out what was said, along with any recommendations or consensus that may have been reached by participants.

The published proceedings of the National Round Tables will help to inform the general public about the issues addressed there. It is anticipated that publication of the round table proceedings will prompt further consideration of the ideas and debate captured in the reports and encourage Canadians to come forward at the public hearings or to make written submissions with further thoughts and recommendations.

We are deeply indebted to all participants in the National Round Table on Aboriginal Health and Social Issues for their input and advice, and to Dr. John D. O'Neil, who prepared the Round Table report presented in this volume.

This report of the proceedings is intended to stimulate further dialogue and positive changes in policy. Your views and recommendations on this important issue are welcome. We invite you to write to us at the address set out elsewhere in this document and to appear before us when we hold public hearings in your area.

René Dussault, j.c.a.
Co-Chair

Georges Erasmus
Co-Chair

Introduction

*Louis T. Montour**

Elders, Participants, Commissioners and Observers. Greetings and welcome to the National Round Table on Aboriginal Health and Social Issues. It is a great pleasure for me to be here today and to have the honour and privilege of serving as Round Table Chairman. I am thankful for the opportunity to contribute in any way I can to the historic work of this Royal Commission and I look forward to working with all of you. Together with good minds, we can all assist the Commission in completing its important work.

Over the next few days, we will be focusing our undivided attention on a number of important themes relating to health and social issues in Aboriginal communities – issues that have received much press coverage in recent days, but little action over the years. By reviewing your agenda, you will see that our task is significant in terms of our making a major contribution to the work of the Royal Commission on Aboriginal Peoples. This National Round Table is the third in a series of major focus sessions of the Royal Commission. As part of the Commission's public consultation and education process, we have an opportunity to make an historic impact on changing the reality of health and social conditions in Aboriginal communities today. We have an obligation to future generations yet unborn to do our very best.

---

* Dr. Montour, who is the director of professional servces, Kateri Memorial Hospital, Kahnawake, Quebec, chaired the National Round Table on Aboriginal Health and Social Issues.

It is important therefore for us to understand, acknowledge and consider the testimony already provided to Commissioners by individuals and organizations, Aboriginal and non-Aboriginal, right across the country. Although I personally have not previously been involved with the Commission, I am informed of two documents soon to be published by the Commission: one document provides an overview of what was heard during the second round of public hearings; the other document synthesizes those views into a discussion paper.

There have been numerous of reports, studies and surveys completed over the last twenty years, each with their own set of relevant recommendations. To what degree or extent have such recommendations been implemented? And what are the obstacles that must still be tackled? Presenters have referred Commissioners to examples that demand answers. Why must so many studies be undertaken, and what is preventing the implementation of their recommendations?

To cite a few examples:

- The Alberta Mental Health Association (Lac La Biche, Alberta, June 1992) referred to a community that had 26 private consultants coming in, doing work and leaving: 26 people at one time. They wondered why efforts had not been made to instead co-ordinate the expertise needed and focus on preventative measures.
- The Swampy Cree Tribal Council and Health Centre (The Pas, Manitoba, May 1992) described to Commissioners the obstacles they've been encountering for almost 30 years regarding health transfer.
- A study examining the extent and degree of alcohol and drug abuse in urban communities completed by the National Association of Friendship Centres in 1985 is "still being considered".
- And recently, we have seen the pain and suffering endured by the Innu children of Davis Inlet, and what we know about Davis Inlet continues in many Aboriginal communities across the country.

Many presenters noted that although a major impediment is a lack of resources – financial, human and physical – there are other barriers. Aboriginal women appearing before the Commission spoke strongly about family violence issues and about the need for healing the individual, the family, the community and ultimately the nation. But what is preventing the application of these Aboriginal-designed strategies from being implemented? Aboriginal youth have expressed in very clear terms their concerns about their future. Dennis Peters, a student at the Crocus Plains Secondary School in Brandon, Manitoba said, "You should provide children with examples of the right things to do: teach kids how to live, not how to die."

The Commission was also told that there will be no fundamental change unless and until cultural identity and cultural wholeness are restored. The further message that comes through is that no health or social issue can be 'cured' if the problems are approached in a piecemeal fashion. Health and social issues must all be addressed as part of a systematic understanding of the links between oppression and self-destruction. And they must lead to culturally appropriate means and sites for change and recovery.

Over the next three days, we will hear from First Nations, Inuit and Métis peoples sharing descriptions of their initiatives in changing things in their communities. By understanding more about these initiatives and other models, we will have an opportunity to further the dialogue on content and priorities that will shape the recommendations of the Royal Commission.

The Commission has published its second discussion document, *Focusing the Dialogue*; one of its major focuses is healing. Based on what the Commission has heard to date, there appear to be five recurring themes among the approaches to healing:

1. Parity in medical and social service standards
The Yukon Medical Association, appearing in Teslin, Yukon said, "The average Canadian is unaware of the degree of ill health in the Aboriginal population in Canada. It is a fact that in many areas of this country, the health of Aboriginal peoples is equivalent to poor third world standards."

2. Focus on self-esteem
Violet Mundy of the Ucluelet Health Committee in Port Alberni, B.C. said that "modern medicine [needs to learn] that self-esteem is an important part of being a healthy human being. By feeling good about yourself, by knowing that you have value, that your life means something, you will have the confidence to lead a healthy life."

3. Recognition of traditional healing and traditional culture
The vision statement of the Native Child and Family Services of Toronto speaks to "providing for a life of quality, well-being, caring and healing for our children and families ... it does this by creating a service model that is culture-based respecting the supreme values of Native people, the extended family and the right to self-determination."

4. Holistic approaches to critical symptoms
Sophie Pierre, administrator of the Tunaxa/Kinbasket Tribal Council, said in Cranbrook: "Wellness encompasses all areas of human development...if any of the facets is in need of healing, a complete range of related solutions is necessary."

5. Aboriginal and community control of programming
Henoch Obed, an addictions counsellor with the Labrador Inuit and Drug Abuse Program, told Commissioners in Nain that "there must be full recognition of [Inuit] Aboriginal rights and promotion of cultural health and pride, and that a strong Inuit identity must be a pre-condition to good effective emotional, spiritual, physical and mental health upon which all services must be provided."

These excerpts from testimony at the public hearings are just a sampling of what the Commission has heard.

And so we come back to our task – why we are here. Although health and social issues are the topic of this Round Table, you must always bear in mind that health problems and social problems in Aboriginal communities are not end-points in and of themselves, but rather are symptoms of a larger ill. The approach to a community with symptoms is no different from the approach to an individual with symptoms – identify and treat the cause, and the symptoms will go away.

What is this illness? To quote Dr. Clare Brant quoting Ramon Cajal in 1899, "Every disease has two causes. The first is pathophysiological; the second, political." As all of you know, Indian medicine *is* political.

It would do us all well to recall that our work and our recommendations – to quote Alma Favel-King in her paper on the Treaty Right to Health – will be achievable only if the federal government is serious in addressing the health and social needs of Aboriginal people.

So, what is the illness?

Loss. Multiple losses. To quote Bea Shawanda, "multigenerational trauma and grief". Loss of ways of life. Loss of language. Loss of ceremonies and traditions. Loss of a land base. Loss of meaningful control over day-to-day life.

Despite this picture of multiple loss, there are reservoirs of strength and pockets of traditionalism still present in Aboriginal communities right across the country. There is mention by several of the presenters of a renaissance of traditionalism burning across the land. It remains for us to nurture and fan this flame. I was trying hard to avoid the word 'culture'. That, too, is one of our losses. As a simple, practical measure, we must remember that *language is culture*, and we should repeat here and from all the rooftops to all Aboriginal communities everywhere, *learn* your language, *use* your language, *save* your language.

Canada must renegotiate a new social contract with its Aboriginal peoples, including a land base, economic autonomy and political self-control. Health improvements and social improvements will assuredly follow.

I hope over the next three days that we can draw on our strengths and develop ideas and that these deliberations can be directly and practically applied to the benefit of all Aboriginal people.

With your knowledge, expertise and wisdom, we have an opportunity to address the fundamental questions facing us and suggest concrete measures to contribute to a path of reconciliation in this country.

Report from the Round Table Rapporteur

*John D. O'Neil**

This paper was commissioned by the Royal Commission on Aboriginal Peoples to provide a summary of the proceedings of the National Round Table on Aboriginal Health and Social Issues, held in Vancouver March 10-12, 1993. Portions of this summary were provided to participants at the Round Table in an oral presentation at the end of the conference. Ideas first presented there have been developed further in this paper. A draft of this paper was circulated to the Commission Co-Chairs and others involved in organizing the Round Table, and their comments have been incorporated.

The National Round Table on Aboriginal Health and Social Issues brought together approximately 80 people from across the country actively involved in health development in Aboriginal communities. Most of participants were Aboriginal health workers, including physicians, nurses, CHRs, social workers, administrators, and scholars. Four Aboriginal elders representing Inuit, Métis, and other First Nations communities provided guidance to the discussion. The remainder of the participants were either non-Aboriginal health workers and scholars active in the field of Aboriginal health development, or representatives from the federal and provincial ministries responsible for health development in Aboriginal communities.

* PhD, Associate Professor of Medical Anthropology and National Health Research Scholar, Northern Health Research Unit, Department of Community Health Sciences, University of Manitoba.

The program included the presentation of eleven background papers commissioned by the Royal Commission. The background papers were reviewed and the principal ideas are included in this summary. In addition to these discussion papers, eight community projects were described detailing community-based developments in health and social services from across the country. These also inform the summary in an essential way.

Keynote addresses by Dr. Harriet Kuhnlein on Global Nutrition and the Holistic Environment of Indigenous Peoples and by Professor Robert Evans on global health economics further informed the Round Table discussions.

The Round Table could be characterized as generating two powerful and seemingly opposed feelings among various participants. These feelings were sometimes expressed formally during the discussion periods and at other times informally over coffee in the hallways. On the one hand, participants shared a sense of frustration with the inability of various levels of government and the health care system to respond adequately to the desperate needs of some Aboriginal communities. This frustration also extended to some extent to the Round Table process, in that many participants felt that further discussion and study of the issues was not moving us closer to solutions.

At the same time, however, a strong sense of optimism and confidence was apparent at the Round Table, reflecting the remarkable accomplishments of many Aboriginal communities in the health development field. This optimism was also stimulated by the obvious recognition that Aboriginal health is increasingly in very capable Aboriginal hands. Again, optimism was reflected in the consensual spirit of the Round Table, despite the ongoing frustration experienced by most participants with an external environment that reinforces conflicts among different Aboriginal groups and different paradigmatic approaches to health and healing. For example, this Round Table provided a rare opportunity for the joint consideration of diverse approaches to health and healing representing various Aboriginal traditions as well as western medical practices.

Major Thematic Concerns

Theme 1: Fourth World Health Conditions

In developing this summary of the Round Table, my first draft did not include a health conditions theme because, by and large, health conditions in the various and diverse Aboriginal communities were absent from most of the discussion. With the exception of my own background paper, Dr. Brandt's discussion of suicide rates and mental health conditions, Professor Larocque's identification of the proportion of women who are victims of violence in Aboriginal communities, and Ms. Sinclair's and Mr. Tomkins' description of Aboriginal people with disabilities, there was little attention to the underlying health problems and their distribution in Aboriginal societies. For example, no one described the problem of diabetes during formal discussions. While this absence of discussion might be considered surprising and seen as a flaw in the Round Table discussions, in fact I believe an awareness of these conditions was just below the surface of many presentations and commentary. Indeed, as I pointed out in my oral report, I believe Round Table participants were keenly aware of the 'ticking clock' and the number of otherwise preventable deaths that were occurring in Aboriginal communities even as the conference proceeded.

The chief characteristic of health conditions in Aboriginal communities is that mortality and morbidity from both infectious and chronic disease (e.g., deaths and sickness from diseases such as tuberculosis and diabetes) exceed Canadian averages in most areas. Even for diseases such as cancer or heart disease, where current conditions are similar to Canadian standards, there is growing evidence that these problems may increase dramatically in the not too distant future. A further characteristic of fourth-world health conditions is the high prevalence (i.e., the proportion of people suffering from the problem) of socially derived problems such as domestic violence, suicide, and alcohol abuse, which reflect typically urban conditions of poverty, political alienation and racial discrimination.

Despite these conditions, it is important to note that the illness care system (as described by Professor Evans) was initiated historically in Aboriginal communities in response to high rates of infectious diseases, such as tuberculosis, but has remained largely unresponsive to changes in the pattern of health problems reflecting chronic illness and social problems. In particular, many of the problems now confronting Aboriginal communities can be addressed more effectively in a health promotion framework (rather than from a curative approach), but this shift in focus has been difficult for an illness care system oriented to the treatment of infectious disease.

A final concern expressed at the Round Table by many participants is the problem of adopting a universal and status-blind approach to the description of Aboriginal health conditions. Most of the current epidemiological literature is based on data derived from status populations (Inuit and First Nations people living on reserve) for whom Medical Services Branch and the Department of Indian Affairs and Northern Development are responsible for service provision. Round Table participants argued that for the roughly two-thirds of Aboriginal people living off reserve, and particularly in urban areas, these data do not accurately reflect the health conditions for most Aboriginal peoples in Canada. Further, some Aboriginal regions and communities suffer from health and social problems at far higher rates than others; indeed many Aboriginal communities should be characterized as healthy. Clearly, an accurate picture of health conditions off reserve and outside the Territories is required if health service planning is to be grounded in the real needs of Aboriginal communities.

Theme 2: Environmental Context

At times understated, but nonetheless consistent throughout the Round Table, was the recognition that health is determined by much more than services provided by professional caregivers. In his presentation describing conditions surrounding suicide in Aboriginal communities, Dr. Clare Brandt specifically identified poverty, despair, poor housing and political alienation as the root causes for the traumatic mental health problems that plague many Aboriginal communities. Other speakers, such as Professor Evans and Dr. Kuhnlein, further distinguished between the relative contribution that environmental conditions and medical (or illness) services contribute to improvements in health. Historically, in society generally, health improvements have come about as improvements in the social infrastructure and the economy have changed; where water supply, sanitation, housing, economic and recreational opportunities have improved, so has the health of the general population.

Other participants reflected on the paradigm shift, outlined by Rosemary Proctor, required to shift our energies from a narrow illness service model to a more holistic, integrated, multi-disciplinary, and multi-sectoral approach to improving Aboriginal health conditions. Some participants emphasized, however, that the Euro-Canadian concept of holistic health care, while an important development within western society, is only a pale reflection of the holistic approaches to health that characterize Aboriginal traditions. These traditions, which emphasize the multi-dimensional nature of people as physical, mental, emotional and spiritual beings, must inform Aboriginal health development. Indeed, many participants emphasized the conceptual sophistication of Aboriginal approaches to holistic health, which western approaches are increasingly attempting to incorporate.

Participants also acknowledged the important point made by Professor Evans, who demonstrated graphically that illness care services are using up financial resources that might be directed more profitably to broader community development.

From both the Aboriginal and the Euro-Canadian perspective, however, participants agreed that basic changes in the political and economic conditions of Aboriginal community life are essential for long-term health development. These changes must include secure access to traditional lands and food resources, as well as self-governing structures that remove the yoke of colonialism, which has damaged the spirit of many Aboriginal people.

Theme 3: Aboriginal Cultural Foundations to Understanding Health

Guided primarily by the elders' wise contributions to the Round Table, many participants articulated the important premise that Aboriginal healing is a way of life rather than a segregated or specialized activity. A particularly poignant example illustrating this premise was provided by Dr. Brandt, who described one of his patients whose life had been turned around by a traditional healer. The healer's recommendation was to host a clan feast to resolve a curse. The effort required to organize the feast led to the reintegration of the 'patient' into the community. Other participants spoke of the higher authority that underlies Aboriginal healing practices and that must characterize efforts to integrate health institutions within Aboriginal traditions.

Participants also spoke of the significant contribution that various aspects of Aboriginal medicine have made both to Aboriginal communities and to the larger society and of the need to develop a legislative and institutional framework that both supports and protects ongoing activity in this area. While some participants, such as Dr. Connors, argued that institutions such as western hospitals and health care professions need to develop strategies for further integration of traditional medicine into institutional life, others expressed concern that the natural self-regulation that currently protects the clients of Aboriginal medicine might be disrupted by increased involvement with the external western medical system. Elder Douglas, in particular, expressed concerns that Aboriginal plant medicines must be protected from scientific and commercial expropriation.

Participants also concurred that different Aboriginal societies have different traditions and approaches to health and healing that must be respected. Aboriginal members of the medical and nursing professions expressed a further concern that Aboriginal people pursuing training in western health care professions must be encouraged and have the opportunity to further their understanding of Aboriginal healing traditions in order to be effective practitioners in Aboriginal communities. Several examples were provided of institutions where traditional and western medicine is integrated (such as Anishnabe Health, Toronto) but there was consensus that this is an important area for policy development.

Theme 4: Understanding Aboriginality and Aboriginal Rights

Many participants articulated a concern about the diverse ways in which the rights of Aboriginal people in Canada are interpreted and institutionalized by both the external society and other Aboriginal people. Indeed, several participants raised fundamental questions about the term 'Aboriginal' and the tendency to discuss Aboriginal health issues from a status-blind perspective. Métis participants in particular expressed the view that while their communities share some common experiences and concerns with other Aboriginal communities, they are distinctive in several key areas. Foremost among these distinctions is the fact that Métis communities have negotiated service arrangements primarily with provincial governments and have been ignored historically by the federal government. Other important differences are the extent to which Métis communities have supported the development of mainstream institutions in the wider Canadian society. Several participants described the importance of education, and particularly professional education, to the current character of Métis communities, and one participant described the contribution that Métis society in Manitoba had made to one of the foremost tertiary teaching hospitals in the country (St. Boniface Hospital in Winnipeg). Inuit participants also described important differences in their traditions as well as the unique nature of the political and administrative structures in the Territories where Aboriginal people have obtained a degree of self-government not found elsewhere. Other participants articulated concerns that the all-encompassing term 'Aboriginal peoples' may inhibit recognition of the important differences among Aboriginal peoples living on reserve across the country, as well as the externally imposed differences (in terms of access to resources particularly) between people who live on or off reserve.

Alma Favel-King and Ron George made the important point that treaty rights (and Aboriginal rights generally) should not be confused with legal discussions of status and entitlement provisions. Specifically, the interpretation of the intent of the 'medicine chest' clause in Treaty Six and Aboriginal interpretations of other treaties underlie ongoing concern that the federal government in Canada recognize and respond appropriately to its obligations to protect the health and welfare of Aboriginal peoples throughout Canada. Confusing status with treaty rights blurs and obfuscates the contention of all Aboriginal people that a constitutional recognition of Aboriginal rights as understood from an Aboriginal perspective is fundamental to health development.

Theme 5: Political Support of Health Concerns

Several participants spoke of the problem of isolating health issues from broader developmental concerns related to self-government. Implicit in these discussions was a concern that Aboriginal political organizations from the band to the national level have not identified health issues as a high priority and have not devoted adequate resources to policy development in this area. Recent initiatives are changing this historical picture, but participants expressed concern that further development is needed.

Concern was also expressed that the problem is sometimes more serious than simply lack of political support or leadership for health development but can sometimes be characterized as political interference in the health development area. Several participants described the sometimes chaotic administrative structures at the band level that inhibit health and social program development, while others expressed concern about post-colonial governing structures, which sometimes fail to acknowledge the serious abrogation of women's and children's rights in some communities.

However, participants were also careful to point out that the current political problems in some Aboriginal communities are not the inherent fault of Aboriginal people but are a legacy of the *Indian Act* and colonial history.

While changes in the constitutional recognition of First Nations as self-governing societies will contribute substantially to health development in many communities, participants also emphasized that new governing structures in First Nations communities must shed the vestiges of a paternalistic colonial administration and be embedded in cultural traditions that are often matrilineal in structure. Without such change, the violence and abuse experienced by eight out of ten Aboriginal women, according to Professor LaRocque, may be perpetuated.

Other participants spoke of the significance of the political leadership respecting healing efforts within their communities through their own behaviour. The Alkali Lake model was widely acknowledged as providing a superlative example of the broad health effects that occur when the political leadership in a community embraces a healing perspective. Another participant addressed representatives from external institutions and asked that individual and community healing efforts by Aboriginal people be respected through both individual and institutional behaviour. For example, it was suggested that health professionals working with Aboriginal communities must exercise limits on their drinking behaviour, and conferences such as this Round Table should refrain from serving alcohol to participants.

Finally, participants agreed that political will in support of Aboriginal health must originate in the prime minister's office. Without leadership at this level and recognition of the priority that Aboriginal health must assume in the country, it is unfair to expect that the Aboriginal political leadership will assume these responsibilities unsupported.

Theme 6: Jurisdictional Frustration and Innovation

A common theme heard through many of the formal and informal presentations at the Round Table was frustration with the often piecemeal and buck-passing nature of funding opportunities for health development. Although reserve and Territorial communities are at some advantage because most of their needs are the responsibility of either two federal departments or the Territorial governments, approximately two-thirds of Aboriginal people in the country who live off reserve are consistently frustrated in their attempts to secure resources from various federal, provincial and municipal sources. This frustration was particularly evident for urban Aboriginal people, as was expressed in presentations describing the situation in Vancouver and Toronto.

However, I was also struck by the similarity of experience between Aboriginal people living in inner-city Vancouver and the Innu frustration with jurisdictional responsibility in northern Labrador. Despite dramatically different situations, these two communities with excessive levels of health problems are similarly stymied in their efforts to develop community-based approaches to meet the needs of their people.

In this context, participants also expressed frustration with the evaluatory structures characteristic of federal and provincial bureaucracies, which seem to reflect the needs of the administration more than the needs of Aboriginal communities. Specific reference was made to the transfer initiative of Medical Services Branch and the perceived inappropriateness of departmental evaluation philosophy.

Also mentioned in this context was the lack of consultation and co-ordination among federal departments such as Indian Affairs and Health and Welfare, and particularly among Health and Welfare and provincial departments of health. While some communities understand funding structures and are able to exploit opportunities, other communities are ill-informed about the various protocols in place and often miss out on program opportunities because of an overall lack of co-ordination on the part of institutional funders.

Nonetheless, several examples of attempts to alleviate these jurisdictional nightmares were presented by government representatives from Ontario and Quebec particularly. An Ontario initiative based on a fundamental recognition of Aboriginal rights has developed multi-sectoral and multi-disciplinary committees focused on 'healing the family'. This initiative appeared to be a significant move toward simplifying the institutional-community relationship. Efforts in Quebec to respond on a multi-sectoral basis, where housing, education and mental health counselling were considered together as part of a broad health development strategy, are also encouraging developments in this area.

Theme 7: Practice Before Policy (or, Just Do It!)

In the Euro-Canadian political environment, the standard approach to structural change is linear and begins with a period of consultation followed by a period of policy development with, it is hoped, a period of implementation leading to structural change in society. This philosophy is also consistent with theoretical models, which identify structural change in the social environment as a necessary pre-condition to changes in the lives of individuals, families and communities. This theoretical orientation could be characterized as an effort to level the playing field, so that all players have an equal opportunity to take advantage of the opportunities available in that society. Indeed the Royal Commission process is embedded within this structure where an interest in long-term policy initiatives will lead, it is hoped, to a restructuring of the relationship between First Nations communities and the wider Canadian society. This restructuring will eventually contribute to improvements in the environmental conditions that underlie the health problems in Aboriginal communities.

However, some participants at this Round Table articulated a different model for structural change in society that embraces the grassroots development philosophy of scholars such as Paulo Freire. This perspective was outlined effectively by Mr. Bill Mussell, who argued that social change occurs through communicative action and a dialogic process between individuals, communities and societal institutions. Other participants described efforts in their own communities to address health problems through institutional change, where barriers in the Canadian institutional structure were simply ignored or overridden as new programs and services were implemented. Particularly good examples of this process were the health developments in Kahnawake around the Kateri Memorial Hospital and the development of an indigenous midwifery program under the direction of an Inuit women's organization in Povungnituk, northern Quebec. Similar processes were described for the Grand Lac Victoria Band Council in northern Quebec and the remarkable achievements of the Mi'Kmaq AIDS Task Force in Nova Scotia.

Participants in these developments sympathized with the frustration experienced by other participants whose attempts to develop culturally appropriate and responsive services have been frustrated by institutional inertia, but they argued that Aboriginal people must not wait for broader social structural change but must instead force that change to occur through community-based initiatives.

Theme 8: Community Healing as a Fragile Process

Although there was consensus among participants that efforts by elders, medicine people, community health workers and other Aboriginal health professionals to heal communities from within deserve accolades, there were also concerns expressed regarding the scale of the problems in relation to the human resources available. Many examples were provided of the powerful contribution that traditional medicine makes to the well-being of individuals, families, and communities, but participants were also keenly aware of the stress these contributions place on the individuals involved. People involved in facilitating community healing, from organizations such as the Alkali Lake Group and Bear Woman and Associates, are required to commit extraordinary amounts of time and personal energy to travelling and consulting across the huge and difficult-to-access territory of northern Canada.

The genocidal effects of the *Indian Act* and other colonial monsters such as residential schools have thinned the ranks of elders and other healers within Aboriginal communities who are willing to make their knowledge and abilities available in even an Aboriginal public context. Their efforts are limited further by inconsistencies in the financial and philosophical support from external agencies and institutions such as federal and provincial health departments, professional medical associations, universities, etc. Other Aboriginal health workers experience similar demands on their time and energy, and several participants commented on the problem of burn-out that afflicts the relatively small cadre of Aboriginal community health workers, social workers, nurses, physicians, and administrators.

Although this Round Table provided ample evidence that these individuals are making extraordinary contributions in the field of Aboriginal health development, the Round Table was also provided evidence that extraordinary responsibilities and demands are also being placed on these people at very early stages in their careers. It is not at all uncommon for recent Aboriginal health professional graduates rapidly to assume wide responsibilities in the areas of policy, administration and program development while simultaneously being expected to develop their service skills.

Finally, considerable discussion was devoted to the issue of how to assess the effectiveness of a variety of community healing initiatives, from traditional medicine to community mental health programs, in ways that do not interfere with their cultural autonomy and integrity, but at the same time ensure that other Aboriginal communities have access to a critical understanding of the strengths and weaknesses of these initiatives. Many participants argued that the internal peer review process characteristic of Aboriginal societies is sufficient to ensure that individuals and communities are aware of situations where traditional healers break the cultural rules appropriate to their activities. However, participants also emphasized that formal supports are required to ensure that knowledge regarding effective community programs is more readily available to the wider Aboriginal society other than through government reports or academic publication. Externally imposed evaluation structures in the area of community healing may do little to facilitate the development of an accessible knowledge base in this area.

Theme 9: Recognition of Special Needs and Priorities

The final and perhaps most important theme that emerged at the Round Table discussion was that in the context of fourth-world health conditions, where people suffer from a variety of infectious and chronic diseases as well as social violence and mental health problems, some particular groups and needs require targeted attention and specific policy frameworks. These groups are listed below in no particular order:

- victims of residential schools
- Aboriginal people with disabilities
- victims of sexual abuse and domestic violence
- Aboriginal people with AIDS
- children with fetal alcohol syndrome

Victims of Residential Schools

Although the impact of residential schools on Aboriginal society must be considered in broader terms than health consequences, many participants at the Round Table linked their own and others' experience in the residential schools to problems of alcohol abuse, suicide, and family violence in Aboriginal communities today. While significant efforts are under way within Aboriginal communities to heal the wounds inflicted by residential schools, broader policy for compensation must be developed and provided to individuals, families, and communities whose lives have been disrupted by this particular historical experience.

Aboriginal People With Disabilities

Although federal inquiries into the needs of people with disabilities have included Aboriginal people, several participants indicated that the specific needs of people with disabilities in Aboriginal communities have been largely ignored by administrative authorities at all levels, including band, provincial, and federal authorities. In particular, people with disabilities often suffer many of the other health and social problems in Aboriginal communities, such as sexual abuse, domestic violence, and chronic illness, but are in double jeopardy because of their disabilities.

Victims of Sexual Abuse and Domestic Violence

Professor Larocque provided a powerful indictment of a system that remains insensitive to and unresponsive to the needs of women when it is estimated that eight Aboriginal women in ten have experienced sexual abuse or violence. Programs and facilities to protect and heal victims of abuse are clearly essential. Other participants expanded this issue and identified that healing is also necessary for men as perpetrators of domestic violence.

People with AIDS and Children with Fetal Alcohol Syndrome

These two conditions were identified as a growing concern in Aboriginal communities and as problems that may not have been considered in the medical service transfer process, which limits flexibility both for developing additional services and expanding services for individuals suffering from either of these conditions. Participants indicated that current rates of alcohol abuse and sexually transmitted diseases will likely result in epidemic conditions for AIDS and fetal alcohol syndrome. If this occurs, the service needs will far exceed the resources currently available to Aboriginal communities that have assumed responsibility for delivering health services on behalf of the federal government.

The themes just described characterized much of the discussion at the Round Table, but it is important to remember that health issues reflect the broader social, economic, political, and cultural conditions of Aboriginal life and cannot be addressed effectively as a circumscribed and specialized area of interest, as is often the tendency in modern industrial societies. This understanding is particularly important for people who do not work in the so-called health field and who may view it as an area defined largely by medicine, with the attendant belief that it is an area requiring highly scientific and technical solutions. While illness services are admittedly complex and require sophisticated professional and administrative expertise for both efficacy and universal application, it is important to keep illness services in proper perspective with respect to the more holistic approach to health. I will close this section with two stories which are well known to people working in the health field but may help those outside the field understand the connectedness of health to other social issues. One is the often quoted truism that the measure of a society is its ability to protect and care for its most vulnerable members – in this instance the children, people with disabilities, and the chronically ill.

The second anecdote is widely quoted in the public health literature in many variations and is known as the 'upstream downstream story'. This story goes something like this: A man is fishing on the banks of a river when suddenly he sees a person struggling out in the river. He leaps in, rescues and resuscitates the person on the banks of the river and goes back to his fishing. As the morning passes he rescues and resuscitates several more people. Finally the fisherman decides to investigate where these people are coming from and works his way through the bush upstream to discover a village perched on the edge of a cliff beside the river. As he stands watching, he realizes that the local bar is built on the edge of the cliff, and as people stumble out, a good proportion of them slip and fall down the cliff and into the river. Clearly the solution to the problem is to build a fence or perhaps close the bar, but our fisherman finds that building a fence is not within the mandate of government agencies responsible for drowning people. However, he is able to convince the local population to drag all their broken-down automobiles to the edge of the cliff to create a temporary barrier.

DISCUSSION PAPERS

Aboriginal Health Policy for the Next Century

*John D. O'Neil**

In October of 1991, I sat listening to a nationally respected anthropologist argue that medical understandings of alcoholism as a disease were inadequate to the task of developing effective health policy for alcohol problems in Aboriginal communities. She argued instead for a socio-historical approach that situated Aboriginal alcohol problems in the context of both local cultural conditions and colonial history. At the end of her presentation, the moderator for the workshop took issue with her presentation and suggested instead that models that situate alcohol problems as symptoms of social and cultural conditions serve only to justify government refusals to fund alcohol treatment programs run by Aboriginal people. The moderator further argued that alcoholism was a devastating disease contributing to overwhelming morbidity and mortality in Aboriginal communities that could be addressed only through aggressive treatment programs oriented to individual well-being.

The most significant aspect of this debate was that it occurred in Alice Springs, Australia, and the moderator for the workshop was Eric Shirt, co-founder of the Nechi Institute and Poundmaker's Lodge in Alberta, Canada. Mr. Shirt had been invited to Australia by the Central Australian Aboriginal Congress to assist them in their efforts to develop community-controlled alcohol treatment centres. The workshop also took place in the context of the Australian Public Health Association meetings where Mr. Shirt and other representatives from

* Associate Professor of Medical Anthropology and National Health Research Scholar, Northern Health Research Unit, Department of Community Health Sciences, University of Manitoba.

Canadian First Nations were keynote speakers. Many members of the audience were Aboriginal people from different regions of Australia, with the remainder drawn from public health academics and professionals.

My purpose in describing this incident is threefold. First of all, Aboriginal health policy in Canada as well as Australia is the product of a dialogue among health professionals, Aboriginal communities and, to a lesser extent, social scientists. As a non-Aboriginal social scientist without clinical health care experience, I am highly conscious of my position as an outsider at this conference. Although I have directed large research initiatives into health policy issues in various Aboriginal communities in Canada (and Australia), I am without a direct stake in the outcome of the policy deliberations we are undertaking over the next few days. Neither will my children die, nor will I go without sleep for a week of on-calls, if our recommendations do not result in the reduction of alcohol-related violence that plagues many Aboriginal communities. While this outsider status may confer a degree of objectivity useful when assessing complicated and conflicted policy issues, it may nonetheless be a limitation when desperate times require passionate ideas.

A second reason for describing this anecdote is that it points to the importance of developing health policy well-grounded in scholarly conceptual work, while also underscoring he contentious theoretical and political debates that often structure multidisciplinary discourse. Not only do medicine, public health and the social sciences promote sometimes contradictory models for explaining disease and illness, but these models are subject to critiques from Aboriginal scholars and health care professionals. While Aboriginal and other minority scholars argue convincingly that prevailing scientific models in any discipline are grounded in Eurocentric philosophic traditions, Aboriginal and non-Aboriginal health professionals alike demand 'workability' if conceptual approaches are to be useful in improving health conditions. Thus, 'colonialism' as a central explanation for current Aboriginal health conditions may have limited applicability.

The most important reason for introducing this paper with this anecdote is because I believe it may serve as a signpost for future development of Aboriginal health policy. The most startling thing about the meeting in Alice Springs was that international collaboration between Aboriginal societies to confront common health concerns was occurring under the noses of the public health community who were by and large ignorant of its implications. Taken together with the international Healing the Spirit Worldwide conference, held in Edmonton in July 1992, which drew more than 3500 Aboriginal participants from 14 countries (including a delegation of 150 Aborigines from Australia), these First People consultations are without doubt the most significant contemporary initiative in the Aboriginal health arena. Indeed, as I began to review the literature for this paper, it struck me as quite ironic that many reports written by non-Aboriginal scholars continue to conclude with a plea for "greater involvement by Aboriginal communities in solutions to health problems" when in fact the volume of this activity is now probably greater than mainstream non-Aboriginal research and planning activity.

This paper will develop these perspectives through a review of literature related to the health status and development of health services in Aboriginal communities. This review will rely on published material in government documents (including federal, provincial and Aboriginal) and scientific publications. The paper will first of all review major trends in social health conditions and then discuss the various policy and planning initiatives that provide a context for considerations of future efforts.

Social Health Conditions[1]

Although historical epidemiology is largely a speculative science and is plagued by inconsistent debate, most scholars agree that European-introduced disease was a major factor in the catastrophic decline in the North American Aboriginal population. Thorton, for example, estimates that the Aboriginal population of the United States was more than five million at the beginning of the sixteenth century.[2] This population was halved every 100 years and reached its nadir of 250,000 (less than 5 per cent of the pre-contact population) by the end of the nineteenth century. Although other factors such as warfare and extermination of the bison contributed to this decline, infectious diseases introduced by Europeans were by far the major factor.

A similar global assessment of historical epidemiology in Canada is not available; however, most scholars would agree the picture is not markedly different. Norris estimates the pre-contact Aboriginal population in Canada at 210,000, dropping to about 80,000 in 1870 and recovering to 120,000 in the early 1900s.[3] Relative to the U.S. experience, there is some evidence that Aboriginal populations in some regions of the country had much higher survival rates (particularly the west coast and western sub-Arctic), that the overall survival rate was somewhat higher, and that the most significant population losses occurred later; in general, however, the impact of infectious disease in Canada was equally disastrous.

Given the scale of this catastrophe, it is remarkable that Aboriginal culture has survived at all. Oral traditions are threatened by the premature loss of elders, social organizations cannot function when entire families and clans are decimated, and economic dependency on the external society becomes a matter of survival. The consequences of this demographic disaster are long-term. While current historical attention focuses on the destructive social impact of institutions such as residential schools on Aboriginal culture, the impact is likely exacerbating already existing conditions.

It is also important to point out that current epidemiological trend analysis graphically represents Aboriginal societies as if these contact epidemics were an intrinsic characteristic of Aboriginal culture. Figure 1, for example, suggests that

Figure 1

Infant Mortality Rate: Canada, 1925-1988 (Indian, Inuit and national populations)

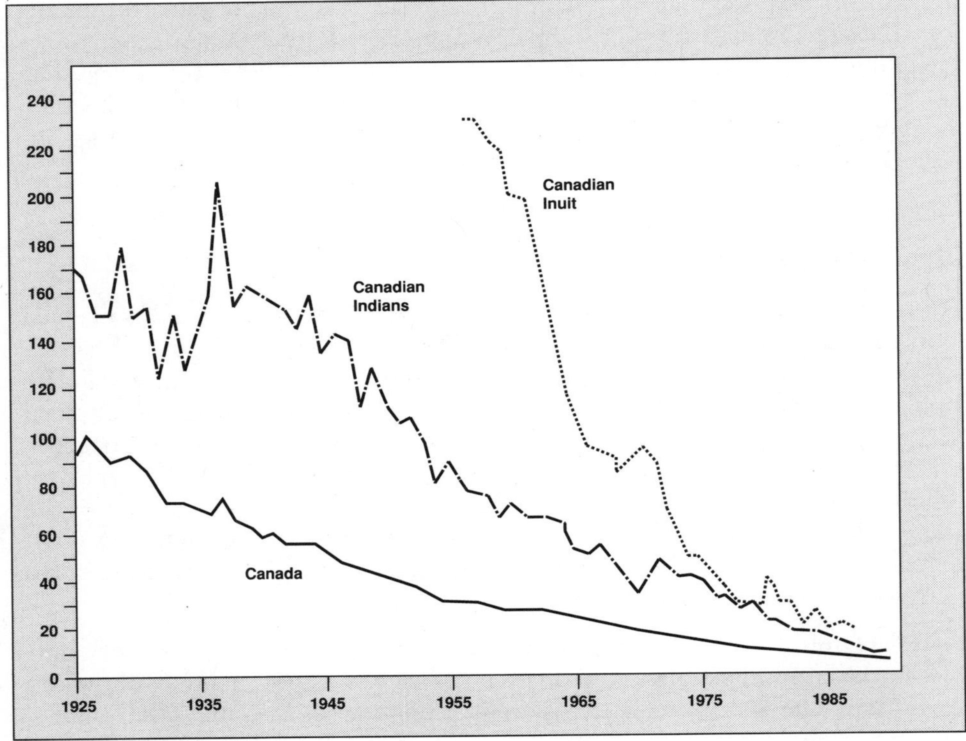

prior to 1925, Aboriginal infant mortality was consistently high when in fact we have no evidence to support this interpretation. On the contrary, the evidence we do have suggests that before contact, morbidity and mortality in Aboriginal societies were probably quite low.[4] However, epidemiological trend analysis is limited to the period when the federal government determined that Aboriginal deaths were worth counting; hence the appearance of time beginning in 1925 for Aboriginal societies.

Although there has been a remarkable recovery of the Aboriginal population since the end of the nineteenth century, largely as a result of very high fertility rates, mortality rates continue to be excessive. Figure 1 illustrates a declining infant mortality rate among status Indians and Inuit but shows nonetheless that these rates remain roughly twice the Canadian average. Recent data from Health and Welfare Canada indicate that while the Canadian infant mortality rate has stabilized at 7.8 deaths per 1000 live births over the period 1984-88, the Inuit rate remains at 19.9 and the registered Indian rate is at 17.7.[5] Infant mortality rates are generally considered to be a powerful reflection of underlying disparities in socio-economic conditions and health care services. Table 1 confirms this by demonstrating that for Inuit, most infant mortality is due to low birth weight, pneumonia and meningitis, and 'unexplained sudden deaths' (mostly accidents, but also suggesting a lack of medical capacity for diagnosis). These are a reflection of poverty, sub-standard and overcrowded housing, and an underdeveloped infrastructure.

Table 1

Infant Mortality Rates by Cause (Inuit in the Northwest Territories, 1981 to 1988, and total population of Canada, 1986)

		Rate (per 1000 Live Births)		
		Inuit		Canadian
Cause of Death	**ICD-9 Codes**	**81-84**	**85-88**	**1986**
Sudden unexplained	798	4.0	4.7	1.0
Premature, low birth weight	764-769	6.3	2.1	0.5
Congenital anomalies	740-759	2.2	1.8	2.5
Septicaemia, perinatal infections	038,771	0.8	1.8	0.1
Birth asphyxia, anoxia, hypoxia	768-770	4.0	1.5	1.7
Pneumonia, bronchitis	466,480-486, 490-491	2.5	1.4	0.1
Meningitis	036.0,320-322	0.4	1.1	0.1
Gastrointestinal disorders	008,009, 557,558,777	0.4	0.7	0.1
Injury and poisoning	E800-E999	2.6	0.4	0.2
All other causes		3.2	5.9	1.8

Source: Medical Services Branch, Health and Welfare Canada, in-house statistics; Northwest Territories Department of Health; Statistics Canada, Vital Statistics, Vol. 1, *Births and Deaths*, cat. 84-204, and Vol. 4, *Causes of Death*, cat. 84-203.

The picture for overall population mortality is also disturbing. Table 2 shows that for almost every age group, death rates for the registered Indian population are at least twice and sometimes four times as high as the Canadian average. Particularly at risk are young children, teenagers and young adult males. The mortality picture for registered Indians and Inuit shows other alarming differences from the Canadian population. Figure 2 shows that while diseases of the circulatory system (heart disease and stroke) and neoplasms (cancer) are the major killers of most Canadians, Aboriginal people die primarily from injuries or poisonings, causes that are clearly related to socio-economic conditions and hence, preventable. Additionally, Young and others have shown that diabetes is increasing as an important threat to all Aboriginal people in Canada, and there is disturbing evidence that death due to heart disease and cancer is also increasing.[6] AIDS is also recognized as a potential devastating threat for Aboriginal communities.[7]

Table 2

Age-Specific Death Rates (registered Indian population served, 1984-1988, and population of Canada, 1986)

Age (Years)	Death Rate per 1000 Population in Age Group Indian*	Canadian
1	39.69	7.89
01-04	1.60	0.46
05-09	0.44	0.23
10-14	0.69	0.23
15-19	2.45	0.74
20-24	3.47	0.87
25-29	3.16	0.85
30-34	3.80	0.97
35-39	4.02	1.24
40-44	5.66	1.87
45-49	7.04	3.12
50-54	9.38	5.30
55-59	14.96	8.44
60-64	21.09	13.23
65-69	30.50	20.74
70-74	39.69	32.63
75-79	59.10	51.75
80+	90.10	114.89

*Five-year average rates.

Source: Medical Services Branch, Health and Welfare Canada, in-house statistics; Statistics Canada, Vital Statistics, Vol. 4, *Causes of Death*, cat. 84-203.

Table 3 presents a very disturbing picture of suicide trends in the registered Indian population. Although the overall rate has dropped slightly in the past decade, it remains twice the national average, and in some locations there is evidence that the rate is increasing. These data are difficult to interpret because of very small absolute numbers in different regions. It is clear, however, from other studies in Inuit communities that suicide rates are increasing, and that the group most at risk are young men (ages 15-25).

Clearly, these data tell only part of the story. While national and regional databases provide a comprehensive picture of mortality for on-reserve Indians and Inuit, the picture is much less clear for morbidity patterns (particularly in relation to the impact on health of social problems such as family violence and child abuse). Our understanding of social health conditions for Aboriginal people living off-reserve and particularly in cities is almost negligible.

Figure 2

Leading Causes of Death (registered Indian population served and Inuit in the Northwest Territories, 1986-1988, and population of Canada, 1986)

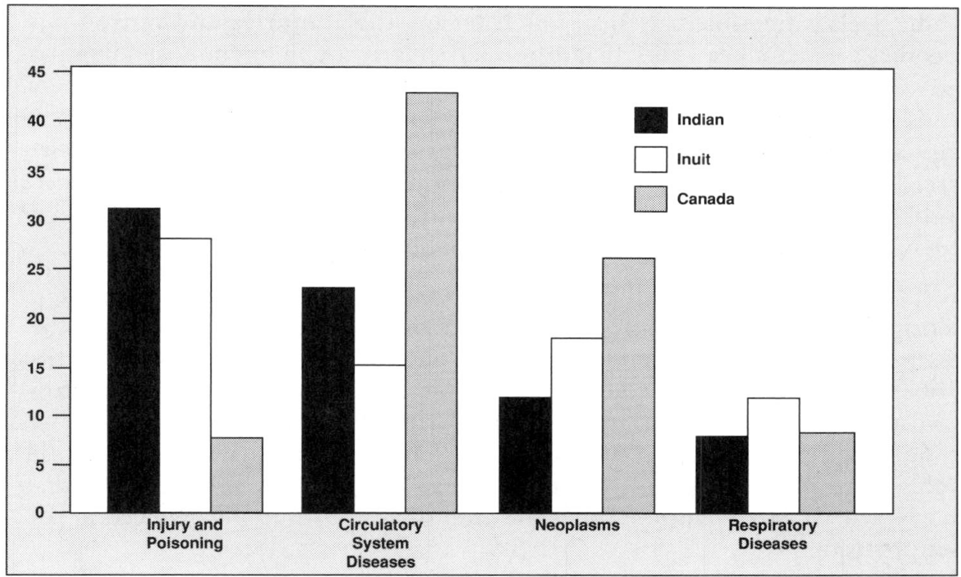

Table 3

Suicide Death Rates by Sex and Region (registered Indian population served, 1980-1988, and population of Canada, 1986)

	Suicide Rate per 100 000 Population					
	Indian*				Canadian	
	Male		Female		Male	Female
Region	**80-84**	**84-88**	**80-84**	**84-88**	**1986**	**1986**
Atlantic	48.8	70.6	2.9	15.6	16.3	3.7
Quebec	70.4	47.2	13.8	4.2	27.5	7.9
Ontario	55.6	52.4	18.4	11.6	19.1	6.0
Manitoba	62.6	43.5	6.3	14.6	22.9	6.1
Saskatchewan	85.0	52.1	35.1	18.3	21.2	6.1
Alberta	72.8	86.8	28.8	18.4	28.7	7.0
Pacific	64.6	52.0	16.6	13.3	23.6	6.0
Yukon	178.3	112.5	26.8	9.7	65.0	17.9
N.W.T.	21.8	53.6	00.0	8.8	47.5	8.1
Total	67.5	57.8	18.9	14.5	22.8	6.4

* Five-year average rates.

Source: Medical Services Branch, Health and Welfare Canada, in-house statistics; Statistics Canada, Vital Statistics, Vol. 4, Causes of Death, cat. 84-203.

These epidemiological data are also limited in what they tell us about health conditions in Aboriginal communities for a variety of methodological reasons. First of all, only those events considered significant by non-Aboriginal health scientists are counted. For example, mortality is classified according to standard medical classification systems, which means that 'injuries and poisonings' becomes a catch-all category that is not particularly useful in understanding patterns of social violence in Aboriginal communities. Mental health in general tends to be ignored. Despite widespread recognition that mental health is an important issue in Aboriginal communities, provincial and national reports rarely provide more than a rudimentary estimate of the distribution of these problems, partly because of jurisdictional debates over whether the provincial or federal government is responsible for mental health.

Despite the limitations inherent in the epidemiological understanding of Aboriginal health, the systems of surveillance that produce the data are nonetheless powerful social instruments for the construction of Aboriginal identity, problem identification and resource allocation. Indeed, one reason that epidemiologists are attracted to working with data derived from Aboriginal communities is the comprehensiveness and relative completeness of the database. Given the highly centralized surveillance systems of Medical Services Branch and Indian and Northern Affairs, little escapes the attention of institutions involved in service provision.

International research has shown that public health surveillance systems perform disciplinary and regulatory functions in society independent of their overt purpose of tracking health conditions.[8] This analysis points out how knowledge is constructed about sectors of society that reinforces unequal power relationships; in other words an image of sick, disorganized communities can be used to justify paternalism and dependency.

The external agencies and academics that analyze the data also have the power to interpret the data and to construct an image of Aboriginal communities as desperate, disorganized and depressed environments. This image is created ostensibly to support lobbying efforts to secure a larger share of national resources for community development. However, this image is reflected through the Canadian media and general public and is to some extent internalized by Aboriginal communities, reinforcing dependency relationships.

Resistance to the totalizing effect of surveillance systems is emerging in Aboriginal communities who are undertaking independent research on health issues. Many of these initiatives have occurred in the context of the federal government's transfer initiative (discussed below), where community health assessments are required as a preliminary phase prior to transfer negotiations. Although these assessments are often conducted by external consultants, they are unique for several reasons. First of all, most are designed from a holistic perspective more reflective of Aboriginal cultural traditions. Not only do they integrate standard medical interests with broader social, emotional and spiritual concerns, but there is also an expanded interest in 'health' as opposed to the 'sickness profiles' common to mainstream epidemiology. Issues such as family violence, addictions, and mental and spiritual health are fundamental rather than secondary concerns.

Perhaps more important, these studies are regarded as the property of the bands and tribal organizations that have commissioned them and are generally not available outside the context of negotiations with the federal government for transfer of health services. Ownership of health information has clearly been recognized by Aboriginal communities as a component of self-determination in health care. Interpretation of the information is protected by maintaining the holistic integrity of the documents guaranteeing a more balanced picture of community health. For example, I have selectively borrowed tables from scientific and government publications in order to substantiate my own perspectives on Aboriginal health conditions. If the data contained in community health assessments were generally available, I would have relied more extensively on those documents, but my use of that data would have been selective and beyond the control of the communities that generated the information.

While many people might argue that free and democratic access to scientific information precludes interpretive control over data, the fact is that most health scientists are members of an elite and dominant sector of society and cannot help but reflect the normative assumptions of that group in scientific work. Until Aboriginal communities have proportional representation in the institutions that structure public interpretations of community information (i.e., universities, health professions, scientific journals, media, etc.), their only recourse is to attempt to control the dissemination of information that reflects their everyday lives.

This does not mean that interpretations are biased in the scientific sense. Although some scientists claim that scientific work is value-free, this claim is usually made from a position firmly situated in the context of a white, male, middle-class, Eurocentric background. Aboriginal, other minority, and feminist scholars have argued convincingly that so-called value-free science in fact supports the central values of the dominant ideology in society and that claims to independent objectivity are central to maintaining control over definitions of the normal and abnormal, and appropriate and inappropriate social behaviour.

I have made reference on several occasions to problems of family violence and mental health in Aboriginal communities. Recognition of the magnitude of these problems is not usually based on academic assessments, although some information is available,[9] but is expressed instead through the experience of people living in communities where their everyday lives are continually affected by the pain that these problems inflict. This experience is documented in the many regional and national conferences that have been held in the past decade oriented toward community healing.[10] These reports (examples are included in the notes) underscore two simple facts: one is that the magnitude of a problem can be understood without the elaborate statistical analysis common to scientific work, and the other is that Aboriginal women are at the forefront of efforts to heal their families and communities. I will return to both these issues later in the paper after a discussion of health service development.

Health Service Development

Recently, several medical historians in Manitoba (who will remain nameless) set out to write a history of medicine in Manitoba. After completing six or seven chapters describing the heroic efforts and brilliant discoveries of the "elders" of the Manitoba medical community, one author decided it would be appropriate to begin the book with a chapter on "Indian medicine". An early first draft of this chapter, which drew loosely on traditional anthropological interpretations of Indian healers as shamans who practised psychotherapy, was sent to a medical colleague with "cultural inclinations" who in turn asked me to review it. My advice was polite, but I suggested dropping the project – a less ambitious book describing the more limited accomplishments of scientific medical men might be warranted. Unfortunately, the project has gone ahead, and I expect publication will generate some controversy.

The problem of course is that medical history in Manitoba, as in the rest of North America, is incomplete without an integrated consideration of both Aboriginal medicine and the colonizing impact of western medicine on Aboriginal society. Aboriginal medicine is no more an appended first chapter than is western medicine the modern saviour of Aboriginal society. The relevance of this understanding should become apparent in our consideration of contemporary issues in health service policy for Aboriginal communities.

Young and Smith[11] provide a useful summary of health service developments in Aboriginal communities over the last several decades, and I am indebted to their scholarship in developing this section of the paper.

Although many Aboriginal communities are attempting to build a community health model that integrates traditional and western medicine, I believe these approaches need to be addressed separately. The distinctly colonial character of so-called western medicine has been the subject of much negotiation in terms of political and fiscal control over existing medical institutions. This process can be understood only in the context of broader negotiations toward self-government, as many scholars have argued.[12]

Traditional medicine on the other hand has always been in the control of Aboriginal communities and is evolving separate from the negotiation of institutional control over western medicine. This does not mean that the two systems cannot be integrated, or indeed in some cases are not already integrated at the community level. However, even where community control over both systems is most developed, the systems continue to operate to some extent in isolation from one another.[13] For these reasons, I will discuss developments in these areas under separate sub-headings and then describe current efforts toward integration, or at least collaboration, in the conclusions to this paper.

Traditional Medicine

Canada is one of the few countries in the world where medical pluralism is not a taken-for-granted aspect of everyday life. The medical monopoly in Canada has assumed greater control over healing activities then anywhere else in either the industrialized or the developing world. Perhaps the best example of this is the situation of midwifery, which is defined as a medical act in Canada, whereas midwifery is a separate, legal, and widely used professional service in the rest of the world (including the United States, Europe, and Australia). Other healing systems such as homeopathy, chiropractic medicine, acupuncture, and naturopathy are well established, professional and, in some instances, state-supported through health insurance in Britain and other parts of Europe. Ayurvedic and Chinese medicine are ancient and well-established healing systems for most of the world's population (in India and China respectively). While it is beyond the scope of this paper to address the social history of Aboriginal medicine in Canada, traditional medicine has been and continues to be misunderstood by mainstream health care providers. Indeed, 'misunderstood' is a polite way to describe the systematic discrimination that characterizes the history of the relationship between the two systems in Canada.

While traditional Aboriginal medicine has always fascinated external observers (particularly anthropologists), and much has been written that purports to describe and analyze beliefs and practices, very little of this literature is useful to understand traditional medicine in either historical or contemporary perspective. Much that has been written is from what anthropologists refer to as an 'etic' perspective; that is the phenomenon is understood according to the explanatory frameworks of the external observer. For example, traditional medicine is described as a mechanism of social control, in an effort to provide a 'rational' explanation for a phenomenon that to the western scientific mind is 'irrational' and unintelligible. Rarely have 'emic' explanations been attempted – that is, explanations that attempt to understand Aboriginal medicine in its own terms according to the world view of its practitioners.

Aboriginal medicine is also an oral tradition (unlike some of the other pluralistic traditions described above, which have huge literatures documenting the knowledge base). Oral traditions require a social environment that is supportive of knowledge transmission and protection from generation to generation. The catastrophic population losses described above, combined with federal legislation and religious oppression, served to threaten severely the knowledge base of Aboriginal medicine.[14]

Traditional Aboriginal medicine in Canada should also be understood, historically at least, as a diverse and heterogenous phenomenon, albeit with some consistent principles and values such as the importance of spiritual well-being and balance in everyday life. Considerable variation exists from the medicine societies of the Kwakw*aka*'wakw and Anishina'beg to the family-based *angatquq* of the Inuit. Additionally, within each society, other healers such as midwives and herbalists were recognized.

In those Aboriginal societies where traditional healing was organized into a more institutional framework, resistance to the destructive forces described above was possible, whereas in situations where healers functioned independently, such as among the Inuit, resistance was weaker.

The purpose of this brief review is to underscore the historical basis for contemporary differences in Aboriginal response to the renewal of traditional medicine, a process that was prophesied by Albert Lightning in 1976 at a University of Manitoba Native Health Conference.[15] This resurgence of ceremonial activity for healing purposes has made a profound change in the lives of many Aboriginal people and now constitutes a widely utilized alternative to western medicine in many communities, particularly in western Canada.

It would be a mistake to characterize all Aboriginal communities and individuals as participants in traditional medicine. Many communities and individuals have adopted and adapted Christianity to provide a spiritual basis for well-being and remain sceptical of 'Indian medicine'. Inuit and Métis communities particularly regard Christian spirituality as a legitimate and important component of their culture and look to these values as a basis for community healing.

Traditional medicine must also be understood in more holistic terms than western medicine. Attempts to compare the two systems from a western institutional perspective fail to grasp the pervasive way in which Aboriginal medicine is constituted as foundational to cultural practices, which are independent of the state-imposed regulatory structures of contemporary Aboriginal life. Aboriginal medicine 'works' largely because participants accept the authority of medicine people to effect changes in their everyday lives. This authority derives from an altogether different source than the authority delegated from the Canadian state. Aboriginal medicine in this sense is a way of life, complete with guidelines for behaviour, systems of authority and, in some instances, punitive mechanisms.[16] As such, it should also be considered in the context of self-government. It is not a system that can simply be regulated by community, band, and tribal governments in the same sense as the institutions of colonial medicine. It is more likely that various levels of Aboriginal government will be regulated by the authority structure of traditional medicine.

Clearly, the acceptance of this authority outside the regular state-sanctioned environment has largely been voluntary, with occasional exceptions (see the article in the *Victoria Times* described in note 16). However, as Aboriginal societies move towards new systems of self-government and justice grounded in traditional authority structures, the voluntary nature of participation will change. In his summary of the National Round Table on Aboriginal Justice Issues, James MacPherson hints at the potential conflict this may create, particularly for the protection of the interests of women, when new justice systems are an imperfect blend of traditional and state-imposed authority.[17]

Transfer of Control over Colonial Medicine

While some members of the audience may find my insistence on using the term 'colonial medicine' as an alternative reference for western, scientific medicine, I have done so purposely for several reasons. First of all, 'western' and 'scientific' are terms laden with cultural meaning that imply that the medicine they describe is somehow superior to other forms of medicine. To assume that science is uniquely a western phenomenon, or that scientific approaches to medicine are found only in the West, is the epitome of cultural arrogance. Other terms such as 'allopathic', 'cosmopolitan', or simply 'biomedicine' might be appropriate, but either they are too obscure or they obscure the profound cultural context in which the system developed. So-called biomedicine developed historically during a period of colonial expansion of European power into all parts of the world, and the system of medicine that we now rely on not only assisted that expansion, but was assisted in its development and domination by the colonial process of subjugation and resource exploitation.[18]

The history of contact between colonial medicine and Aboriginal communities should not, however, be understood only in negative terms. As recent work by Vanast has shown for the Arctic, the neglect of the local population by the Canadian state was sometimes challenged by a few unquestionably heroic doctors and nurses attempting to alleviate horrendous health conditions under impossible circumstances.[19] Nonetheless, as I and others have argued, colonial medical practice in Aboriginal communities has, perhaps unwittingly, contributed to the "intimate enemy" that Nandy[20] describes as the insidious effect when external institutions transmit new ideologies that convince their recipients that their own values and beliefs are no longer valid.[21]

Resistance to this system was recognized officially in 1979 with the publication of the Indian Health Policy by the government of Canada in response to pressure from the National Indian Brotherhood (now the Assembly of First Nations) to reconsider their position on the provision of non-insured services.[22] Indeed, the Advisory Commission Report written by Justice Berger in that same year provided the first systematic inquiry into Aboriginal dissatisfaction with the health care system. Needless to say, this dissatisfaction had been building across the country for nearly a decade before the Commission was formed. Young and Smith[23] provide a useful chronological summary of the 'transfer' process, which I have appended here (Table 4).

Table 4

Devolution and the Health Program Transfer Initiative: Chronological Development

Time Frame	Selected Policy Statements and Activities
1979	• Government of Canada Indian Health Policy Calls for Native CIH in Canada • Advisory Commission on Indian and Inuit Health Commission (ACIIHC) Appointed • MSB Discussion Paper Endorses 1978 Alma-Ata Declaration and 1979 Indian Health Policy
1980	• Inuit Tapirisat of Canada Resolution Calls for Government of Northwest Territories (GNWT) Control of Health Care Delivery • ACIIHC Final (Berger) Report Recommends Consultative Approach Re Native CIH in Canada
1982	• Baffin Phase I Aspect of Devolution of Health Care to GNWT Initiated • Special Committee on Indian Self-Government (SCIS) Appointed • MSB Community Health Demonstration Program (CHDP) Initiated
1983	• SCIS Final (Penner) Report Recommends Administrative Reform Re Native Self-Government
1984	• Dene Nation Resolution Calls for Formal Native Devolution/Transfer Agreements
1985	• GNWT Establishes Devolution Office • CHDP Terminated, MSB Health Program Transfer Subcommittee Established • MSB Transfer Subcommittee Calls for Consultative, Administrative Approach to Transfer • MSB Mission Statement Endorsing Transfer Circulated to First Nations
1986	• Baffin Phase II Aspect of Devolution of Health Care to GNWT Completed • MSB Program Transfer and Policy Development Directorate Established • Health and Welfare Canada "Achieving Health for All" Major Policy Statement • Minister of Health and Welfare Canada in April Letter Notifies First Nations of Intent to Include Them in Health Program Transfer
1987	• Minister of Health and Welfare Canada Attends 1987 Health Transfer Forum and 7th International Congress on Circumpolar Health • MSB Produces Draft *Health Program Transfer Handbook*
1988	• Devolution of Health Care to GNWT Completed in April • First Health Program Transfer Agreement Signed with a First Nation (Montreal Lake)
1989	• Government of Canada Final Approval in June of MSB Health Program Transfer Initiative • Assembly of First Nations Partially Endorses Transfer at 1989 Health Transfer Forum Attended by Minister of Health and Welfare Canada and 300 MSB and First Nations Delegates • MSB Produces "Community Health Plan Format and Sample" and *Health Transfer Newsletter*
1990	• New MSB Assistant Deputy Minister Endorses Health Program Transfer Initiative • First Health Program Transfer Agreement with a Tribal Council (Attikamek-Montagnais) • 8 Transfer Agreements and 67 Pre-Transfer Planning Projects Since 1989 Final Approval

Source: David E. Young and L.L. Smith, *The Involvement of Canadian Native Communities in their Health Care Programs: A Review of the Literature since the 1970s* (Edmonton: Canadian Circumpolar Institute, 1992).

External to this official history were several health service developments that will be summarized briefly to provide a broader context for contemporary developments. In 1975, the James Bay and Northern Quebec Agreement was signed by representatives of the James Bay Cree, the Inuit of Nunavik, and the federal and Quebec governments, in the process creating the first Aboriginal health and social service boards in Canada. While debate continues as to whether this agreement serves as a model for Aboriginal self-determination,[24] there have been significant changes in approach to health and social services as a result. In Povungnituk, for example, the Inuit-controlled hospital board has established an indigenous midwifery program in which Inuit midwives provide a full range of care. The program is unique not only in Aboriginal communities but also for the whole of Canada, as Ontario is the only province in which midwifery has been recently legalized. Povungnituk also provides a model for Inuit in other jurisdictions who regard the expropriation of childbirth from their communities by external authorities as possibly the most significant contemporary threat to community development.[25]

One of the first federal health programs to be devolved to Aboriginal administrative authority was the National Native Alcohol and Drug Abuse Program (NNADAP), established in 1975 and responsible for the creation of hundreds of community-based alcohol prevention and treatment projects across the country. Since the early 1980s, this program has contributed to the emergence of some of the most significant Aboriginal health initiatives in the country, including the Four Worlds Development Project, the Nechi Institute, the Alkali Lake prohibition strategy, and the recent Healing the Spirit Worldwide conference in Edmonton. However, recent evidence suggests that despite the remarkable efforts and success of Aboriginal organizations involved in community mental health and alcohol treatment, frustration remains with the extent to which this program is truly responsive to community needs.[26]

Other non-transfer based initiatives have emerged in the last decade that further provide a framework for understanding the transfer initiative. Some of these are particularly significant because they include non-treaty, urban and Métis communities. For reasons of space I will list some of these briefly here and refer the reader to the bibliography by Young and Smith for more detail:

1. The Alberta Indian Health Commission (AIHCC) was established in 1981 to promote First Nations health concerns in the province and was recognized, together with the Blood Tribe Board of Health, as a First Nations health authority at the 1989 Health Transfer Forum. In addition to consultation and liaison with various Aboriginal and provincial organizations, the AIHCC also provides urban community health representatives in Edmonton and Calgary.[27]

2. The Labrador Inuit Health Commission (LIHC) was created in 1979 in response to the specific exclusionary policies of the International Grenfell Association which refused to recognize Aboriginal rights. The Labrador Inuit

Association refused to witness the signing of the 1986 Canada Newfoundland Native Peoples of Labrador Health Agreement and established the LIHC instead, concentrating on CHR-delivered health education and promotion.[28]

3. The Kateri Memorial Hospital Centre (KMHC) was established in 1955 (!) when a local Mohawk woman elder secured funding from the Mohawk Council of Kahnawake and the Quebec government to continue operating the local hospital. Through 35 years of tumultuous relations with federal, provincial and university (McGill) agencies, KMHC now provides curative and preventative services out of a new building to Aboriginal residents of the Kahnawake reserve and nearby Montreal.[29]

4. Anishnawbe Health Toronto (AHT) was funded in 1988 by the provincial government as a multi-service urban community health centre, grounded in the principles of the Medicine Wheel and mandated to continue a 13-year history of providing services to the off-reserve, non-status and Métis population of Toronto.[30]

However, the majority of community health development in Aboriginal communities in Canada is occurring under the auspices of the transfer initiative, which refers to the transfer of 'control' over reserve health services from Medical Services Branch to Aboriginal authorities, and the devolution of responsibility for health care from the federal to the territorial governments. Culhane Speck[31] argues that transfer initiatives may be driven by federal efforts to off-load programs and contain costs rather than an interest in responding to Aboriginal community needs. Her concerns are reflected in various Aboriginal assessments and evaluations.[32] However, many First Nations have entered into the transfer process, albeit with reservations. This cautious acceptance is perhaps best articulated by the Swampy Cree Tribal Council:

> Overall, this policy direction has been criticized as an attempt to abrogate treaty rights and have Indian people administer their own misery. Nevertheless, we entered the transfer process – but with our eyes wide open. We saw transfer as a way to achieve some of our objectives and we felt we could look after ourselves in dealing with government.[33]

In this context of misgivings and caution, as of September 24, 1991, there were 79 pre-transfer projects (representing 244 bands) and 14 signed transfer agreements (representing 55 bands), as reported in the Gibbons evaluation.[34] The Gibbons evaluation concludes that while most First Nations are generally satisfied with the transfer process, concerns remain. These concerns can be summarized as follows:

1. Unclear relationship with self-government.
2. Lack of recognition of treaty rights to health.
3. Lack of legislative authority to enforce public health laws.
4. Need for program enrichment to meet new needs.

Gregory et al. provide a more scholarly and critical evaluation of one First Nation experience; they conclude that the policy does little to address the wider socio-economic and environmental sources of ill health and argue that the transfer policy reinforces the dominance of a medical model of health, which by definition maintains relations of power over Aboriginal people.[35] These authors report that the Gull Lake First Nation has suspended transfer proceedings and is developing a more comprehensive community health development plan that includes economic incentives.

Devolution of health services to the Northwest Territories was initiated in the early 1980s in response to pressure from the Inuit Tapirisat of Canada (although the Dene Nation expressed serious reservations about the impact of devolution on land claims). By 1988, transfer of authority for health to the territorial government and regional health boards was complete. Evaluations of this process have been largely critical. I have argued elsewhere that little real empowerment of regional health boards has occurred, resulting in increasing tension and alienation between Yellowknife and Inuit in the regions.[36] I argue further that Inuit are concerned that control over health services be embedded in the context of self-government, and particulary the creation of Nunavut, while the territorial government seems resistant to facilitating this process. A recent audit of the health devolution process by the Auditor General of Canada echoes these concerns.[37]

Clearly self-determination in health care is not entirely satisfied by government-mandated transfer programs, and I will return to this issue in the conclusion of this paper. Before addressing these conclusions, brief mention must be made of the human resource component of Aboriginal health. Clearly, the colonial 'face' of the health service system can be altered only partially through administrative and political control of the system. Since health and social service interactions are by definition intimate, the colonial character of the system will be maintained until the majority of services are provided by Aboriginal persons.

Direct Aboriginal participation in the provision of health and social services has been unacceptably slow in developing, largely because opportunities for professional education have been limited. Early development of the Community Health Representative program and other intermediary paraprofessional roles has been demonstrated greatly to improve the quality of Aboriginal experiences in the health care system.[38] The Indian and Inuit Nurses Association of Canada now has more than 300 members and has become an important lobby organization on behalf of Aboriginal communities.[39] Aboriginal physicians and health scientists remain small in number, however, although a dramatic increase in Aboriginal graduates from medical school are beginning to have both a clinical and an academic impact.[40] Clearly, these trends are critically important for the human face as well as the politics of health care for Aboriginal people and must be sustained.

Concluding Remarks

When the Royal Commission asked me to write a 25-page paper that was at once provocative and provided an overview of Aboriginal health conditions and services, I worried that 25 pages was either too long or too short – too long for nothing but personal opinion but too short for a scholarly review. As I complete the paper, these concerns have not changed. This review is selective in its references to trends, issues and events, yet at the same time, my opinions about Aboriginal health are at times undeveloped. Nonetheless, I believe the paper serves the purpose for which it was intended; to provide a framework for addressing and resolving major policy issues in Aboriginal health.

It is obvious from the review that there are some major gaps in our knowledge of Aboriginal health, particularly in regard to off-reserve, urban and Métis communities, although recent work by McClure, Boulanger, Kaufert and Forsyth[41] provides an initial attempt to fill this gap. However, the demand for health information describing the needs of these populations must be understood within the context of control over knowledge production. Health assessments must conform to community standards and definitions regarding the context of health and illness, and the resulting interpretations should be subject to community regulation.

It is also clear from the review that there has been enormous change in the last decade in the field of Aboriginal health. When I entered this field in the mid-1970s, Aboriginal health was defined in narrow biomedical terms, and services were controlled almost exclusively by a rigid and hierarchal federal bureaucracy. Nonetheless, self-determination in health is still a goal, particularly in relation to the broader socio-economic and environmental conditions that produce most of the current health problems in Aboriginal communities, wherever they are located. In the late 1970s, several young solvent abusers from Shamattawa were sent to a treatment centre in Philadelphia; in 1993 young solvent abusers from Davis Inlet are fortunate to be sent to Poundmaker's Lodge, but the conditions producing these situations have obviously not changed.

It would appear that although the transfer initiative occupies most of our attention (and most of our resources) in the development of community-controlled health systems, true self-determination involving broad intersectoral collaboration in the context of sustainable economic development is occurring outside the transfer initiative. Northern Quebec and several urban health initiatives are cases in point.

The concept of community healing, which integrates traditional medicine and professional services, is probably the most significant development in the Aboriginal health field. Although partially supported by NNADAP funding, Aboriginal communities across the country (and indeed around the world) are making huge progress against enormous odds on the problems that are most significant at the community level – alcohol, domestic violence and child abuse. While these problems are clearly linked to historical conditions, such as residential schools, and compensatory programs are demanded, community efforts to resolve problems deserve far greater attention and support by the public health community.[42]

Finally, traditional Aboriginal medicine clearly is undergoing a renaissance in the country and is making an enormous but undocumented contribution to community well-being. While documentation should be done only by Aboriginal scholars according to elders' regulations, I believe it is in the context of traditional medicine that issues of self-government, socio-economic development and environmental protection are best integrated with community health development for most Aboriginal communities. Even in situations where traditional medicine has been severely colonized, the underlying principles of balance, harmony, and respect, common across the Aboriginal world, provide the foundation for development.

Notes

1. The term 'social health' first appeared in the literature on Aboriginal health in the work of the Joan Feather (1991), *Social Health in Northern Saskatchewan* (Saskatoon: University of Saskatchewan). Members of the Working Group on Health Conditions in Northern Saskatchewan developed the term as a way of integrating ideas about health drawn from family and community medicine, mental health, and Aboriginal ideas about holistic health and the medicine wheel.
2. R. Thorton (1985), *American Indian Holocaust and Survival: A Population History Since 1492* (Norman, OK.: University of Oklahoma Press).
3. M.J. Norris (1990), "The demography of Aboriginal people in Canada", *in* Ethnic Demography: Canadian Immigrant, Racial and Cultural Variations, ed. S.S. Halli, F. Trovato, and L. Driedger (Ottawa: Carleton University Press), pp. 33-59.
4. H.F. Dobyns (1983), *Their Numbers Become Thinned: Native American Population Dynamics in Eastern North America* (Knoxville, TN: University of Tennessee Press).
5. Health and Welfare Canada (1991), *Health Status of Canadian Indians and Inuit – 1990* (Ottawa: Minister of Supply and Services Canada).
6. T.K. Young, E. J. Szathmary, S. Evers and B. Wheatley (1990), "Geographical distribution of diabetes among the Native population of Canada: a national survey", *Soc Sci Med* 31:129-39; T.K. Young and G. Sevenhuysen (1989), "Obesity in northern Canadian Indians: patterns, determinants, and consequences", *Am J Clin Nutr* 49:786-93; Y. Mao, H. Morrison, R. Semenciw, and D. Wigle (1986), "Mortality on Canadian Indian reserves 1976-1983", *Can J Pub Health* 77:263-68; D.C. Gillis, J. Irvine and L. Tan (1991), "Cancer incidence and survival of Saskatchewan northeners and registered Indians, 1967-1986", *in* Circumpolar Health 90: Proceedings of the 8th International Congress on Circumpolar Health, ed. B. Postl et al. (Winnipeg: University of Manitoba Press), pp. 447-51.
7. McGill AIDS Centre (1992), *First Quebec Native Aids Conference* (Montreal).

8. D.A. Armstrong (1983), *Political Anatomy of the Body: Medical knowledge in Britain in the twentieth century* (Cambridge: Cambridge University Press).

9. Cariboo Tribal Council (1991), *Faith Misplaced: Lasting Effects of Abuse in a First Nations Community; Manitoba Keewatinowi Okimakanak (1993), Solvents Poison Reserves: No facility for northern addicts* (Winnipeg Free Press, February 9, 1993).

10. Indian and Inuit Nurses of Canada (1990), *Annual Assembly Report for 1990 on Child Sexual Abuse in Aboriginal Communities*; Femmes Autochthones du Quebec (1991), *Domestic Violence in Aboriginal Communities: reference manual* (Quebec: Government of Quebec); Pauktuutit (1990), *No More Secrets: A Report on Child Sexual Abuse.*

11. D.E. Young and Leonard L. Smith (1992), *The Involvement of Canadian Native Communities in their Health Care Programs: A review of the Literature since the 1970s* (Edmonton: Canadian Circumpolar Institute).

12. Dara Culhane Speck (1989), "The Indian Health Transfer Policy: A step in the right direction or revenge of the hidden agenda?", *Native Studies Review* 5/1:187-214; John D. O'Neil (1990), "The Impact of Devolution on Health Services in the Baffin Region, NWT: A case study", *in* Devolution and Constitutional Development in the Canadian North, ed. G. Dacks (Ottawa: Carleton University Press).

13. J.D. O'Neil (1988), "Referrals to Traditional Healers: The role of medical interpreters", *in* Health Care Issues in the Canadian North, ed. D. Young (Edmonton: Boreal Institute for Northern Studies); L. Garro (1988), "Resort to Traditional Healers in a Manitoba Ojibwa Community", *Arctic Medical Research* 47/Suppl. 1:317-320.

14. R. Titely (1989), *A Narrow Vision* (Toronto: University of Toronto Press). Titely describes the amendments proscribing traditional healing ceremonies to the Indian Act, which were sponsored by missionaries and Indian agents concerned that these ceremonies were a threat to the conversion of Aboriginal populations to 'hard-working' Christian farmers.

15. A. Lightning (1976), "Sources of Healing", *University of Manitoba Medical Journal* 46/4:123-125.

16. Victoria Times Colonist, July 18, 1992, "Couple Caught in Cultural Crunch". This somewhat biased article describes the practice of initiating new members into a longhouse community, sometimes against their will, as a form of remedial action when families determine a member is acting inappropriately. In this instance the individual brought charges against the band and spirit dancers for unlawful confinement.

17. James C. MacPherson (1993), "Report from the Round Table Rapporteur", in *Aboriginal Peoples and the Justice System: Report of the National Round Table on Aboriginal Justice Issues* (Ottawa: Royal Commission on Aboriginal Peoples, 1993). Oddly, MacPherson never mentions traditional medicine in his summary of the Justice Round Table, although he acknowledges the arguments of several Aboriginal scholars that Aboriginal societies have their own internal mechanisms of social control and dispute resolution, which are compromised by state-imposed systems.

18. David Arnold, ed. (1988), *Imperial Medicine and Indigenous Societies* (Manchester: Manchester University Press).

19. Walter J. Vanast (1991), "Hastening the day of extinction: Canada, Quebec, and the medical care of Ungava's Inuit, 1867-1967", *Etudes/Inuit/Studies* 15/2:55-85.

20. Ashis Nandy (1983), *The Intimate Enemy: Loss and Recovery of Self under Colonialism* (Delhi: Oxford University Press).

21. J.D. O'Neil (1986), "The Politics of Health in the Fourth World: A northern Canadian example", *Human Organization* 45/2:119-128.

22. Government of Canada (1979) "Indian Health Policy", *in* Report of Advisory Commission on Indian and Inuit Health Consultation, T.R. Berger, commissioner, Appendix 2 (Ottawa: Health and Welfare Canada).

23. David Young and L. Smith, The Involvement of Canadian Native Communities in their Health Care Programs.

24. For contrasting perspectives on this debate, see R. F. Salisbury (1986), *A Homeland for the Cree: Regional Development in James Bay 1971-1981* (Montreal: McGill-Queen's University Press) and S. Weaver (1990), "Self-Government Policy for Indians 1980-1990: Political Transformation or Symbolic Gestures", paper presented at the 1989 UNESCO Conference on Migration and the Transformation of Cultures (Calgary: October 1989).

25. J. D. O'Neil and P. Kaufert (1993), "Irniktakpunga!: Sex Determination and the Inuit Struggle for Birthing Rights in Northern Canada", *in* Conceiving the New World Order: Global and Local Intersections in the Politics of Reproduction, ed. F. Ginsberg and R. Rapp (Los Angeles: University of California Press, forthcoming).

26. Concerns about NNADAP have been expressed in Four Worlds Development Project (1990), "Survival Secrets of NNADAP Workers", *Four Worlds Exchange* 2/1:24-39; Alberta Indian Health Care Commission (1990), "All Chiefs Health Conference Resolutions" (Edmonton); and L. Bird (1991), "Presentation: Montreal Lake", in First Nations Health Transfer Forum, November 28-30, 1989 (Ontario: Union of Ontario Chiefs).

27. For a description of history and activities see the reports of the AIHCC (1983-1992) and R.N. Nuttall (1982), "The Development of Indian Boards of Health in Alberta", *Canadian Journal of Public Health* 73/5:300-303.

28. See W. Anderson and M. Baikie (1988), "Factors Affecting Health and Social Conditions in Labrador", *Arctic Medical Research* 47/Suppl. 1:63-65, and I. Allen (1990), "Community Health Representatives Working in Labrador Inuit Communities", *in* Circumpolar Health 90, ed B. Postl et al. (Winnipeg: University of Manitoba Press).

29. See L.T. Montour and A. Macaulay (1988), "Diabetes Mellitus and Atherosclerosis: Returning research results to the Mohawk community", *Canadian Medical Association Journal* 139/3:201-202, and A.C. Macaulay (1988), "The History of Successful Community-Oriented Health Services in Kahnawake, Quebec", *Canadian Family Physician* 34:2167-2169.

30. See Anishnawbe Health Toronto (1988), *A Proposal to Establish a Community Health Centre.*; V. Johnston (1990), "Health: Yesteryear and Today", in Multiculturalism and Health Care: Realities and Needs, ed. R. Masi (Ontario: Canadian Council on Multicultural Health); and C.P. Shah (1988), "A National Overview of the Health of Native Peoples Living in Canadian Cities", *in* Inner City Health – The Needs of Urban Natives: Proceedings, ed. Y. Yacoub (Edmonton: University of Alberta).

31. Dara Culhane Speck (1989), "The Indian Health Transfer Policy".

32. See Assembly of First Nations (1989), "Draft Discussion Paper: Health Program Transfer Proposal of Medical Services Branch"; Union of Ontario Indians and Assembly of First Nations (1991), "First Nations Health Transfer Forum", November 28-30, 1989 (Nipissing First Nation: Union of Ontario Indians); M. Dion-Stout (1991), "The Role of Participation in First Nations Health Development: Is Transfer an Empowering Process?" *Synergy* 3/3:1-2.

33. G. Connell, R. Flett and P. Stewart (1990), "Implementing Primary Health Care Through Community Control: The experience of the Swampy Cree Tribal Council", *in* Circumpolar Health 90, ed. B. Postl et al. (Winnipeg: University of Manitoba Press).

34. Adrian Gibbons and Associates (1992), *Short-Term Evaluation of Indian Health Transfer* (Ottawa: Health and Welfare Canada).

35. David Gregory, C. Russell, J. Hurd, J. Tyance and J. Sloan (1992), "Canada's Indian Health Transfer Policy: The Gull Lake Band Experience", *Human Organization* 51/3:214-222.

36. J.D. O'Neil (1990), "The Impact of Devolution on health services in the Baffin Region, NWT: a case study", in Devolution and Constitutional Development in the Canadian North, ed. G. Dacks (Ottawa: Carleton University Press); and J.D. O'Neil (1991), "Democratizing health services in the Northwest Territories: Is devolution having an impact?", *Northern Review* 5:60-82.

37. Auditor General of Canada (1992), *Comprehensive Audit of the Department of Health: A report to the Legislative Assembly of the Northwest Territories.*

38. For a review of the CHR program see E. Paul, V. Toulouse and E. Roberts (1988), "The Role of Canadian Native Health Workers in Achieving Self-Government", *Arctic Medical Research* 47/Suppl. 1):66-69; and Assembly of First Nations (1988), "Community Health Representatives, Proposals for Enrichment and Expansion: Background Paper". For a critical discussion of the advocacy roles of other paraprofessionals such as medical interpreters, see J. Kaufert, J.D. O'Neil and W. Koolage (1985), "Cultural Brokerage and Advocacy in Urban Hospitals: The impact of Native language interpreters", *Sante/Culture/Health* 3/2:3-9; J.D. O'Neil (1989), "The Cultural and Political Context of Patient Dissatisfaction in Cross-Cultural Clinical Encounters: A Canadian Inuit Study", *Medical Anthropological Quarterly* 3/4:325-344.

39. J.C. Goodwill (1988), "Organized Political Action: The Inuit and Indian Nurses of Canada", *in* Canadian Nursing Faces the Future: Development and Change, ed. A.J. Baumgart and J. Larsen (St. Louis: C.V. Mosby Company).

40. A. Gilmore (1990), "Educating Native MDs: 'Always go back and serve your people in some larger way'", *Canadian Medical Association Journal* 142/2:160-162.

41. L. McClure, M. Boulanger, J. Kaufert and S. Forsyth (1992), *First Nations Urban Health Bibliography: A Review of the Literature and Exploration of Strategies* (Winnipeg: Northern Health Research Unit).

42. For examples of a largely undocumented area of development, see Assembly of Manitoba Chiefs (1991), *Family Violence and Community Healing: A Plan of Action* (Winnipeg); W.J. Mussell, W.M. Nicholls, and M.T. Adler (1991), *Making Meaning of Mental Health Challenges in First Nations: A Freirean Perspective* (Chilliwack, BC.: Sal'i'shan Institute Society); S. Hume (1991), "The Champagne/Aishihik Family & Children's Services: A unique community based approach to service delivery", *Northern Review* 7:62-75; and A. Kamin and R. Beatch (1991), "A Community Development Approach to Mental Health Services", *Northern Review* 7:92-111.

Challenging the Way We Think About Health

*Rosemary Proctor**

On January 10 this year, the *New York Times* contained an article announcing that the prestigious National Institutes of Health is establishing a new Office of Alternative Medicine. This new office will "begin seeking proposals from researchers who want to explore the merits of therapies outside mainstream healing." The *Times* noted that "some researchers hail the initiative as visionary, but others liken it to governance by horoscope". The first director of the office is a paediatrician who is familiar with American Aboriginal medicine through his Mohawk mother and through work on the Navajo Reservation.

When I saw this article, it seemed to me a very significant step on an important debate about understanding health and health policy. I hope the content of this paper will explain this significance.

Our society is really actively engaged right now, and has been for some years, in changing the way we think about health, illness, curing and caring. What we are doing is changing the paradigm that defines health and disease, how we think about health and what we do about illness.

I have chosen to use the idea of a paradigm in this discussion, because I continue to think it is useful in analyzing and understanding the subject. I want to acknowledge from the outset that there are many authors who disagree with this way of analyzing the course of events, who think this approach too restricted.

* Deputy Minister, Ministry of Community and Social Services – Ontario.

Nonetheless, I think it is useful to help us understand the changes in our approaches to health and medicine if we cast it in the language of paradigmatic thinking. In this sense, a paradigm is a shared body of theory and practice that defines a certain science. This means that the people who operate in the particular science agree upon what are the important theories, experiments, and bodies of fact for that science. They also agree about what are outstanding issues they need to investigate. The paradigm defines their intellectual world.

Occasionally, scientists operating in one paradigm change the dominant way of thinking and replace it with a new framework. The process of changing from one dominant body of theory to another has been likened to a revolution. An example is the change Galileo precipitated for western thinking when he 'discovered' that the earth revolves around the sun, rather than the sun around the earth. It certainly took a while for people to accept and digest that change. It meant looking at the world, and describing things people observed, in completely different ways.

About 30 years ago, Thomas Kuhn wrote a very influential book called *The Structure of Scientific Revolutions*. While Kuhn's book is about the history of science, it provides a useful way to think about human health.

What Kuhn says is that a revolution in scientific thinking occurs when the theories scientists use to explain reality, and the ways they practise their science, become unable to deal with critical questions or issues relevant to that science. The existing ways of thinking and working do not explain things that happen, do not explain observations that scientists make. The results of experiments somehow don't fit the expected pattern.

When this begins to happen frequently, scientists start trying to reformulate their theories to try to get more accurate or complete answers to their questions. They also go back over other contradictory evidence that has accumulated over the years but has been neglected. They reassess it. But they don't abandon the existing paradigm – the body of theory and practice – until a new one emerges to replace it.

This process of developing a new paradigm takes time. And since it is essentially a process of redefining how one sees the world (or that part of the world in question), it is often resisted by people who prefer the old definitions. Adopting a new paradigm is a sort of conversion to a different way of thinking.

What happens when we apply this framework to the issue of human health?

In the western world – that is, the white western world – starting in the early 1800s, scientists began developing what we call the 'germ' theory of disease. This theory explained that illnesses are caused by specific germs or other causal agents. It helped to explain smallpox and tuberculosis and other significant diseases of the day.

This theoretical framework, or way of defining and explaining disease, was successful in many different ways. It fostered rigorous training of physicians, objective interpretation of symptoms, and extensive research into the causes and cures of disease. Over many years, the causation paradigm has been able to deal with ever more challenging questions or demands, including organ transplants and *in vitro* fertilization.

A really important aspect of the causation paradigm is the way it defines disease. In this framework, disease has tended to be defined as a dysfunction or inability to function, the cause of which originates outside the individual. In short, it's not your fault that you are sick. The sickness comes from outside you. Health is then defined as the absence of disease, a relatively neutral state.

Over time, these definitions have also resulted in the tendency to identify everything that is not health as disease. Addictions have become illness, bizarre behaviour has become illness, disability and aging have become illnesses. All these conditions are then supposed to be treated by the medicine or intervention prescribed by the dominant paradigm.

For nearly two centuries, this paradigm has developed and has increasingly influenced the way people throughout much of the world think about health and disease. It fundamentally influences what we call health care and what we call something else – such as social services or religion.

However, the paradigm has not been without challenges. In fact, over the past 30 years or more, people have been criticizing many aspects of the causation paradigm, suggesting that it is not necessarily or always valid or that it is too narrowly conceived. It is not able to deal adequately with the experiences of illness in contemporary society.

For example, at one time the development of scientific medicine was generally credited with a substantial improvement in life expectancy. More recent studies suggest that the decline in the mortality rates actually started before the rise of modern medicine. Increases in life expectancy can be explained more accurately by improvements in nutrition, housing, contraception and sanitation. Other population studies indicate that patterns of illness and morbidity are more successfully explained by environmental facts such as occupation, socio-economic status and gender than by access to health care or treatment of disease.

In several areas, recent studies have identified trends toward greater disparity in mortality and morbidity rates within societies. That is, there is a trend toward reduced mortality in the higher socio-economic classes and increasing mortality in the lower socio-economic or occupational groups.

In the mental health field, critics question the utility of the causation paradigm in understanding behaviour or in prescribing effective treatment. Including so-called mental illness in the purview of the paradigm is seen as misrepresenting the nature of human experience and problems of living.

The causation paradigm was never situated in a social or economic context. It is generally seen as being timeless, and without boundaries, because it is rooted in proven scientific evidence and physiological facts. It does not acknowledge that as modern medicine has spread around the world – has become the dominant paradigm – it has engulfed, and in many cases discredited and eliminated, traditional forms of thinking about health and health care in different parts of the world. Much as dominant western, industrialized culture has spread its hegemony, the subculture of health care and thinking about individual and community health has also spread.

Dr. David Skinner, of the Yukon Medical Association, whose presentation to the Royal Commission I read, has articulated this clearly:

> What we have to remember here is, we have a white ethnocentric health care system which we have brought to the native people, and we are asking them to see it and do it our way.... It is our belief, though, that because our white man's medicine is very technical-oriented, very symptom-oriented, very drugs- and surgery-oriented, it lacks something that native medicine has and which we desperately need but don't practise: spirituality, or a spiritual component.

One criticism of the paradigm is its narrowness: human experience is being fit into too tight a mould. The paradigm began to be constructed at a time when European living standards were improving dramatically. The newly developing paradigm was not necessarily aware or conscious of the significance of these improvements. Nor did the causation paradigm confront the problems associated with efforts to eradicate a culture. It can explain little about the associated problems of family breakdown, violence, suicide, alcohol and drug use. It does not embrace the compounding problems of poverty, lack of employment, and powerlessness.

Gradually, a new or modified paradigm is emerging to challenge the firm premises of specific causation. I tend to think of this emerging body of work as an environmental paradigm, because it explains illness and disease in terms of all aspects of our world environment and of our bodies themselves. In this environmental paradigm, health and illness are no longer opposites, but more like points along a continuum.

The environmental framework sees human beings as adapting to their environment in effective and ineffective ways and simultaneously altering their environment in beneficial and harmful ways. The environmental framework includes the psychology of human beings and society, the vulnerability of individuals to specific diseases, the interaction of people and their environment. Health has become a goal statement: the presence of physical, social and mental well-being. The question has become not what is the cause of disease, but what are the determinants of health.

Disease is seen less frequently as being caused by specific agents and identified more as emerging from the interaction of the individual and the social environment (the concepts of risk, the effects of pollution) and the individual (genetic vulnerability to certain illnesses, lifestyle or life experience). The emphasis is more on defining wellness.

In turn, the mediating forces, those that promote health and prevent illness, include social supports, employment, reduced environmental pollution, and so on. These, as well as health care, are seen as legitimate subjects for research in the areas of health and illness. The individual's social and physical environment may be more appropriate for intervention than the nature of the specific illness. Sophie Pierre made this point in her presentation to the Commission at the Cranbrook hearing: "Wellness encompasses all areas of human development that affect the physical, emotional and spiritual wellness of our people. If any of these facets is in need of healing, a complete range of related solutions is necessary."

The process of reconsidering an old paradigm, rejecting it, and developing a new one is filled with conflict. There is a strong tendency for people working in one paradigm to ignore evidence that contradicts their version of reality. One obvious example is the well documented iatrogenic effects of medical treatment, that is, the fact that drugs and treatments can and do cause illness. There is a tendency for the medical treatment system to adopt medical procedures and continue to use them despite documentation that they are ineffective or harmful.

Conflict over public policy occurs as practitioners or proponents of the two paradigms compete for support and resources. This is a paradigm shift that is not limited to scientists and laboratories. It engages the public individually and collectively. It engages us in our communities, in our particular historical and social consciousness. Consider the strength of the causation paradigm and the professions and institutions it has engendered. Consider the importance of health to people generally. The struggle for power – for the influence to define the meaningful questions, methods and theories – is understandable.

However, this may sound too much like a conflict between two quite opposite ways of viewing reality. Rather, the situation is probably closer to creating a new paradigm by incorporating aspects of the specific causation framework and aspects of the new insights into a larger whole. This process enables us to test what more effectively answers the perplexing questions of our time and our communities. It will also enable us, one would hope, to add a sense of cultural and historical reality to our so-called 'scientific' knowledge.

Health promotion and prevention have become key concepts in the new paradigm. Initially, the definitions of prevention were highly individualistic. They reflected a linear relationship between, for example, 'lifestyle' and a person's risk for illness, e.g., the relationship between cigarette smoking and lung cancer. Over time, health promotion and prevention are becoming more social in nature. They are seen as community, group and collective efforts. The issues of lifestyle are recognized as being very complex.

In the new paradigm, there is scope for individual responsibility for health, certainly in terms of personal health but also more generally. For example, when the occurrence of disease is correlated with lack of exercise, the individual is seen to bear some responsibility for this behaviour and to some extent for the presence or duration of disease. In the more general case of morbidity that is correlated with environmental factors, such as poverty and lack of nutrition, the paradigm suggests that society as a whole is able to affect health. Collectively, we have a responsibility to prevent disease or improve the chances of achieving health. Efforts to recover or rediscover aspects of traditional healing and bring these to bear on modern afflictions are also expanding the new framework. Healing circles, for example, may illustrate the more effective linkage of people's spiritual and social well-being with the physical and emotional problems they experience.

In efforts to develop a new paradigm, the dominant culture is searching for new ideas. People may well be too conditioned by the dominant mode of analyzing and explaining reality, and this itself may be a barrier to thinking creatively about alternatives. Nonetheless, this creative work is going on in communities in Canada and elsewhere. The work of the Aboriginal communities in finding ways of integrating traditional understanding and healing with modern medicine may not only assist the people in these communities, but also help to further the development of new ways of understanding human health and the challenges of caring and curing.

Which brings me back to the *New York Times* article. To me it represents a successful challenge to the power of the established paradigm, because it recognizes that there are other questions to pursue. It helps bring mainstream resources to answering questions that are important to the new paradigm. It illustrates the importance of the bridge between traditional understandings and approaches to health and those that are embodied in the dominant culture. While it certainly may threaten the firm views of some researchers, to others it represents the creative challenge of addressing questions that are important to our communities. It shows that the definition of health and illness is an open question, one in which many of us may usefully and creatively engage.

Suicide in Canadian Aboriginal Peoples: Causes and Prevention

*Clare Clifton Brant**

> The greatest evil...and the worst crime is poverty. Our first obligation to ourselves is not to be poor.
>
> – *George Bernard Shaw, playwright, 1907*

> Every disease has two causes. The first is pathophysiological; the second, political.
>
> – *Ramon Cajal, pathologist, 1899*

The suicide rate for Aboriginal people in 1984 was 43.5 per 100,000 population. This compares with an overall Canadian suicide rate of 13.7 per 100,000 that year. The Aboriginal suicide rate in 1984 showed a substantial decline from 64 per 100,000 in 1981, but was still three times the Canadian rate. Reliable statistics are not available for para-suicides and suicide attempts. There also is some difficulty in documenting the actual incidence of suicide in Aboriginal populations, since non-status Indians may not be included in some statistics. The method of identification of Aboriginal people varies from location to location across the country.

* M.D., F.R.C.P.(C). Mohawks of the Bay of Quinte #1484, Box 89, York Road, Shannonville, Ontario, K0K 3A0; (613) 966-0888.

Suicide in the Aboriginal population tends to occur in clusters. Dr. Jack Ward (1977) reported a suicide rate of 267 per 100,000 in 1975 for a twelve-month period at Wikwemikon – astronomical in comparison to the average suicide rate in Canada overall, which is fairly constant at 14 per 100,000 population per year. Other reserves and settlements, however, report a zero suicide rate per year. These clusters of suicides and suicide attempts often attract intense scrutiny and media reporting that borders on sensationalism.

The suicide rate for Aboriginal people is highest in the age group 15 to 24 years. Among the demographic characteristics of suicides and suicide attempters are those identified by Travis (see Table 1) and Dizmang et al. (1971):

- non-parental caretakers
- caretaker arrests
- early age of first arrest
- arrest in previous 12 months
- recent break in relationship through conflict or death.

These demographic characteristics seem to be fairly constant in other studies. (Ward, 1977; May, 1974)

Table 1

Suicides and Suicide Attempters (North-West Alaska, 1970-1980)

Characteristics	Male	Female
Age	23.2 years	22.0 years
Education	10.5 years	9.5 years
Unemployed	78%	82%
Never married	92%	77%
No occupation	61%	79%
Household income less than $10,000/year	77%	88%
Alcoholic or alcohol abuse	77%	65%

Source: Travis, 1983.

A significant demographic characteristic identified in Travis's study and supported by other studies is that suicides tend to be slightly better educated then their non-suicidal Aboriginal peers but still less educated than the non-Aboriginal population. This would suggest that they may have had ambitions about participating in mainstream society but may have encountered difficulties competing for jobs or recognition because they were behind in terms of educational achievement. Ninety-two per cent of male suicides were never married. Some of the studies break down the 'never married' category into single and common-law relationships.

Single people in the general population are more vulnerable to suicide, but when you think of the importance of being connected in a family for Indian people, that figure is very significant; in many Indian traditions a young man does not become recognized as an adult until he takes a wife and establishes a self-sustaining family unit. Sixty-one per cent of suicides and suicide attempters had no occupation. Annual household income compared to the average income in the region was substantially lower in households of suicides. Alcoholism or alcohol abuse was present in 77 per cent of cases.

Another factor that has been identified in other studies, in particular one done by Dizmang in 1971, is the frequency of non-parental caretakers or foster care. Young people who had been suicidal frequently had been cared for in their early lives by persons other than their parents or family. Dizmang also found that the caretakers themselves had been arrested more frequently than a similar group of Aboriginal people who were the same age, tribal background and community experience. He found that the suicides tended to have caretakers who had troubled personal situations as well.

In 1985, the Canadian Psychiatric Association Section on Native Mental Health, known now as the Native Mental Health Association of Canada, had a three day meeting in Sainte-Foy, Quebec, on suicide. The following paradigm was established as a framework for understanding the distressingly high incidence of self-destructive behaviour in the Aboriginal population.

1. Poverty		1. History of disturbing childhood experiences		1. Alcohol abuse
2. Powerlessness	+	2. Recent separation or loss	=	2. Depression
3. Anomie				3. Suicide

Poverty

Dr. Fred Wien, who discussed the contribution of poverty and its relationship to suicide at that meeting, gave us the chronology of the economic history of the Micmacs shown in Table 2 (next page).

The centralization policy worsened a trend toward higher unemployment that began with the depression of the 1920s and 1930s.

Although this is the economic history of the Micmac Nation, it can be applied at different times and at different levels to other First Nations. Looking at the Micmac economic history, one has to be impressed with the variation in their economic fortunes, ranging from self-reliance to complete destitution and various points in between in the several centuries since European contact.

Table 2

Major Periods in Micmac Economic History

Approximate Dates	Principal Characteristics
1. Up to 1500	Aboriginal subsistence patterns; community production and consumption
2. 1500-1783	Early European contact and the fur trade
3. 1784-1867	Transition to settlement and subordination
4. 1868-1940	Labour in the industrial economy
5. 1941-present	Centralization, welfare and government dependence

1. An Aboriginal period dating from some 10,600 years ago and lasting to about 1500 A.D., at which point European contact became a significant factor. The period prior to 1500 can be characterized by the pursuit of Aboriginal subsistence patterns, based on the hunting, fishing and gathering of natural food sources and organized on a community basis.

2. A period dating from the early 1500s to 1783, which was characterized by early contact with Europeans and increasingly by the exploitation of the fur trade. European diseases and other forms of interference in traditional patterns took their toll. However, the Micmac could adapt fairly readily to the demands of the fur trade, since it did not represent a sharp break from Aboriginal hunting patterns and they were certainly important, necessary participants in the fur trade economy. They had, therefore, some leverage over the situation and no doubt they used their influence to advantage.

3. By the late 1700s the fur trade had given way to an economy based on settled agriculture, pursued by a rapidly growing number of European and American immigrant settlers. This period, which lasted until Confederation, was a disaster for the Micmacs of the province because it was completely incompatible with the Indians' preferred and accustomed way of making a living. It also provided few opportunities for Micmac participation.

4. With Confederation came a shift in adminstration to a more activist federal government and a continuation of Micmac efforts to achieve a toehold in the prevailing economy of the region. To a considerable degree, they were successful; for much of the period to 1940 they worked on the fringes of the white economy, achieving a largely self-reliant economic base although one that was precarious and not prosperous.

5. The final stage extends from 1940 to the present day and is characterized by at least three significant features. First, the Indian Affairs Branch, in its wisdom, decided to centralize the many Indian reserves scattered across the province into two locations, at Shubencadie on the Nova Scotia mainland and at Eskasoni in Cape Breton. While their intentions were not fully implemented and some families trickled back to their original locations after a period of time, still many hundreds of people were uprooted in the process and along with them were destroyed the tenuous economic adaptations that they had made to their local environment. While a short employment boom occurred in the centralization locations, much of it occasioned by the need to build housing for the new arrivals, this was not to last more than a decade.

There has always been a widely recognized and accepted statistical correlation between socio-economic class and suicide in the North American culture. The highest suicide rate is in the fifth and lowest socio-economic class, which includes those on public assistance and welfare. Aboriginal people are part of this fifth class. The next highest incidence occurs in the first socio-economic class, though at a lower rate. This author has never heard a satisfactory explanation of why lower classes in an upwardly mobile capitalist democracy frequently engage not only in self-destructive behaviour but in substance abuse.

Accounts of early settlers and missionaries described the Aboriginal people of Canada at the time of early settlement as living in the stone age as self-reliant, innocent, peaceful and joyful. Using Dr. Wien's summary of Micmac history, one cannot fail to see the parallel between economic independence followed by dependency and subjugation with the erosion of self-esteem and the rise of social problems. Canada is not the only country in the world where foreign settlers deliberately displaced, overwhelmed, subjugated and humiliated the indigenous population. A similar pattern occurred in New Zealand, Australia and South Africa. The Aboriginal people of Canada had no concept of land ownership. They did feel entitled to exclusive hunting rights to certain areas but these were fluent and flexible.

A capitalist democracy was established in North America with an allegedly classless society. This was different from the European aristocratic society, which was based on heredity, title and land ownership. North American 'meritocracy' promises success, wealth, fame and fortune to all who are born in the country and even to new immigrants. However, these aspirations are pie in the sky hopes when one's family is hungry and one's heating oil tank is empty. Most Indian reserves are placed in areas where economic development is impossible, thus excluding most Aboriginal people from the job market. Approximately 3 per cent of the budget of the department of Indian Affairs is spent on economic development. Television programs, via satellite, have made even the most remote Aboriginal peoples aware of the luxuries available to the citizens of Canada. We who live in more prosperous areas have come to terms with the fact that programs like *Dallas* and *The Brady Bunch* do not, in fact, represent the ordinary or normal way of living for most North American citizens, but if one is in an isolated setting, this is held up as the norm. To take one's eyes off a television program depicting the grandeur of the residence at South Fork and to survey one's own poorly heated and insulated hovel can only have a deleterious effect on self-esteem. As far as this author knows, there has been no study relating the invasion of satellite television to the suicide rate. Aboriginal people have, however, been included in the global village of Marshall McLuhan and are daily reminded of their poverty, despair and hopelessness. North American Aboriginal people do not have the career aspirations of Donald Trump, but they are not alone in their disappointed aspirations. There is also an epidemic of suicide and para-suicides as well as suicide attempts in disaffected youth in the non-Aboriginal population because education, the original ticket to prosperity, has been invalidated. Doctors of philosophy are driving taxis in Toronto.

Powerlessness

Dr. Marlene Brant-Castellano, in her presentation at the suicide conference in 1985, spoke to the issue of powerlessness and power as a contributing factor in Aboriginal suicide. Three dimensions of power and the lack thereof are described:

1. Personal power (I'm okay)
2. Interpersonal power (I am related)
3. Functional power (I can do)

Characteristics of Powerful and Powerless Persons

Powerful	Powerless
1. Personal Power	
• childhood experience of being nourished and guided • knowing and valuing their gifts • having a sense of perspective	• unstable relationships in early life • uncertainty that life and their place in the world will give them what they need • questioning whether the frustration and deprivation they experience are their fault • hopelessness
2. Interpersonal Power	
• maintaining caring relationships with a variety of persons • mature sexuality	• inability to sustain relationships in which they care for others and are cared for • unrealistic expectations of others • expecting rejection and acting in a way that invites rejection
3. Functional Power: Knowing things and knowing how to do things	
• effective in work • providing for family • taking on and fulfilling responsibility • recovering from failure and learning from experience	• lack of training and job skills • unemployment • aggressive behaviour without a positive goal • impulsive crime • reckless driving • fighting

At a personal level, powerful persons generally are those who have had childhood experiences of being nourished and guided. They come through the stormy time of adolescent transition from childhood to adult responsibility and as adults they know and value their gifts and their particular place in the world. When they experience setbacks, they have confidence that after a period of mourning, they will be able to get up and go on with the battle of life again with energy and purpose. On the other hand, people who are personally powerless frequently report unstable relationships in early life. They are uncertain that they will get what they need even at the most fundamental level of physical survival. They experience uncertainty about whether the frustration and deprivation they experience are external or internal in their causation. This generates a feeling that there is nothing they can do to change the unfortunate situations in which they find themselves. This hopelessness about themselves, if triggered by mechanisms of alcohol abuse, a broken relationship, grief over the loss of someone close or even the suicide of someone they hear about, can push them over the edge from hopelessness to self-destruction.

At an interpersonal level, powerful persons are able to establish and maintain caring relationships with a variety of persons. That is to say they feel connected to and loved by a number of people in their environment and are able to return this love in a responsible way. A lack of connectedness or interpersonal power can lead to a feeling of indifference about the feelings of the survivors of their own suicide. Since no one cares, no one will grieve. They have lost or not established what Jean Vanier considered most valuable when he said, "I think the most important thing in life is to feel that you are loved, to feel that if you are not there, you will be missed and that if you die, someone will weep for you."

The functional dimension of power and powerlessness is "knowing things and knowing how to do things", a phrase borrowed from Erik Eriksen's *Youth Identity and Crisis*. Functionally powerful people demonstrate effectiveness in work, in providing for family, in taking on and fulfilling responsibility, in recovering from failure and in looking at those failures as the basis for learning. When one reviews the demographic characteristics of suicides and suicide attempters, one notices the poverty, unemployment, poor education and lack of family responsibilities. (Travis, 1983) In summary, Dr. Brant-Castellano, in her review of the research, reported that persons whose hopefulness about themselves, hopefulness about their relationships, and hopefulness about their competence to do something worthwhile is under repeated assault from an early age are particularly vulnerable to suicidal thoughts, gestures, attempts and completed suicides.

Anomie

Anomie is a term that conveys the opposite of complete institutionalization. When an individual is institutionalized in a convent or the army or a mental hospital, the things in life are decided for them. Their relationships, their values, what they do during the day, who they relate to, who the heroes are, who the villains are, are all prescribed. Anomie is the exact opposite – a state or condition where all societal values lose structure and meaning. One of the early sociologists and still extensively quoted suicidologists was Emile Durkheim who, in his 1897 book *Le Suicide*, divided suicide into three categories:

1. Altruistic suicide. This is done for love of one's country, nation, family or other organization. It occurs occasionally in the Aboriginal population. This author recalls a particularly effective and charismatic young Aboriginal leader who hanged himself out of frustration and as a protest against the bureaucratic system of Indian Affairs.
2. Egoistic suicide, corresponding to Dr. Brant-Castellano's outline of powerlessness, in which life no longer has meaning in terms of the meaning of existence for the individual.
3. Anomic suicide, resulting from lack of regulatory factors in life.

In his book Durkheim says that "anomie indeed springs from the lack of collective forces at certain points in society; that is, of groups established for the regulation of social life. Anomie results from the same state of disintegration from which the egoistic current springs."

Nothing could better describe the state of social disorganization on many Indian reserves. The old methods of coping, the old philosophies and religions, which taught resilience, survival and a sense of being at one with nature, have been denigrated and destroyed by the dominant culture and discarded by many Aboriginal people. There is a wellspring of hope coming from re-establishment of Aboriginal traditions, such as sweat lodges, sweet grass ceremonies and the establishment of departments of Aboriginal studies at various universities where young people can rediscover the old ways.

Rediscovering or establishing one's Aboriginal identity and the normative rules of Aboriginal society is not without risk. The parents of the students in the Aboriginal studies programs, raised in traditional Christian churches, often chastise their children for studying "demonic religions". These parents have identified with and become like the oppressors. In a review of suicides at the Prison for Women in Kingston, Ontario, one of the precipitants of suicide, whose importance could not be fully assessed in the overall stressful environment facing Aboriginal women in that institution, was thought to be in part their entering an Aboriginal awareness program by way of an Aboriginal women's group with outside medicine people, sweat lodges and sweet grass ceremonies. Some of these women, who had lived anti-social lifestyles to the point where they had to be locked up for their own safety and the safety of others, became aware that life had meaning, purpose and direction; but when they returned to the cells and the ranges and were confronted with the harsh realities of the oppressive and cruel prison structure, the change was too abrupt and overwhelming. Suicide was their escape from this mind-splitting discrepancy between the inner peace they had acquired and the unspeakable cruelties of the prison system. In some respects, their suicides could be classified as containing altruistic, egoistic and anomic features.

General Causes of Psycho-Social Stresses

A list of the general causes of psycho-social stress was compiled from 600 non-directed interviews with Aboriginal people across Ontario. (Technical Assistance in Planning Associates, 1979) These causes were identified by Aboriginal people without prompting:

1. inadequate housing
2. lack of employment and other income support, including adequate welfare benefits
3. absence of recreation facilities and programs
4. poor access to education and health resources
5. disorganized band administration
6. absent or inadequate transportation
7. disorganization and inadequacy of social services, including family and children's services
8. absence of counselling services for Indian people

Housing on most Indian reserves across Canada is in a state of crisis. Two or three families sometimes live in a three-bedroom bungalow designed for a single family. These crowded conditions serve as a hothouse for irritability and family violence. One of the most serious crimes that can be committed on an Indian reserve is arson, because the community is outraged that precious housing has been destroyed, sometimes leaving three or four families literally out in the cold.

The list of stressors contains, of course, chronic unemployment and under-employment, resulting in the social problems outlined by Dr. Wien.

There are very few recreation centres on reserves and those that do exist are poorly maintained and equipped. Young people, idle and bored, are frequently seen hanging around outside with no real goal or purpose to their activities. The old adage that "the Devil finds work for idle hands" applies in that young people get involved easily in thrill-seeking and risk-taking behaviour, solvent inhalation and other forms of substance abuse out of sheer boredom.

Statistics are not immediately available as to what percentage of Aboriginal students have to leave home to obtain a secondary school education, but there are very few high schools close enough to Indian reserves to allow daily transportation, particularly in the North. It is necessary for young people to go into boarding situations, in strange communities, at the tender of age of thirteen or fourteen years when they are most vulnerable to societal prejudices against pigmented skin and lack of fluency in the English language. Many Indian reserves are provided health care services through a fly-in physician, and many are not large enough to warrant the establishment of a nursing station.

Disorganized band administration, which is patterned on the bureaucracy of the department of Indian Affairs, is a daily thorn in the flesh of every Indian person. Band office staff, who are often inadequately trained, have no job descriptions, no sense of empowerment or responsibility and little opportunity to learn, terrorize the reserve residents with their oppositional behaviour. Frequent appeals are made to the chief and councillors, who intervene in ordinary day-to-day decisions of the band administration, further eroding and undermining staff confidence and their ability to make useful decisions. The chief and councillors are also distracted from important issues by wasting their time on minor administrative matters.

One does not often think of transportation as being a psycho-social stress – at least those of us who own several vehicles don't. If one had the qualifications for a job in the city, and if one could afford the air fare to get to the interview and muster the fluency of language to obtain the job, one would still be faced with the unhappy decision of having to establish two residences, thereby reducing one's income to less than the welfare benefits that would be available if one stayed home. A return air ticket to the closest settlement in the far North can cost $600. Food that is flown in is exorbitantly expensive and of poor quality.

There is a patchwork of Aboriginal family and children's services funded by the federal government and mandated by provincial governments to do prevention work with children and families on reserves. The mandate for protection remains with the provincially funded agencies. As a psychiatrist, this author has frequently been involved in jurisdictional disputes between prevention and protection services, and the level of tension that this generates is remarkable.

Identifying the absence of counselling services as a stressor means that Aboriginal people wish to be spoken to in their own language by indigenous counsellors. Outside consultants, even eminent psychiatrists who are worthy and venerable in their own communities, often bring more mischief than assistance when parachuted into our Aboriginal communities.

This list of stressors, added to the poverty, powerlessness and anomie already outlined, compounds levels of psycho-social stress and tension to the point where one wonders how any Aboriginal person has survived at all without resorting to substance abuse or self-destruction.

The foregoing outline of the contributing causes of suicide among Aboriginal peoples in Canada is far from complete, but it should be adequate to give readers a sense of the contributing factors. Because of space and time constraints, it is now necessary to move on to prevention strategies.

Prevention Strategies

These can be divided into primary, secondary and tertiary. Tertiary prevention refers to dealing with actual suicide attempts, which usually involves temporary hospitalization to deal with the physical injury, crisis intervention counselling on an emergency basis, evacuation to a locked psychiatric facility, treatment of depression and other mental illnesses, alcohol detoxification and rehabilitation, pharmacotherapy and psychotherapy. Suicide attempters usually get the treatment they need. There seems to be a bottomless pit of funds from different sources to mop up blood. The reader should not take this sarcasm as ingratitude for the emergency assistance offered to Aboriginal suicide attempters by the dominant culture. The wish in making this remark is to draw attention to the need for secondary and primary prevention.

Secondary prevention consists of early identification of those people at risk. One might say that the entire Aboriginal population of Canada is at risk, and this would be partially true. However some are facing an acute risk. This intervention would mean education in the early recognition of suicidal risks in the community by the general population of the reserves. The typical Aboriginal person at risk for suicide is a 23-year-old male who has had a failed attempt at higher education, is unmarried, unemployed and poor, and who abuses alcohol. A previous history of suicidal attempts and gestures is often present. There is a problem with early identification and treatment of at-risk persons because Aboriginal societies are generally non-interfering; if such a person were identified and approached to ask whether he was having problems, the probable response would be “Nothing I can’t handle”, because self-reliance in one’s internal emotional world is expected.

Beatrice Shawanda, speaking at the 1985 suicide conference, outlined social programs in the Manitoulin Island area, which could be classified under the rubric of secondary prevention. After the 1975 suicide epidemic on Wikwemikon Reserve, the Rainbow Lodge for local treatment of alcohol abuse was established. The lodge became a spark plug for the rest of the community, in that numerous community programs were run by the staff. Ms. Shawanda has published a book, which is available from the Rainbow Lodge at Manitoulin Island. Some of these interventions were innovative to say the least. Bea Shawanda felt it important that the community get together on a regular basis just to socialize and re-introduce themselves to each other. Feasts were held to honour prominent citizens in the community. The cooking and washing up was done by volunteers who were invited from the community to do so; thus most of the people on the reserve were included in one way or another, even those who continued to abuse alcohol. Bea went as far as to hold a dog show, complete with prizes and a banquet. These social occasions assisted in developing a sense of community, purpose, direction and belonging. Other events, such as political or religious gatherings, tend to split communities rather than unite them in a common purpose.

All, however, are effective when they unite the members of an Indian reserve into one large family.

It is easier to do this with an agricultural people such as the Iroquoian groups. We have been least affected by the exploitation of the white man, since we had already established large villages and a village economy. The hunting and gathering tribes who used to live in groups of 15 to 25 people have still not adapted to living in large communities of up to 1,500 people.

Primary prevention, which would remove the causes of poverty, powerlessness and anomie, are infrequently discussed and rarely implemented. At a general level, according to Dr. Fred Wien, the following general considerations need to be addressed around poverty:

1. just settlements of Aboriginal land claims in order to affirm historical rights, resist external incursions, and expand the resource base of Indian communities to permit future development;
2. the furtherance of Indian control over their institutions and programs, but not as an excuse for the federal government to wash its hands of the problems that have been created and reduce funding in the process. Full and relevant training of the staff involved in program takeovers and the redesign of programs to meet Indian needs are essential;
3. undertaking serious, long-range employment and economic development initiatives supported by Indian-controlled development institutions and aimed at expanding economic opportunities for all segments of Indian communities;
4. enhancing the adaptive capacity of Indian communities by continuing to improve the opportunities for and the quality of education available to persons in all age groups;
5. encouraging the development of political structures at the band level that are seen to be legitimate, that encourage the involvement of all band members, and that resist the abuse of power and the development of sharp inequalities;
6. developing and implementing an approach to community development that is both consistent with the components mentioned above and that, in terms of process, is effective in Aboriginal communities.

Prevention and Treatment of Powerlessness

The expert in this area, William Mussell, is already on the program and undoubtedly will deal in detail with empowerment. In 1992, at the Canadian Mental Health Association meeting in Ottawa, he stated that "people who have been oppressed for generations have a great fear of responsibility. We must learn to approach and interact with people who are afraid of responsibility." (Mussell, 1992) This reminded me of a clinical anecdote told by Dr. Jack Ward before his untimely death in 1990. He reported that in one of the communities where he served as a visiting psychiatrist, a 12-year-old girl had lost her 15-year-old sister to suicide. This young girl, to whom he gave the name Elaine, began to feel hopeless and wished to join her sister in death. She began by collecting some of her mother's pills and taking them. She then threw a rope over a rafter in their home and put the noose around her neck. At about that time, her brother looked in the window; Elaine noticed him, and this stopped her suicide attempt. However, the parents were notified and she was assessed at the mental health clinic. It was not entirely clear to Dr. Ward what had happened at the clinic, because one person reported that there was nothing wrong with the girl. The other report from the clinic was that she refused to talk and because she would not talk, nothing could be done for her. She was sent home. Subsequently over the next two months, Elaine would continue to get upset, drink alcohol and slash her arms. She had a number of scars on her arms from where she had carved away at them. Her parents knew of about least three of the five slashing episodes. There was no attempt to get help. Finally one night, Elaine went outdoors, sometime around 11 p.m., and joined some friends; they consumed the better part of a 26-ounce bottle of spirits. Elaine said to her friend, "Would you help me find a place, because I want to go out and hang myself?" The girlfriend hugged her and said, "We love you" but let her go. An hour later, Elaine turned up at her home and said to those present, "Good-bye, I am going to hang myself." She left the house but turned up again perhaps a half-hour later, saw another girl, and again said good-bye to her and that she was going to hang herself. At 4 a.m. they found her body hanging from a tree in the bush.

Dr. Ward counted 21 people to whom Elaine had talked about suicidal ideation and plan. No one responded to her cry for help. Can the reader imagine himself or herself in such a desperate situation and what it must have been like to have the door slammed in one's face when one is in such a state of hopelessness and despair. When confronted at a coroner's inquest about the lack of interest or intervention in this young girl's distress, most of the 21 people reported that they did not want to discuss suicide with her because then "she would go out and do it".

This gruesome anecdote is recorded to point out the necessity for public education around suicide, not only as a secondary prevention, but as a primary prevention to encourage Aboriginal people to discuss their inner feelings without fear of being put down for not being self-reliant.

It has been estimated that the language skills of most Aboriginal people are at about the grade seven level. (Ward, 1985) We often assume that because they speak Cree or Ojibwa or Mohawk, that they can discuss difficult and complex existential and emotional issues in their Aboriginal language. The reality in most cases is that they are no more fluent in their Aboriginal language than they are in English and struggle to express themselves in either language. Thus they are unable to communicate inner feelings or to name and understand the inner workings of their own minds.

It is important to develop the language skills of our young Aboriginal people to the point where they can name, identify and express feelings and internal processes and thus establish interpersonal connectedness and communication. (Mussell, 1992) This could occur in discussion groups established at recreational facilities, church meetings, leisure activities and formal therapy and healing groups. There is a common myth among many Aboriginal people that to discuss depression, other bad feelings and suicidal thoughts, is to give evil a space in one's mind and in the community. To listen to another's complaint of hopelessness, psychological torment and despair is to be reminded of one's own, and so a denial process is rampant. Bad feelings are, in fact, contagious. If my brother is in pain and he tells me in a way that I can relate to, I will experience his pain as well which, added to my own, might tip me into hopelessness, despair and suicide. Thus Aboriginal people, as illustrated by Dr. Ward's story, pussyfoot around seriously depressed and suicidal members of their community for fear of getting in touch with their own psychological torment. I suppose the catastrophic event would be a mass suicide of the entire community; the price for not speaking up, however, or listening actively, is to wall off the desperate suicidal members of the community with a conspiracy of silence and denial.

Dealing With and Preventing Anomie

Only during the last ten years have Aboriginal studies been introduced into the public school system. When the students of a school are predominantly Aboriginal, they are taught their heritage, ceremonies, legends and even have a block of days set aside for festival activities honouring the history of their own tribes. This author's children, aged nine and ten, are far better informed about the Mohawk culture than he was at their age. In this setting, self-esteem as an Aboriginal person can develop in a fashion parallel with the dominant culture. Previously one's self-esteem depended on the degree to which one could acculturate oneself and give up the old Indian ways in favour of an allegedly more progressive culture. Throughout the period of colonial suppression of traditional Aboriginal ways, a few people have held fast to the dignity and the wisdom that they received from their fathers and mothers and grandfathers and grandmothers. Over decades and even centuries, these people who have held firm held intact the integrity of Aboriginal traditions, have become resource persons, elders, role models and real inspirations to those of us who have been trying to recreate or discover an understanding of what it means to be Aboriginal, what it means to be Mohawk, Ojibwa or Cree. These elders who recall or have preserved the old methods of resilience, recovery and survival are not given as prominent a position in our societies as they deserve. Aboriginal people themselves must ask and insist, "Teach us grandfather, teach us the old ways of thinking."

It is a principle of psychoanalytic theory that when a group of people, even if they are of diverse backgrounds and aspirations, get together on a regular basis, a group process will evolve. The group will establish for itself an identity, become a living organism made up of individual cells (persons), and establish for itself and its members purpose, direction and belonging. In order to deal with anomie in our Aboriginal communities, the solution is simplistic. We need places, times and opportunities to get together, speak to each other, develop a language among us to talk about our inner feelings and to establish new methods of coping using the old Indian ways. This probably would be best done under the supervision and direction of an elder. It initially, I suppose, would contain a great deal of psychotherapeutic work, but eventually it would evolve into a sense of community. Sweat lodges and healing circles are now serving this function in some communities, but they should be expanded, financed, allowed and facilitated by Aboriginal people themselves, using external resources of funding and occasionally, professional consultation. If a group of Aboriginal women gets together to sew a quilt, they do more than make stitches. They establish a sense of purpose, direction, belonging and continuity when younger members are added to their group. The Indian need for and fascination with gossip in these groups is satisfied, contained and sometimes even controlled by the correction of misinformation about community members.

Morrison (1981) partially corroborated the list of psycho-social stresses from the Indian perspective in her compilation of suggested solutions to mental health problems among Canadian Indians. She listed them as follows:

1. parenting skills, training courses (100 per cent of respondents)
2. increased recreation (97.7 per cent)
3. improved housing (97.7 per cent)
4. long-term job opportunities on and off the reserve (96.5 per cent)
5. on-reserve counselling services (95.3 per cent)

It is remarkable that 100 per cent of the people Morrison interviewed indicated to her that they felt ineffective in dealing with behavioural problems, communicating with, guiding and nurturing their children. The cause of this feeling of parental incompetence could be the subject of an entire thesis. The development of parenting skills was interrupted by the residential school system, so that there were two or three generations of Aboriginal people who were 'parented' by religious institutions and subjected to coercion and verbal, sexual and physical abuse. Even those people who did not have the residential school experience reported that the old childrearing practices of non-interference and permissiveness no longer were relevant in twentieth-century Canada.

Items two, three, four and five above correspond to the previous study by the Technical Assistance and Planning Associates (1979). A culturally appropriate parent effectiveness training course should be developed, disseminated and implemented. Aboriginal parents are desperate for input into the management of their children. In this author's clinical practice, few Aboriginal adults present on their own for treatment. They tend almost exclusively to bring their children, who are experiencing substance abuse, behaviour problems and depression. When psychological distress is identified in the parents, the response is almost unanimously, "Forget about me, Doc, do something for my kids." In most Aboriginal communities children are still the priority, but the parents know not what to do for them.

Summary and Conclusion

The author wishes to remind the reader of the original paradigm on which this paper is based: the triad of poverty, powerlessness and anomie, mixed with memories of disturbing childhood experiences and a recent separation or loss, results in depression, substance abuse and suicidal ideation and plan. Each of the factors has been alluded to briefly. It is this author's firm belief that the Aboriginal people of Canada have the emotional and intellectual resources to deal with these difficulties. The solutions would be different for each band and tribe because of location, culture, language and custom. Trust the assessment of local Aboriginal leaders and indigenous helpers to say what the local interventions ought to be. "Send us the tools and we will finish the job", to quote an eminent Anglo-European statesman. The non-Aboriginal helpers should serve as a source of funding, resources, training, manpower and backup networking for indigenous helpers.

References

Brant Castellano, Marlene. *Suicide in The North American Indian Causes and Prevention*. Transcribed and Edited Proceedings of the Canadian Psychiatric Association Section on Native Mental Health. Native Mental Health Association of Canada, 1985.

Dizmang, L.H., and Reznick. "Observations on Suicidal Behavior Among American Indians". *American Journal of Psychiatry* 127/7 (January 1971).

Durkheim, Emile. *Suicide*. Glenco, Illinois: Free Press, 1951.

Morrison, J. "A Mental Health Needs Assessment of the Kenora and Fort Frances Area Indian Reserves". Unpublished report. Medical Services Branch, Health and Welfare Canada, 1981.

Mussell, William. "Healing the Wounds of the Native Family". Keynote Address to a Native Mental Health Association of Canada meeting. Ottawa: 1992.

Shawanda, Beatrice. Transcribed and Edited Proceedings of the Canadian Psychiatric Association Section on Native Mental Health. Native Mental Health Association of Canada, 1985.

Technical Assistance and Planning Associates. "A Starving Man Doesn't Argue". Report Prepared for Policy, Research and Evaluation Division, Department of Indian Affairs and Northern Development, 1979.

Travis, Robert. "Suicide in Northwest Alaska". *White Cloud Journal* 3/1 (1983).

Ward, J.A. and J.A. Fox. "A Suicide Epidemic on an Indian Reserve". *Canadian Psychiatric Association Journal* 22/8 (December 1977).

Wien, Fred. Transcribed and Edited Proceedings of the Canadian Psychiatric Association Section on Native Mental Health. Native Mental Health Association of Canada, 1985.

Ward, Jack. Transcribed and Edited Proceedings of the Canadian Psychiatric Association Section on Native Mental Health. Native Mental Health Association of Canada, 1985.

Violence in Aboriginal Communities

*Emma D. LaRocque**

The issue of domestic violence in First Nations and Métis communities is one that demands urgent study and action. There is every indication that violence has escalated dramatically. For example, studies show that among Indians "the single most important group of health problems in terms of both mortality and morbidity is accidents and violence".[1] The goal of this paper is not to comment on family violence generally, though it does require further comment. This paper will focus on family violence as it affects Aboriginal women, teenagers and children. And since much family violence involves sexual assault, special attention is given to sexual violence within the Aboriginal community.

While domestic or family violence clearly affects all members within a family, the most obvious victims are women and children. A 1989 study by the Ontario Native Women's Association reported that 8 out of 10 Aboriginal women were abused. While this study focused on northern Ontario, it is statistically representative of other communities across the country. There is growing documentation that Aboriginal female adults, adolescents and children are experiencing abuse, battering and/or sexual assault to a staggering degree. A 1987 report by the Child Protection Centre of Winnipeg stated that there is "an apparent epidemic of child sexual abuse on reserves". And just recently, it was reported by the press that on one reserve in Manitoba, 30 adults were charged with having sexually abused 50 persons, many of them children.

---

* Professor, Department of Native Studies, University of Manitoba.

Since it is considerably more difficult to get precise statistics on Métis people, it is virtually impossible to say with any exactness the extent of sexual violence in Métis families or communities. However, as more victims are beginning to report, there is every indication that violence, including sexual violence, is just as problematic, just as extensive as on reserves. In November 1992, the Women of the Metis Nation of Alberta organized an historic conference near Edmonton dealing specifically with sexual violence against Métis women. The interest shown by Métis women from across Canada was overwhelming. The stories shared by the 150 or so conference participants indicated that Métis women, no less than Indian women from reserves, have been suffering enormously – and silently – from violence, including rape and child sexual abuse.

In accordance with the request by the Royal Commission, this paper will address the following: (1) women's perspectives on factors that generate and perpetuate domestic violence and (2) strategies proposed to reduce and eliminate violence. Barriers to implementing these strategies are implied within this discussion.

I understand that the Royal Commission wants policy recommendations more than an extensive analysis of violence. However, I believe it is of value to take some time to think about the possible reasons for violence against women. Not only is analysis an inherently indispensable tool in working toward proposed solutions, but it is also part of the educational process we all need in order to address this horrific issue with comprehension and compassion.

Naturally, this paper cannot and does not propose to look at all possible reasons for family or sexual violence. There are a number of works that provide useful but fairly standard views on sexual violence, especially in regard to treatment and to 'offenders'.[2] I wish to provide additional perspectives, some of which may disagree with commonly held beliefs about the nature of sexual violence and the reaction to 'offenders'.

Colonization

Colonization refers to that process of encroachment and subsequent subjugation of Aboriginal peoples since the arrival of Europeans. From the Aboriginal perspective, it refers to loss of lands, resources, and self-direction and to the severe disturbance of cultural ways and values. Colonization has taken its toll on *all* Aboriginal peoples, but it has taken perhaps its greatest toll on women. Prior to colonization, Aboriginal women enjoyed comparative honour, equality and even political power in a way European women did not at the same time in history. We can trace the diminishing status of Aboriginal women with the progression of colonialism. Many, if not the majority, of Aboriginal cultures were originally matriarchal or semi-matriarchal. European patriarchy was initially imposed upon Aboriginal societies in Canada through the fur trade, missionary

Christianity and government policies. Because of white intrusion, the matriarchal character of Aboriginal spiritual, economic, kinship, and political institutions was drastically altered.

Racism, Sexism, and the Problem of Internalization

Colonization and racism go hand in hand. Racism has provided justification for the subjugation of Aboriginal peoples. While all Aboriginal people are subjected to racism, women further suffer from sexism. Racism breeds hatred of Aboriginal peoples; sexism breeds hatred of women. For Aboriginal women, racism and sexism constitute a package experience. We cannot speak of sexual violence without at once addressing the effects of racism/sexism. Sexual violence is related to racism in that racism sets up or strengthens a situation where Aboriginal women are viewed and treated as sex objects. The objectification of women perpetuates sexual violence. Aboriginal women have been objectified not only as women but also as Indian women. The term used to indicate this double objectification was and is 'squaw'.

A complex of white North American cultural myths, as expressed in literature and popular culture, has perpetuated racist/sexist stereotypes about Aboriginal women. A direct relationship between racist/sexist stereotypes and violence can be seen, for example, in the dehumanizing portrayal of Aboriginal women as 'squaws', which renders all Aboriginal female persons vulnerable to physical, verbal and sexual violence.

One of the many consequences of racism is that, over time, racial stereotypes and societal rejection may be internalized by the colonized group. The internalization process is one of the most problematic legacies of long-term colonization. It is not well understood, but it is certainly indicated by various oppressed or minority groups in North America. Many Black, Chicano and Aboriginal writers have pointed to this problem. Understanding the complex workings of the internalization process may be the key to the beginnings of understanding the behaviour of the oppressed and the oppressive in our communities.

In his book *Prison of Grass* (1975), Howard Adams referred to the problem of "internalization". By this he meant that as a result of disintegrative processes inherent in colonization, Aboriginal peoples have subconsciously judged themselves against the standards of white society, often adopting what he called the White Ideal. Part of this process entails 'internalizing' or believing – swallowing the standards, judgements, expectations and portrayals of the dominant white world. Many other Aboriginal writers have pointed to the causes and consequences of having struggled with externally imposed images about themselves and the policies that resulted from them. The result was/is often shame and rejection not only of the self but also of the similar other, i.e., other Aboriginal people.

A lot has changed within the Aboriginal community since Adams wrote *Prison of Grass*. A lot more Aboriginal people are aware of the whys and wherefores of their position in Canadian society. As more Aboriginal people grow in political awareness, they are less prone to judge themselves or act by outside standards. However, the damage has been extensive, and the problem of internalization does still exist. It is still of value to study how Aboriginal internalization of racist/sexist stereotypes may be at work in the area of violence.

One of the central questions we need to address is this: we know there has been violence by white men against Aboriginal women, but what do we make of the violence by Aboriginal men against Aboriginal women and children?

Too often the standard answer or reason given is that Aboriginal 'offenders' were themselves abused and/or victims of society. There is no question that this answer may be partly true for some of the abusers, especially the young. However, it is hardly a complete answer and certainly should not be treated as the only or final answer to this problem.

There are indications of violence against women in Aboriginal societies prior to European contact. Many early European observations as well as original Indian legends (e.g., Wehsehkehcha stories) point to the pre-existence of male violence against women. It should not be assumed that matriarchies necessarily prevented men from exhibiting oppressive behaviour toward women. There were individuals who acted against the best ideals of their cultures. Even today, all the emphasis on Mother Earth has not translated into full equality and safety of women.

There is little question, however, that European invasion exacerbated whatever the extent, nature or potential violence there was in original cultures. Neither is there much question that Aboriginal men have internalized white male devaluation of women. As one scholar observes:

> Deprived of their ancestral roles...men began to move into areas that had previously been the province of women, adopting some of the white attitudes toward women and treating them as inferiors rather than equals.[3]

How might this internalization work with respect to violence generally and sexual violence specifically? Consider this: what happens to Aboriginal males who are exposed not only to pornography but also to the racist/sexist views of the 'Indian' male as a violent 'savage' and the Aboriginal female as a debased, sexually loose 'squaw'?

Pornography in popular culture is affecting sexual attitudes and behaviour within Aboriginal communities. And given the lengthy and unrestricted mass media projection and objectification of 'Indians' as violence-crazed savages, the problem of internalization should come as no surprise.

But it is disturbing. Aboriginal internalization of racist/macho views of Aboriginal men and women has contributed to violence generally and to sexual abuse specifically.

Defence of Offenders Perpetuates Violence

It is difficult to say whether there is more sexual violence in Aboriginal communities than in white ones, for we know that sexual assault is also prevalent in white homes and neighbourhoods. But I don't think we should defend either community in this regard. Rather, we should expend our energies in showing categorical disapproval appropriate to the crime and seeking solutions to what is an intolerable situation.

I have been troubled by a number of things relevant to the discussion on sexual violence. It is distressing to observe apathy by both Aboriginal and non-Aboriginal populations concerning sexual violence. The Aboriginal leadership, in particular, must be called on to address this issue. Nor should the general public or governments walk away. The onus for change cannot rest solely on Aboriginal shoulders. White people in positions of power must share the burdens of finding answers, as they have been part of the problems.

I have also been concerned about the popularity of offering 'cultural differences' as an explanation for sexual violence. When the horrifying story of the Lac Brochet teenager came out in the late 1980s, I was stunned by comments and attempted explanations around me. The numerous males who had attacked this 14-year-old girl (who had been repatriated against her will in the name of 'culture' to begin with) were being defended with tortured and distorted notions of Aboriginal culture.

Erroneous cultural explanations have created enormous confusion in many people and on many issues. Besides the problem of typecasting Aboriginal cultures into a static list of 'traits', 500 years of colonial history are being whitewashed into mere 'cultural differences'. Social conditions arising from societal negligence and policies have been explained away as 'cultural'. Problems having to do with racism and sexism have been blamed on Aboriginal culture. When cultural justifications are used on behalf of the sexually violent, we are seeing a gross distortion of the notion of culture and of Aboriginal peoples. Men assault; cultures do not. Rape and violence against women were met with quick justice in original cultures. And if there is any culture that condones the oppression of women, it should be confronted to change. But sexual violence should never be associated with Aboriginal culture! It is an insult to healthy, functioning Aboriginal cultures to suggest so! Would one entertain using 'racial differences' as an explanation for sexual assaults? Is it any less racist to resort to 'cultural' ones?

As long as offenders are defended in the name of culture, they will continue to avoid taking any personal responsibility for their actions. And this will only perpetuate the problem.

Equally troubling in the defence of offenders is popular advancement of the notion that men rape or assault because they were abused or are victims of society themselves. The implication is that as 'victims', rapists and child molesters are not responsible for their actions and that therefore they should not be punished – or, if punished, 'rehabilitation' and their 'victimization' must take precedence over any consideration of the suffering or devastation they wreak on the real victims! Political oppression does not preclude the mandate to live with personal and moral responsibility within human communities. And if individuals are not capable of personal responsibility and moral choices (the things that make us human), then they are not fit for normal societal engagement and should be treated accordingly.

Obstacles Facing Real Victims

And what do victims of sexual assault face within Aboriginal and mainstream communities? The following is a brief but realistic scenario. Aboriginal victims face obstacles that come with all small communities. There is a lack of privacy. Fear of further humiliation through community gossip and fear of ostracism and intimidation from supporters of the perpetrator may all be at work. Often a victim is confronted with disbelief, anger, and family denial or betrayal. Secrecy is expected and enforced. There is, in effect, censorship against those who would report sexual assault or even other forms of violence.

But if a victim does proceed with reporting, who will want to hear? And if she goes out of the community, she faces racism/sexism in the form of judgement, indifference or disbelief. Many non-Aboriginals in positions of social service or power either have little knowledge of what circumstances confront the victim, or they do not take complainants seriously. The stereotype that Aboriginal women are sexually promiscuous is still quite prevalent. Also, in many communities women cannot trust policemen since some policemen, especially in previous generations, were also doing the attacking! This is not to mention that the entire process of reporting is itself a formidable challenge.

If the victim goes as far as the courts, a whole new set of problems emerges. It is well-known that even for white middle-class women, rape trials are torturous, with no guarantee of justice at the end of it all. If only 10 per cent of white women report sexual assault, then considerably less than 10 per cent of Aboriginal victims report. And of course, the conviction rate is dismal.

The other problem, a problem I believe perpetuates sexual violence, is the fact that the courts are wantonly lenient with regard to sentencing. As a rule, thieves and minor drug dealers receive way stiffer penalties than do child molesters, rapists or even rapist-murderers! This in itself is a chilling message regarding societal devaluation of human dignity. Many Aboriginal communities have expressed concern that courts are especially lenient with Aboriginal offenders who assault other Aboriginal people. The easy parole system, along with lenient sentencing, further sets up Aboriginal victims.

If the victim succeeds in sending her assailant to prison, she may expect quick retaliation. Sexual offenders may come out of prison within three weeks, perhaps six months. These men usually go straight back to their small settlements and proceed to wreak further violence and intimidation.

When all is said and done, what of the victim? Where is the help for her? Where is the concern for *her* rehabilitation?

The whole judicial process reflects privileged, white male definitions and experience. It also reflects tremendous naïvete – naïvete often found in white liberal social workers, criminologists and justices. These lenient sentences are consistent with the growing heroification of rapists and child molesters as 'victims'. Today there is persistent sympathy for sexual offenders with little, of any, corresponding concern for the real victims. It is a bizarre situation!

Questions About the Causes of Sexual Violence

Given the popularity of presenting rapists as victims, and given that such a notion has not in any way resolved the problem – and in fact may be perpetuating sexual violence – is it not time for new and hard questions here? While it is sociologically apparent that poverty and marginalization can play havoc in a community, it is difficult to accept without question that being a so-called victim causes one to be a victimizer. If that were true, millions of women would take to victimizing. Further, if poor social conditions necessarily breed 'offenders', this raises more questions than it answers. Why, when the chips are down, do men turn on women and children? What are we saying here about the nature of man? What are we saying of Aboriginal men – that when conditions of oppression, poverty or abuse exist, they cannot think of anything else but to turn on innocent women and children? And this should then be met with sympathy? And what about the other statistics – what about all the poor men and abused men who do not turn to violence?

Sexual violence is global and universal. Men of all backgrounds, cultures, classes and economic status assault women. Indeed, history is replete with examples of rich, powerful and privileged men who abused women and children. This suggests that the origin of sexual violence is considerably more disturbing than we might like to admit. Maybe it is not as mysterious as we make it out to be.

Most adults who violate others do so from a place of awareness and choice. As one article on child sexual abuse, written by a group of concerned Aboriginal women, states: "Offenders are aware of what they are doing and they know it is wrong."[4] I believe sexual violence is best explained by sexism and misogyny, which are nurtured in our society. North American popular culture feeds off the objectification and degradation of women. Women are presented as sexual playthings who must conform to male needs. Stereotypes of female sexuality are concocted as a rationalization for violence. It is about male maintenance of power, but it is a conscious and deliberate form of power, not one that is necessarily caused by 'abuse' or other traumas. Obviously power brings all sorts of advantages. It has been in the interests of men to keep women down. Society supports all this with its tolerance of violence against women. The criminal justice system reflects its bias through its laws and judgements.

Rape in any culture and by any standards is warfare against women. And the degree to which any community tolerates sexual violence is an indication of concurrence in this warfare against women.

The point is, we may never know for certain what exactly causes sexual violence. But whether we know or not, we should never use any 'explanation' – be it psychological, personal or political – as absolution for the offender. We should never justify or tolerate sexual violence. The criminal justice system must do its duty and serve 'justice' not only because justice is essential to a victim's healing, but also because a message must be given that sexual violence is insupportable. Justice and concern for rehabilitation must not be seen as mutually exclusive.

The other point, and perhaps more to the point, is why all this concern with finding reasons or explanations for what causes men to be rapists and child molesters? Given that we may never know, should we not turn our attention to the real victims?

Recommendations

Strategies to reduce and eliminate violence would, of course, include addressing the issues that contribute to violence. Perhaps we can approach the strategies under three headings: prevention, services for victims and judicial action with respect to offenders.

Toward Prevention

I believe a preventive approach is necessary. How can we ever stem the tide of all this violence? It surely will not happen overnight. Meanwhile, we have young people to attend to. If we can reach the Aboriginal youth, we may see some light on a number of fronts. The first set of recommendations concerns young people.

Obviously, a multi-faceted, comprehensive approach is required. Socio-economic revitalization is a must. Human beings need to have meaning in their lives; one of the avenues for meaning lies in economic bases/activities. This issue of economy is crucial to young people who are currently caught within a socio-cultural vacuum. They are looking for vocational opportunities in a world that has stolen their land-based ways, yet has not prepared them for urbanization/industrialization.

The miseducation of Aboriginal youth must be addressed. One of the enduring legacies of colonization is the mistreatment of Aboriginal history and issues in schools. Schools must stop presenting Aboriginal history, cultures, peoples and issues in biased, ethnocentric or racist ways. Along with correcting the social studies aspect of the curriculum, schools must make every effort to stop alienating Aboriginal youth by providing skills and knowledge relevant to both cultures. Also, understanding and attitudes toward Aboriginal culture itself must change. Aboriginal cultures should not be presented only in terms of the past (often stereotyped at that). Young people often feel paralyzed: how can they move toward the future if their culture is defined in terms of the past? Young people need help in clarifying what is heritage and what is culture. They also need to be reassured that it is within Aboriginal cultural definitions to change and to make bridges from the past to the future. Aboriginal young people should not have to feel that in order to be loyal to their personal identities they have to sacrifice vocational choices of the future.

Another large problem in many Aboriginal communities is that of boredom. Boredom is a problem that has not received the attention it should. Boredom is often the cause of a lot of difficulties young people get into, including drugs, alcohol, sexual experimentation, mob behaviour, violence and suicide. Community leaders must make every effort to provide qualitative recreation for young people. Funding and resources must be made available for the development of recreation facilities, sports programs and other projects. I have often wondered, what is everybody waiting for? Why haven't there been massive efforts to provide recreation facilities for youth in Aboriginal communities? There is so much untapped potential for excellence in our youth. Every time I watch any national or international sports event, I think of all the Aboriginal youths who could be participating. Is it not time to move in that direction?

With respect to sex and violence, education and sexual enlightenment may be our best hope for our future. One of the biggest problems in Aboriginal homes and communities is lack of qualitative sex education. As a rule, parents and other adults are not providing sex education to their young. Children and adolescents are left to their own devices and to the influence of popular culture, misguided peers or even abusers to learn about sex. In this sense, sexual problems are recycled. Aboriginal children and teenagers are desperately in need of solid sex education. Schools (preferably in co-operation with community initiatives and programs) should step in by providing qualitative sex education to children and teenagers.

Such education must include not only the physiological aspects of sex and sexuality but must also promote respect for persons. There must be special emphasis on respect for female persons, respect for each other's sexuality and self-respect. There must also be education about safe sex, birth control, pregnancy, reproductive choice and sexual responsibility. Schools must also provide education on drugs, alcohol, smoking, glue-sniffing, etc.

A special word needs to be said about Aboriginal teenage girls. Little has been documented thus far, but many of the stories of sexual abuse reveal that Aboriginal women were often attacked as teenagers. Teenage girls with little or no sex education in an environment conducive to alcohol abuse and violence are particularly vulnerable to adult male sexual seductions/attacks. Rape can devastate teenagers. There is growing documentation that following sexual assault, teenagers turn to substance abuse, prostitution, self-mutilation and/or suicide. This is not to mention that they can get pregnant and/or contract sexually transmitted diseases. The suicide rate is five times the national average in the 15 to 24 age group among Aboriginal youth. One book analyzing the death of an Ojibwa community in northwestern Ontario links female suicide with sexual assaults.[5]

Teenagers are perhaps among the most susceptible to sexual assault. They are sexually sensitive yet immature; they are often unmindful of what adults are capable of doing to them. This is another reason why silence must end. Often, adults who know who the offenders are keep such information away from others. If there could be disclosure, exposure and open discussion between victims and other youth, it would help protect the unsuspecting. Adults such as parents, grandparents, teachers, ministers, counsellors and so forth must take special care to protect, educate and prepare teenagers about sex and sexual violence. And if violence takes place, there must be emotional, psychological, medical and legal support services in place. All Aboriginal youth should also have access to counselling services. They also need safe houses for those times when their homes or communities do not feel safe. Some youth may be in need of psychological or psychiatric services – these too should be made accessible to them. There should also be some attention to young people's spiritual needs. Aboriginal young men and women have dreams and hopes for their futures and their well-being. Every effort must be made by all parties concerned to protect these young people and to facilitate their aspirations. I think Aboriginal communities could organize conferences, guest speakers, and seminars that could address their needs as well as present role models.

If young people enjoy their daily existence, and if they can have dreams that are attainable, I do believe their daily activities would change substantially. I do believe they would respond to a creative environment and move away from destructive influences and destructive behaviours. If we wish to eliminate violence, we have to substitute constructive, creative and meaningful alternatives to it. Our children deserve nothing less.

Better Responses for Victims

The silent suffering of girls and women who have been subjected to rape and other assaults demands immediate attention. Silence must end. Support systems must be created. Aboriginal victims of violence need safe houses, rape crisis centres, counselling services and clinics. They need family and institutional support. They need therapists who are skilled in dealing with post-traumatic stress syndrome. They need a society that cares about them and that values their safety, their dignity and their rehabilitation. Laws must be changed and enforced. The whole judicial process of dealing with complaints of violence must be changed.[6]

It cannot be emphasized enough how very desperately long-term qualitative counselling/therapy and community programs are needed. Long-term therapy programs are required. Rape and early childhood abuse cause lifetime devastation. As concerned Aboriginal women put it, "...sexual abuse is a reality and a hell that must no longer be ignored.... We have felt the pain and anger...for damaging a child's life forever."[7] An indication that Aboriginal women are suffering from post-traumatic stress syndrome can be seen in the level of female violence, alcoholism and extent of incarceration.

Studies show that rural Aboriginal women move to urban centres to escape family or community problems. Most Aboriginal communities are small, making the situation that much more difficult for victims. Apathy and lack of leadership or family support effectively chase victims from their own communities. This should not have to happen. No one should ever have to leave home in order to feel safe!

The Aboriginal leadership at the federal, provincial and regional levels must take a strong stand against violence, and certainly against sexual violence. The message and modelling must be clear and firm that sexual violence against women, teenagers and children is inexcusable, intolerable and insupportable. In effect, the Aboriginal leadership must take the initiative in raising the consciousness of communities about the destructiveness inherent in violence. Violence must be raised as the social problem it is, a problem requiring urgent attention. Forums for discussion, education, and information must be set up to facilitate awareness and social concern. Every effort must be made by the leadership to prevent abuse and to help those who have been abused.

All Aboriginal and non-Aboriginal agencies involved with Aboriginal family problems, i.e., hospitals, police, lawyers, judges, social workers, therapists, child care organizations, etc., should be required to attend workshops and/or conferences geared to addressing the issue of sexual violence. Again, the Aboriginal leadership must initiate such forums; the government must provide the resources.

Aboriginal women must be free to address unwieldy and unpopular issues such as violence, equality, patriarchy, political leadership, etc. They also must receive support to create forums through which they can gather to discuss issues of mutual concern. But there must be recognition of issues/concerns that pertain to Indian women and those that pertain to Métis women. To these ends, Aboriginal women need their own organizations and must be funded separately from the larger, umbrella organizations.

As discussed earlier, a large portion of the root of our problems lies with our colonization. Again, Aboriginal leaders and educators must make every effort to facilitate forums for discussion on the legacies of colonization in our lives, in our homes and communities. Perhaps Paulo Friere's ideas on the 'pedagogy of the oppressed' could be adopted. Raising the consciousness of the Aboriginal grass-roots is one of the important tasks in moving toward wholeness and can be seen as 'service' to victims of violence. People need to understand the disintegrative processes of colonization; they need to know the consequences of having been defined outside of themselves, of being powerless. Aboriginal people need to understand the institutional forces of invasion in their worlds and what that has done to their lands and economies, their relationships, their cultural values and symbols, their self-determination and self-confidence. They also need to believe that restoration is possible. They need to believe that they can act to make changes and that by acting on issues they are empowering themselves. People may best be able to make changes once they can articulate the places of invasion in their lives and in their histories.

We may need years to help Aboriginal peoples understand and resolve the violence; meanwhile, we must deal with the everyday realities of it. Even if we agree about what causes sexual violence, we could not immediately, if ever, end it. Besides the social, economic and educational programs we can pursue, we are forced to look at the criminal justice system with respect to protection and justice.

Victims, the 'Offender', and the Criminal Justice System

In terms of change in the judicial process, it would be redundant to repeat the extensive and generally excellent recommendations offered in the Manitoba *Aboriginal Justice Inquiry Report* (1991). Anyone working in this area must consult this report. I also recommend the handbook *The Spirit Weeps*, published by the Nechi Institute, (1988) which offers useful information on the characteristics and dynamics of incest and child sexual abuse with an Aboriginal perspective.

The criminal justice system is, of course, a whole field of study. I wish only to emphasize certain (and to me more bothersome) aspects of it, namely, its sympathetic posture toward sexual offenders and other hard-core violent criminals. Since the mid-1960s, the criminal justice system has increasingly exhibited wanton leniency in the trying and sentencing of sexual offenders. Such leniency amounts to negligence. What feeble laws exist regarding sexual assault are routinely diluted by the judicial process and decisions. In the case of Aboriginal people against Aboriginal people, victims of aggravated sexual assault (the majority being female, a great number being teenagers) are set up to live lives of silent pain, fear and continual victimization. For example, the leader of those gang rapes against the Lac Brochet girl received only four years – with virtual apologies from the judge! I believe such an irresponsible sentence makes a mockery of all women and certainly of the girl's trauma and what will surely be her lifelong post-traumatic stress syndrome.

Obviously, there are no easy answers. Nor am I suggesting any simplistic solutions, but I do believe that we have so over-complicated the issues surrounding violence that the laws and the exercising of these laws have become absurd and have played into the hands of child molesters, rapists and calculating murderers. This has resulted in the devaluation of human dignity in the whole system. Property and liquor/drug offences mean more to the system than violation of one's person.

I do suggest the corrections system, be it Aboriginal or mainstream, take the following direction. A dual structure should be set up to accommodate the types of crimes and criminals being addressed. Distinctions must be made between non-violent and violent offences. There is a world of difference between, say, stealing a VCR and brutalizing a human being!

People committing certain non-violent crimes could become involved in community-oriented programs instead of jails to compensate for their offences. Here, 'meet-the-victim' models might apply. Also, we must draw on alternative-to-jail programs that are in existence in Canada, the United States and elsewhere.

There are also various degrees and forms of violence, and the system of punishment must make a distinction between a slap, a minor brawl and gross violence such as battering, stabbing and shooting, or wilful and callous violence such as sexual assault and premeditated murder.

Those involved in minor scuffles should receive help via community-based education/renewal programs. Personal, family and community counselling with an educational and/or therapeutic focus might be considered.

Those involved in gross violence should receive stiff custody penalties along with strong education/therapy programs.

Those involved in gross and wilful crimes should receive very lengthy jail sentences and, in specific cases, should also be permanently removed from their communities. In cases of brutalization, rape and ruthless murder, removal may be the only effective measure of protection for victims and their families, especially in small and/or remote settlements. Indeed, many northern communities have requested removal and stronger penalties.

All forms of sexual assault are on a continuum of violence; therefore, most forms must fall under the category of violence. Those, including boys, who commit 'minor' sexual offences must be considered potentially dangerous.

Those who commit violence and plead no-sentencing on the basis of insanity, drunkenness, youthfulness, or even poverty, must be placed in custody away from their victims. The law must also change from 'not guilty by reason of insanity' to 'guilty but insane' and proceed to sentence such parties to custody appropriate to their crime and condition.

As well, the *Young Offenders Act* must be changed. I think it is atrocious that a 13-year-old can brutally kill two women and be sentenced to only three years.[8] There is no question that our colonial, negligent, violence-crazed, misogynist popular culture is culpable for violent (usually male) children; still, innocent people should not be sitting ducks for such violence.

There are degrees of youth and knowledge. There are large differences even between two 12-year-olds. Surely, the law (and psychiatrists) must profile and reflect these differences. The law must also reflect the changing times – children today are much more street-wise than those of yesteryear.

On every level of sentencing, whether in the non-violent or violent category, there must, of course, be extensive efforts toward rehabilitation. A word again must be said about rehabilitation. Often, lenient sentences have been promoted on this basis. The problem here is that there has been a blanket assumption that justice and rehabilitation are mutually exclusive. Yet statistics show that sexual offenders, for example, are rarely 'rehabilitated'.

But the point that seems to be missed in this discussion is this: primary consideration as to sentencing should not be whether the offender is going to be rehabilitated. Rather, the primary consideration should be justice on behalf of the victim. Interrelated with concern for justice must be an unequivocal message to the offender and to society that sexual violence is not acceptable and that it is punishable by law.

While I support the ideals of rehabilitation, I believe that it is incumbent upon any criminal justice system first to dispense justice, then to concern itself with rehabilitation. But rehabilitation must never be at the expense of justice.

All ancient cultures have had traditions of justice, and Aboriginal cultures no less so. Aboriginal cultures used a range of penalties, depending on the nature of the offence: ridicule, shunning, payment or violence in kind (in the tradition of 'an eye for an eye'). We may disagree with some ancient measures, but we cannot deny that justice is essential to the human psyche. There is no peace or healing without justice. Simply on the basis of providing therapeutic service to victims, offenders must be made accountable.

But places of confinement/custody should have extensive and mandatory rehabilitation programs. Such programs should incorporate not only personal therapy but education with respect to decolonization and spiritual/cultural renewal and a sociological grasp of sexism and its relationship to violence against women.

And of course, there should be long-term rehabilitation programs for victims and their families and communities. The destruction inherent in any violence ripples widely into the families and communities of victims.

I am aware that a number of community programs have been developed that promote offender-victim reconciliation. I have read with careful interest the Aboriginal Justice Inquiry's report on the Hollow Water Resource Group of Manitoba. As the AJI describes it:

> Not only does it provide rehabilitation to the offender, and support and comfort to the victim, but it provides a mechanism to heal and restore harmony to the families and the community.... The Hollow Water model was created to protect people against repetition of the offence and to prevent any new incidents of abuse.[9]

I have to admit, on paper it sounds promising. And the people must be commended for their initiative, courage and vision. But since it is so new and does seem to operate on assumptions of rehabilitation, some further questions are raised. It is perhaps too early to tell whether it is as constructive as it sounds. A number of questions come to mind: are victims in small communities really free to become part of these meet-the-offender programs? How young are the victims? What is the nature of the violence? Are victims agreeing to these models as a result of social pressure and lack of other choices? How are they being affected by all this? Do they have enough political and social awareness to be able to make a choice with such programs? Are offenders really being 'rehabilitated'? And should this be the primary goal for helpers, families of victims, justices and communities? Is it possible that offenders use such programs to get out of sentencing and other responsibilities?

I have some difficulty with the attention given to sexual offenders. Might there be other programs besides having to meet their assailants that would be perhaps more healing and less stressful for victims?

Calls for services for women often contain the phrase 'culturally appropriate'. While the principle behind this phrase is supportable, there is a need for clearer definitions about what is meant. I am afraid that there is some notion at large that it is 'cultural' for Aboriginal women to tolerate violence at all costs in the name of 'family' or 'tradition'. This is reminiscent of some churches that admonish women never to leave 'the sanctity of marriage', even if the women and children are being battered and/or sexually assaulted. Care must be taken that violence of women and children never be advanced in the name of 'culture'.

Family counselling must be encouraged but women must not be made to feel they have to tolerate violence in the name of family or culture. Family means that men must take responsibility and get involved in counselling.

Questions remain as to notions of healing, notions of rehabilitation, and the value of emphasizing family and community unity at the possible expense of victims, many of them children. Studies on abuse of children show that families can be the most dangerous places for them to be. We must take care that we do not advance notions such as the unity of families in any formulaic way because we know, unfortunately, that families are not inherently safe. Each situation must be carefully screened.

Room for Research Questions and Answers

No one has the final answers; we barely have embryonic suggestions. The subject of violence, and particularly sexual violence, is extremely difficult, and made more so because it goes to the heart of personal, family and societal politics. It is also a subject of emotion. While we are beginning to have access to more information and beginning to gain better understanding of the causes and effects of violence, there is room for continued research at all levels.

I think, though, that the focus should move toward prevention, comprehension, support and protection on behalf of the victims. Research monies and energy should be spent there. Services, programs, counselling and long-term therapy for victims should be addressed.

Several times I have referred to post-traumatic stress syndrome. We know that sexual violence causes lifetime problems. Research on the long-term effects of sexual violence must be pursued.

On this note, I wish to caution about some standard usage of terms and notions. Words such as 'healing', 'counselling' and 'family violence' are used a lot. The cumulative effect of using such terms gives the impression that sexual violence causes no great harm and that it is easy to fix. Just go for counselling and the pain will go away. 'Healing' is used so often that it risks promoting the idea that victims of sexual violence can be easily healed. There is every indication that sexual violence is extremely traumatic and destructive and that these effects are long-term. Indeed, is it possible to 'heal' sexual violence? This is not to suggest we should not try, but it is to question the all too hasty use of such terms. We run the risk of trivializing sexual violence by using descriptions and terms that couch and soften the impact.

Words like offender, rather than rapist or child molester, serve to minimize the calculated nature of sexual attacks. Phrases like family or domestic violence also serve to twist the issue: women and children are experiencing brutality to a staggering degree, but it is being reduced and ignored as 'domestic' or 'family' violence. In relation to this, the word 'incest' is also often misused. Incest means that there is consensual sexual intercourse between two people who are too closely related to be married. Sexual attacks on children by male relatives is not incest; it is rape and child molestation. Children, teenagers and women are not consenting to have sex with their relatives; they are being attacked or in some way coerced into unwanted sexual activity.

I believe research would show that as long as softened, couched terms continue to be used, reaction to address this monstrous problem will continue to be slow.

Research specific to Métis families, concerns and data is very much needed. There is such a dearth of specific data on Métis people that no one can even agree as to the population of Métis. How are we going to strategize to eliminate violence unless we have more precise information to work from?

With respect to justice and 'offenders', research into the viability of old notions in new models is also required. We need to follow up on projects such as the Hollow Water Resource Group.

Conclusion

As most of us know, violence has long been rampant in many Aboriginal communities. I know too that we have shied away from dealing with the issue partly because we have had to fend off racism and stereotypes. But given the seriousness of the situation we must confront the problem(s). If we do not, there will be self-government without selves to govern, for people are leaving their places of birth to escape the violence. And it is possible to deal with these issues in an intelligent manner, without having to resort to racist stereotypes.

Finally, lest I be misunderstood, I must emphasize that I am painfully aware of the criminal justice system's dismal record with respect to Aboriginal peoples! I grew up watching police abuse my parents' generation. I saw police rough up and pick up my mother, aunts and uncles for no reason whatsoever. This generation could not defend itself in the courts because of language differences, discrimination and/or poverty. But I also saw or heard of police and courts neglecting Aboriginal victims of Aboriginal violence. This is the ultimate form of racism. It is this latter fact that must be addressed as much as the former. Is it not time for us to take a stand against violence in our midst?

In my community, we were all victims of colonization but we did not all turn to violence. Further, why should Aboriginal victims of Aboriginal violence bear the ultimate brunt of colonization/racism and negligence of the criminal justice system?

My hope, of course, is that our communities will be renewed, that people will find support and restoration.

Thank you for this opportunity; I trust it can have some influence in finding protection and justice for victims and in moving toward some understanding of the issues.

Notes

1. T.K. Young, 1988:54.
2. Hodgson, Daily, Martens, 1988; *Aboriginal Justice Inquiry (Manitoba) Report*, 1991.
3. Dexter Fisher, 1980:13.
4. In *Canadian Women Studies*, Summer/Fall 1989:90.
5. A.M. Shkilnyk, 1985:46-47.
6. For recommendations on these, see the *Aboriginal Justice Inquiry (Manitoba) Report*, 1991.
7. In *Canadian Women Studies*, Summer/Fall 1989.
8. A Manitoba case several years ago.
9. Aboriginal Justice Inquiry, p. 495.

Funding Policy for Indigenous Human Services

*K. A. (Kim) Scott**

This discussion paper was written primarily for the audience of Round Table participants: respected elders, community-based practitioners, the medical community, national organizations and governmental officials. However, consideration was given to the broader Canadian audience who may or may not be involved in health matters and for whom this document will eventually be published. Therefore, although the language may seem pedestrian to some, the goal is to be clear and provocative for all.

For further clarity, a glossary of terms and acronyms has been included. Other terms that do not have the prominence they deserve in the glossary are explained here. These include *Indigenous peoples* and *human services*. Indigenous peoples refers collectively and individually to Métis, Inuit and Indian groups because the term Aboriginal is value-laden. Webster's Ninth New Collegiate Dictionary (1991) indicates that Aboriginal refers to "the first of its kind in a region and often primitive in comparison with more advanced types". Indigenous, on the other hand, refers to that which is of the land or naturally occurring in an environment and hence more accurately reflects the collective of original inhabitants and their descendants.

The term *human services* is used to refer to all that is commonly separated into health (medical services, health education and promotion) and social services (child and family, community development, welfare) in Euro-American terms.

---

* Senior policy analyst, Royal Commission on Aboriginal Peoples.

Euro-American is used not in disregard for Canada but to capture more accurately the continental influences on human services delivery in the Indigenous community. Ideally, the term Indigenous human services encompasses all that affects the person and body, such as land, economy, culture, housing and education, to name but a few. To address these would require resources beyond the scope of this policy paper. Hence, the suggestions contained in this text are limited to addressing those funds channelled into health and social endeavours.

Introduction

Indigenous groups epitomized the state of human health and environmental harmony, with sophisticated systems of kinship and exacting medicinal practices. But with the encroachment of Euro-American influence, captivity and dysfunction resulted. Captivity is a complex web of geographic, economic, legal and social isolation that significantly segregates Indigenous peoples so they cannot benefit from the range and quantity of human services enjoyed by other Canadians. Dysfunction is nowhere more apparent than in the health status of Indigenous peoples.

The primary objective of this paper is to draw attention to current funding policies for Indigenous human services and to stimulate discussion about revising these policies to allow Indigenous health authorities to meet the challenge of providing more holistic health care to their communities. Attention will be drawn to the peculiarities evident in federal and provincial cost sharing arrangements for human services under the Canada Assistance Plan (CAP) and Established Programs Financing (EPF) for health care. The discussion will also consider some examples of administrative transfer agreements between Canadian governments and *Indigenous health authorities* (IHAS: incorporated health and social service boards, band councils, tribal councils) for services commonly provided by either federal or provincial departments.

It is worthwhile noting here that this discussion is based on the fundamental assumption that there should be flexibility in funding policy to allow for the transfer of program and administrative control to Indigenous health authorities where these bodies desire and are prepared to assume responsibility. This paper does not make any assumptions that the suggested policy considerations are universal and could serve the purposes of all Indigenous communities. Rather, the point intended is the following: where communities are ready for change, that change can and should be accommodated in a holistic way by flexible distribution of health resources. In addition, it is assumed that there are three schools of thought on Indigenous human services: one advocates integration with Euro-American models of human services; another advocates the development of separate or parallel Indigenous services; and a third argues for various mixtures of integration and separation.

Federal and Provincial Cost-Sharing for Health and Social Services

On a national scale, funding policies for human services are directed by the Canada Assistance Plan (CAP) and Established Programs Financing (EPF) for health care. CAP defines how the federal government shares the cost with provinces/territories and municipalities for the provision of social assistance and welfare services. EPF directs federal cost sharing of insurable health services (i.e., medically necessary treatment) delivered by the provinces. I am focusing attention on CAP and EPF because it is still not clear to what extent Indigenous peoples benefit from Canada's 'health wealth', by which I mean all the resources available to Canadians generally in human services systems through CAP and EPF. In other words, on a per capita basis, taking all related costs into consideration, is more or less being spent on human services delivery for Indigenous peoples when compared with Canadians generally?

Indigenous health authorities look to CAP and EPF with particular interest because, despite recent administrative transfers, funding policy changes have not been made to ensure that Indigenous communities that choose administrative transfer are funded by formulae comparable to those applied to Canadians generally. In addition, the confusion between federal and provincial governments about who is financially responsible for human services delivery continues. It appears that there is significant variability and confusion about which section of the *Constitution Act, 1867* takes priority – section 91(24), federal responsibility for "Indians, and Lands reserved for the Indians", or section 92, provincial responsibility for establishing and delivering human services. And, in light of the provincial governments' territoriality on matters of health and social services jurisdiction with respect to Indigenous peoples, they are rarely eager to claim financial responsibility.

CAP and EPF revisions could allow human services resources to be directed toward Indigenous health authorities in a more comprehensive way, and these revisions could serve the interests of all Indigenous groups: Métis, Inuit and Indian. Our challenge is to figure out how health wealth and illness risk can be reasonably distributed to accommodate Indigenous health authorities who wish to develop their own locally controlled health models.

Canada Assistance Plan

The Canada Assistance Plan (CAP) allows the federal government to support the provinces in providing institutional care for persons in need and welfare services to "lessen, remove or prevent the causes and effects of poverty, child neglect or dependence on public assistance." (Health and Welfare Canada [HWC], 1992, p. 7) This is done by financially supporting welfare, family services and work activity projects.

For illustrative purposes only, it is useful to consider the range of welfare services provided for under CAP. Included among them are homes for special care; adoption services; casework, counselling, assessment and referral services; community development services; consulting, research and evaluation services; daycare services; homemaker services; rehabilitation services and administrative services. (HWC, 1992) When comparing this range of services with those of Indigenous social services agencies, it is clear that most do not include the full range of services provided to provincial agencies. For example, notably absent in many agreements with Indigenous health authorities are community development, consulting, research and evaluation, homes for special care, daycare, and rehabilitation services. This is clear evidence of a funding policy double standard and does not allow an integrated approach to employment and social development.

Interestingly, Part II of CAP, entitled "Indian Welfare", deals specifically with status Indian populations on reserve. Part II indicates that provinces may enter into agreements with the federal government for the extension of provincial welfare services to status Indians on reserve. The idea behind Part II was to ensure that Indian communities would have social services comparable to those provided to Canadians generally. However, provinces rejected formal agreements under Part II, which would have provided for 100 per cent federal payment of services extended to Indians on reserve by provincial governments, (facsimile, Indian and Northern Affairs Canada [INAC], 15 February 1993) and were able to do so by using the authority of section 91 (24) of the *Constitution Act, 1867*. Still, the 1965 Canada/Ontario Memorandum of Agreement respecting Welfare Programs for Indians (known as the 1965 Agreement or the Indian Welfare Agreement) was an attempt to reconcile section 91 (24), federal responsibility for Indians, with section 92, provincial responsibility for establishing and delivering human services. Under the 1965 Agreement, Ontario is extending social services to Indian communities, and the federal government is paying the majority of the cost. (facsimile, INAC, 15 February 1993) Alberta has a similar agreement, called the Arrangement for the Funding and Administration of Social Services. The problem inherent here, of course, is that there appears to be no mechanism to ensure that if one party does not meets its obligation under section 91 (24) or section (92), the other party will be responsible. Without a provincial/federal agreement for the extension of social services, the federal government is the agent left to establish and provide human services to Indians on reserve, and this is where the funding double standards can originate and develop. The solution would then be for the federal government to ensure that, if it is meeting its obligations under section 91 (24), provincial funding standards are met in social service agreements with Indigenous health authorities on reserve.

Established Programs Financing for Health Care

EPF for health care does not segregate Indigenous peoples in a similar fashion and appears to cover all Canadian residents with the same funding mechanism.

Peculiarly, however, medically necessary treatment is not uniformly covered for all Canadians under EPF. In some cases, treatment is supported exclusively or primarily by Medical Services Branch, Health and Welfare Canada (MSB, HWC). The Moose Factory, Sioux Lookout, Norway House and Fort Qu'Appelle hospitals are examples where MSB provides direct funding for the bulk of operations and the remainder comes from provincial operating grants. (Mark Whitmore, personal communication, 12 February 1993) This is in stark contrast to the provincially funded Kateri Hospital at Kahnawake, Quebec, and the Ungava Tulattuvik Health Centre, Kuujjuaq, Quebec. (Keith Leclaire, personal communication, 4 February 1993; Minnie Grey, personal communication, 16 February 1993) The basis for this variability in funding policy is unclear. It is perhaps rooted in section 91(24) and the residual attempt of the federal government to provide tuberculosis treatment, but it has little political or legal consistency with either EPF or the principle of universality in the *Canada Health Act* (see Appendix A).

It is apparent in cases where the federal government has not honoured its obligations to Indigenous communities under section 91(24) that there is no mechanism to ensure that provincial human services are extended by provincial obligation under section 92. Therefore, the first clear step in human services funding for Indigenous communities is to entrench some form of enforcement mechanism to ensure that at least one party, either federal or provincial, meets its obligations under these sections. It is more politically palatable that the nation-to-nation relationship be maintained and that the federal government assume its responsibility; however, these issues are totally irrelevant to sexually abused children, battered women and people with disabilities.

The principle of accessibility set out in the *Canada Health Act* is of particular interest here. It states that insured health services must be available to all Canadians, regardless of their capacity to pay for the treatment they require. This principle has particular merit. However, accessibility is impeded by factors other than just the economic one; it would be beneficial if, under this principle of accessibility, some consideration could be given to geographic factors. Couldn't a minimum standard of service be defined?

What Are the Grounds for Change?

Perhaps the best way to illustrate why there needs to be closer scrutiny of governmental cost sharing for human services and the fair distribution of health wealth as a result is to cite the following case examples, which are purely fictional.

A small settlement of Indigenous people is located next to a remote Canadian town with limited, though functional, Euro-American human services. The Indigenous community has little or no human services structure of its own. In demographic terms, this Indigenous community (take your pick – Métis, Inuit or Indian) represents 25 per cent of the region's population; yet in the service records of any of these human services organizations, it is clear that only 3 per cent of the clientele is Indigenous. The message is clear. These health agencies are not serving the Indigenous population; therefore, the people are not benefiting from the health wealth provided to these agencies under CAP or EPF. Some of the reasons for under-representation include cultural and linguistic insensitivity and the post-residential school fear of Euro-American institutions. Of course, in some circumstances, the exact opposite may be true. In other words, Indigenous people may be represented as 40 per cent of the service clientele in local Euro-American human services when, in fact, they make up only 10 per cent of the region's population.

Where there is over-representation, it would be interesting to discover Indigenous utilization patterns by service category. In other words, is the over-representation accounted for by tertiary services in which Indigenous participation is under extreme duress (e.g., life-threatening disease) or by force (e.g., foster care)? Or is the over-representation accounted for by Indigenous use of primary care? What about the outflow of preventive health wealth in that region to the Indigenous population or the correlation between representation in treatment and community-based epidemiological investigations? Can we really continue this way? And what about the comparison between housing, employment and education standards for Indigenous groups and Canadians generally in that region?

Indigenous utilization patterns of Euro-American human services are largely unknown on a national basis but can be obtained from human services systems that track their clientele by ethnicity. This will likely be problematic, because under human rights legislation, identifying ethnicity on human services records can only be done voluntarily. (Allan Moscovitch, personal communication, 16 February 1993) I suggest that Round Table participants consider the representation and service utilization issues and their implications for human services funding policies.

Similarly, when examining provincial expenditures on human services as published in provincial public accounts, it would be interesting to determine the amounts per capita spent on provincial populations generally and compare that with the financing arrangements for Indigenous groups. Care must be taken to include the support services enjoyed by mainstream organizations such as accounting, statistics, audit, evaluation, research, legal and administrative support. Invariably, the larger bureaucracies have significantly more resources available to them; these are not included in direct service costs and hence in administrative transfer agreements based on direct service costs. But these hidden costs are, nonetheless, part of the cost of delivering the service. In other words, it seems time to scrutinize closely what is being spent to deliver human services to the Canadian population generally and to compare this, when the services are comparable, to what is being spent to deliver services to Indigenous peoples.

Having considered the apparent variability in jurisdictional priority placed on sections 91(24) and 92 and the important variables of service representation and utilization patterns, I will discuss federal and provincial transfers of administrative control to Indigenous health authorities.

Administrative Transfer

In response to growing pressure from Indigenous groups to move away from paternalistic delivery of human services, the departments of Health and Welfare Canada (HWC), Indian and Northern Affairs Canada (INAC) and, to varying degrees, provincial governments have developed mechanisms to allow the transfer of administrative control of human services to local Indigenous health authorities. Administrative transfer refers to any formal agreement where funds originate from either federal or provincial sources, are administered by Indigenous health authorities and subscription to provincial jurisdiction is imposed.

Administrative transfer is devolution only and not the morally independent, self-directing freedom that Indigenous groups seek in human services delivery. Therefore, any transferred health funds come with imposed legislation, rigid programmatic guidelines and accountability requirements. In cases where transferred administrative control comes with programmatic flexibility, there is room for greater sensitivity to community health priorities. The bottom-line decisions, in any case, remain the sole responsibility of the governments that issue them. These decisions, although not entirely arbitrary, show extreme variation. I will highlight this variation as well as the funding priorities of various transfer initiatives. I will also present the problems inherent in sustaining misguided funding policies and suggest alternatives to facilitate more holistic human services delivery to Indigenous peoples. The first to be considered are transfers offered to Indian communities on reserve by the departments of HWC and INAC.

Medical Services Branch, Health and Welfare Canada

Administrative transfer for a subset of federal health programs is being offered to Indigenous communities through Health Program Transfer (HPT), Medical Services Branch (MSB), HWC. Very simply, HPT gives communities access to funding for the transfer process, which includes pre-transfer planning, a health needs assessment, negotiations and transfer implementation. In the post-transfer scenario, communities administer the funds that MSB was spending on health services personnel, training and support, facilities, vehicles and equipment. In addition, there is an administration budget based not on expenditures incurred by the department in administering the program – which includes departmental executive salaries, policy planning and information, intergovernmental and international affairs, corporate management, personnel administration and communications branches – but conveniently and quaintly on community population. The only post-transfer requirements are that the community continue to provide communicable disease control services, environmental health services, and treatment services and that they maintain an emergency response plan. (HWC, 1989)

In a short-term evaluation of HPT, communities felt HPT allows greater financial and programmatic flexibility to address community needs. (Adrian Gibbons and Associates, 1992) However, HPT funding policy has been criticized primarily because it does not allow for program evolution or enrichment. The problem with evolutionary inflexibility in HPT agreements is best illustrated by the lack of adequate services for Fetal Alcohol Syndrome (FAS) and AIDS cases in the post-transfer scenario. It is shortsighted to expect that 1990s health resources will accommodate the preventive and remedial efforts required to deal with addictions and AIDS into the twenty-first century. In fact, communities have criticized this lack of evolutionary flexibility and interpreted it as a cost containment exercise and a municipalization training program. In other words, when push comes to shove for health resources down the line, communities to which administrative authority has been transferred will then have to look to the province for any additional monies they require, because the federal government has chosen to limit its financial commitment to these communities through the transfer mechanism. And, as illustrated in the discussion on CAP and EPF, this may leave communities in a human services void.

MSB's Community Workload Increase System (see Appendix B), however, is an attempt to assess just how taxed community-based health programs are. Its primary objective is to maintain funding uniformity within the circle of agencies funded by MSB. However, this does not resolve the dilemma of double-standard funding policies between federally and provincially funded systems. This system could be an important funding policy tool, could have wide-reaching post-transfer application, and could facilitate the equal distribution of health resources. Still, to be truly valuable, early developmental stages of this measurement tool should ensure that it would enable comparison with provincial workload measurement systems.

In addition, the HPT package excludes the services of other HWC branches that lend themselves to preventive efforts and are easily divisible, such as Health Services and Promotion, Health Protection, and Fitness and Amateur Sport. Most notably absent, however, are the administrative dollars supporting the bureaucracy of MSB.

Non-Insured Health Benefits

Also not available under HPT are the roughly $214 million being spent annually on non-insured health benefits (NIHB), (facsimile, HWC, 1993) which constitute perhaps one of the most convenient opportunities for reorganization of

Indigenous health resources. I say convenient only because the amount is readily identifiable, unlike resources being provided by provincial human services systems to Indigenous peoples. NIHB cover prescription drugs, prosthetic devices, dental care, eye glasses and medical transportation. Ideally, administrative responsibility for NIHB should be transferred to Indigenous health authorities in a more attractive and flexible way, much like the alternative funding arrangements model (or block funding) offered by INAC. As it stands now, NIHB can be devolved to an Indigenous health authority in a standard contribution agreement that, over the long term, does not allow the retention of surplus monies or their transfer into more preventive health programs, as the HPT agreement does.

Current funding policy for NIHB allows the escalating costs to be demand-driven, not program-controlled: the rate of escalation as depicted in Appendix C is only one good reason why this policy should change. Other practical problems inherent in sustaining a demand-driven funding policy are best explained by example. In the demand-driven situation, clients (as many as demand dictates) must leave the community to seek dental care; their transportation to the dentist's office is paid as well as the dentist's professional service fee. In the program-controlled scenario, the dentist is transported to the community to deliver a dental care program.

Table 1

Comparison of Costs for Demand-Driven Services and Program-Controlled Services

Demand-Driven	*Program-Controlled*
\$24 = Travel	\$24 = Travel
50 = Clients	1 = Dentist
15 = Trips/Treatments	30 = Trips
24 X 50 X 15 = \$18,000	24 X 1 X 30 = \$720
Professional Fee – \$500	Professional Fee – \$500
50 X 500 = \$25,000	50 x 500 = \$25,000
Total - \$43,000	**Total - \$25,720**

It is clear that in the erratically scheduled, demand-driven situation, NIHB costs are \$43,000, whereas the program-controlled scenario, with the dentist travelling to the community two days per week, costs \$25,720.

Taken on a grander scale, if the medical transportation costs of a northern community are hovering at \$2 million annually, how could those dollars be better organized or perhaps merged with provincial health resources to bring services to the people and to prevent treatment in distant medical facilities? After all, even in the best of circumstances, there is no place like home. One of the more dangerous, albeit unintended, side effects of such an ingrained medical evacuation service is that transporters are often seen as part of the medical care system, and are offering medical advice and making referrals!

Other alternatives worth exploring include the U.S. Indian Health Service model of flexibility between contract medicare (program-controlled) and direct service purchases (comparable to Canadian NIHB), or the possibility of establishing an Indigenously controlled health insurance program like the pension plan operations of the Counseil Attikamek Montagnais.

Recent efforts to gain control of the exponential increase in NIHB have had only a marginal impact. An example of cost containment efforts through community-controlled models is the Labrador Inuit Health Commission's administration of NIHB. A review of this arrangement indicates that transfer through contribution agreements does allow for the elimination of abuses, but it does not allow a program-controlled scenario. (Johnson, 1992) Therefore, transfer through standard contribution agreement without flexibility may serve a cost containment objective, but this should not be confused with cost efficiency, which can be achieved more easily in a program-controlled scenario.

Another attempt to curb escalating costs was the elimination of infant formula as an NIHB. This expense has only shifted itself into welfare and family support budgets of social services agencies. (Wayne Helgason, personal communication, 16 February 1993) This is only one of many examples that illustrate the close relationship between health and social services. Others include institutionalization of people with disabilities, elder care, and treatment of child sexual abuse survivors, all of which find their way into the symptom-centred NIHB budget. I urge readers to prepare a blueprint for the greater integration of health and social service budgets, which will accommodate more holistic human services funding policy.

Social Development Branch, Indian and Northern Affairs Canada

Funding policy for Indian Child and Family Services is developed by the Social Development Branch (SDB), INAC. Service funds are devolved to communities through rigid contribution agreements, which may include institutional care for adults and children, homemaker services, prevention of placement, foster care, emergency shelter, group homes and administration. Although the agreement is modeled on a Euro-American notion of social development, the range of services available to Canadians generally is not included. Most notably absent from these budgets are community development and work activity projects. (HWC, 1992) The contribution agreements also generally do not allow for communities to rearrange funds according to their priorities.

However, there have been considerable and promising changes in funding policy for child and family services. Many communities will now be able to establish services that will operate based on Indigenous standards under a new funding policy known as the Management Regime. The disappointing element of this funding policy is that it will not provide for the establishment or operation of services for communities with fewer than 251 children. Understanding limitations in times of fiscal restraint, I am ethically obligated to highlight that this represents the substantive portion of isolated communities where children are at greatest risk. The apparent problem with sustaining this approach is that some children appear to be entitled to protection and some do not.

If it is purely a matter of fiscal limitation for the SDB, then alternatives that could be considered include access to funds generally available to the provincial population for family services. Presumably, if no service exists, the provincial government is under no obligation to provide the services? How can we prevent these children from falling into the jurisdictional void between sections of the *Constitution Act*?

Furthermore, where administrative authority for social development has been devolved to an Indigenous health authority, funds are subject to inflationary increases only. Program evolution or enrichment is unilaterally decided by the SDB; examples that illustrate the dilemma here are the current lack of resources to prevent suicide and sexual abuse of children, as well as mental health services for the recently bereaved.

In all cases of transferred administrative control of social services but one, subscription to provincial jurisdiction is imposed. However, other creative examples of provincial government responsiveness exist in both Ontario and Quebec. Ontario's *Child Welfare Act* specifically recognizes the importance of culture and language in Indigenous childrearing practice. Quebec has offered Indigenous communities the opportunity to write their own youth protection legislation which, if endorsed by the Quebec legislature, would allow communities the savings of professional supervision fees currently paid to the province by Indigenous health authorities. In a small way, Quebec is more removed from the internal operations of family services under this model, and professional supervision monies stay in the community. The ideal, of course, is the Spallumcheen First Nation example, which has jurisdictional control through the bylaw process contained in section 81 (1) (a) of the *Indian Act*.

Provincial Models

There are many examples of administrative transfer to Indigenous peoples on reserve; however, there are very few examples of human services that are culturally appropriate for Indigenous peoples off a land base (e.g., Métis Child and Family Services in Edmonton, Alberta; Anishnabe Health in Toronto, Ontario; Ma Mawi Wi Chi Itata in Winnipeg, Manitoba). These human services are funded by a variety of financial arrangements, all of which represent creative and responsive approaches to Indigenous peoples off a land base but could be improved to facilitate a more holistic and preventive approach in keeping with Indigenous cultures.

Interestingly, the identified problems with provincial human services transfer initiatives are very similar to those of federal initiatives. It is clear that funding comes with rigid program guidelines, inflexibility between program functions, imposition of provincial services policies, and a remedial service volume-driven funding formula. In other words, the critical variable for funding these service agencies is their remedial caseload, which is interpreted by strict provincial definition. (Wayne Helgason, 2 February 1993; Carolyn Pettifer, personal communication, 17 February 1993) In fact, efforts at preventive work are inhibited by policies that make it necessary for self-referred families to sign voluntary child welfare agreements, thereafter being labelled as 'child welfare cases' when they are looking only to extend their support networks to include these agencies. Many families are intimidated by this requirement, fearing that their children will be apprehended, discontinue any contact and hence do not get preventive services. The problem here is that funding policy is clearly based on the number of children in care and provides no incentive for agencies to direct themselves otherwise. The obvious alternative is to redefine who is eligible to be a client and allow total flexibility between family intervention and child welfare budgets.

Some Thoughts for Future Policy Analysis

A fuller explanation of the complex interdependence between policy sectors such as education, land, housing, economy, culture and human services is beyond the scope of this paper but should be addressed in future policy analysis undertaken with the luxury of time and resources. The implications of intersectoral change are most apparent when we consider that individuals become prepared to assume responsibility only with training. Families are ready to nurture only with adequate economic resources and sound cultural foundations. Communities can become self-sufficient only with an adequate land base. But as long as problem orientation dictates funding policy, these fundamentals will not be integrated into human services, and shortsighted, symptom-centred approaches will not produce the greatest cost benefit.

One of the great unknowns on a national scale is just how over- or under-represented Indigenous peoples are in human services. Regionally, some provinces can track service clients by ethnicity. However, there has been no analysis of the data to determine how representation would affect health services financing to Indigenous health authorities. Some examination of Indigenous representation by service type should be done. Key informants now suspect that there is greater representation in remedial or tertiary services than there is in preventive services. In other words, when forced to the last stand, Indigenous peoples are reflected in the service clientele of Euro-American health agencies. However, in early stages of disease, it is by choice, inaccessibility or inappropriateness that Indigenous groups are not reflected service records. When this is the case, the representation issue has grave implications for the funding policy and may hold substantive argument for rearranging resources to provide integrated, accessible, linguistically and culturally appropriate health service. On a very practical level, this kind of flexibility is an ounce of prevention.

Nothing stops interdepartmental human services co-operation. It is already being done with the Family Violence Initiative (HWC and INAC). This co-operation would allow for communities to address the impact of employment, housing, education and culture on health. The inflexibility of current funding arrangements makes the ethnocentric assumption that the western approach to health care and maintenance must be universal. Even in the narrow focus on human services, Indigenous health authorities must deal with several government agents to manage their health programs (INAC, MSB, provincial departments), facilities (Department of Public Works) and personnel (Canada Employment and Immigration). What is preventing more interdepartmental co-operation on these fronts?

My analysis is focused on government funding policies. However, governments are not the only important players in human services. Although many well intentioned bureaucrats have facilitated the changes that have occurred over the last two decades, the most powerful and important players are Indigenous individuals, communities and governments. Still, our task as Round Table participants is not to suggest what Indigenous peoples should do but to revise Canadian systems to allow Indigenous players to orchestrate change that is their own.

Concluding Remarks

Human services funding policy has been developed largely without the involvement of Indigenous peoples, and for those off a land base and in urban centres who must gain access to health services through Euro-American institutions, representation on municipal and district health councils is rare. Our challenge is to develop an interdepartmental mechanism for change with morally independent, self-directing control over the care and maintenance of well-being as the ideal. Rather than Indigenously flavouring models based on remedial, symptom-centred therapies, autonomous Indigenous peoples could aspire to design health care systems that recognize the integration of social and physical elements, where traditional healing is practised freely, where primary prevention is the funding priority, and treatment, when needed, is readily accessible. The goal of Indigenous health efforts is not to replicate highly divisive western approaches to human services, but to provide a holistic approach with community-specific priorities and the financial flexibility to address those priorities.

Administrative transfer models do serve to increase the involvement of Indigenous groups in the delivery and management of health resources. Alternatively, greater local involvement of Indigenous groups through affirmative action by district health councils would be an improvement. The advantage of this approach is clear – greater representation means greater decision-making power over health resources for Indigenous groups. The disadvantage is that this does not serve those who wish to be institutionally complete or distinct with respect to human services. For those that do wish to be institutionally complete, some interdepartmental block funding arrangement should be available. At last, because of their position as the most potent agents of change, the efforts of Indigenous peoples to achieve individual and community healing must be recognized consistently, supported and extended more broadly by responsive and responsible government.

Questions Posed to Round Table Participants

1. How can the responsibilities between federal and provincial governments be reconciled under sections 91 (24) and 92 of the *Constitution Act, 1867*, where few or no services exist for Indigenous peoples?
2. How could federal transfer payments under CAP and EPF be redistributed so that Indigenous health authorities have greater control over health wealth? If Indigenous health authorities gain control over these resources, what accountability mechanisms are necessary? What tax implications would this have?
3. What impact does Indigenous representation in care and service utilization patterns have on funding policy?
4. What prevents the interdepartmental co-operation for funding to Indigenous health authorities?
5. With particular reference to non-insured health benefits, what policy revisions would make NIHB more cost-effective?
6. On a regional or community level, what are the comprehensive, detailed comparative cost analyses of health services for any isolated Indigenous group (Indian, Métis or Inuit) and Canadians generally?

Glossary

CAP – Canada Assistance Plan
EPF – Established Programs Financing
HPT – Health Program Transfer
HWC – Health and Welfare Canada
INAC – Indian and Northern Affairs Canada
Indigenous peoples
– people of the territory, people belonging to the land

Indigenous health authorities
– incorporated health boards on and off a land base, band councils, tribal councils

MSB – Medical Services Branch, Health and Welfare Canada
NIHB – Non-insured health benefits
SDB – Social Development Branch, Indian and Northern Affairs Canada

Appendix A

The Canada Health Act

The *Canada Health Act* is based on the fundamental principles presented below. They are important to understanding the ideals on which the Canadian health care system is based.

The criteria and conditions that each provincial health insurance plan must meet in order to receive full federal cash contributions under the Act of 1977 (*Federal-Provincial Fiscal Arrangements and Federal Post-Secondary Education and Health Contributions Act, 1977*) in each fiscal year are:

(a) Public Administration: Pursuant to section 8, the health care insurance plan must be administered and operated on a non-profit basis by a public authority, responsible to the provincial government and subject to audit of its accounts and financial transactions.
(b) Comprehensiveness: Pursuant to section 9, the plan must insure all insured health services provided by hospitals, medical practitioners, or dentists, and, where permitted, services rendered by other health care practitioners.
(c) Universality: Section 10 requires that 100 per cent of the insured persons of a province be entitled to the insured health services provided for by the plan on uniform terms and conditions.
(d) Portability: In accordance with section 11, residents moving to another province must continue to be covered for insured health services by the home province during any minimum waiting period imposed by the new province of residence not to exceed three months.

For insured persons, insured health services must be made available while they are temporarily absent from their own provinces on the basis that:

- insured services received out of province, but still in Canada, are to be paid for by the home province at host province rates unless another arrangement for the payment of costs exists between the provinces. Prior approval may be required for elective services.
- services out of country are to be paid, as a minimum, on the basis of the amount that would have been paid by the home province for similar services rendered in province. Prior approval may also be required for elective services.

(e) Accessibility: By virtue of section 12, the health care insurance plan of a province must provide for:

- insured health services on uniform terms and conditions and reasonable access by insured person to insured health services unprecluded or unimpeded, either directly or indirectly, by charges or other means;
- reasonable compensation to physicians and dentists for all insured health services rendered;
- payments to hospital in respect of the cost of insured health services.

Appendix B

Community Workload Increase System for Indian and Northern Health Programs at the Community Level

Background

In the past no consistent approach to funding Medical Services Branch activities existed, with the result that major inequities developed with respect to funding. These inequities existed not only among regions but within regions as well.

In 1984 a project called "Costing the Gap" was initiated. Its objective was to identify the requirements to close the gap between existing service levels and health care delivery standards. This project was not successful in producing a realistic and viable tool for justifying resource requirements to Treasury Board.

The Community Workload Increase project was initiated as an alternative approach to "Costing the Gap". The objective was to develop workload ratios that would serve as a tool to justify resource requirements, including incremental requirements as a result of volume and workload, to Treasury Board for current and future years at the community level. Four types of communities were defined to accommodate geographic and demographic circumstances, as the system is predicated on the premise that no community will be financially disadvantaged.

The system considers basic levels of health services, the actual number of clients in the communities, and established schedules for health service delivery required to provide the services.

The system provides an equitable basis for allocation of available resources. Additionally it provides individual communities with some indication of the level of resources that will be available from year to year and will facilitate long-term planning for the transfer process.

Appendix C

Figure 1

Non-Insured Health Benefits
Actual Expenditures by Category

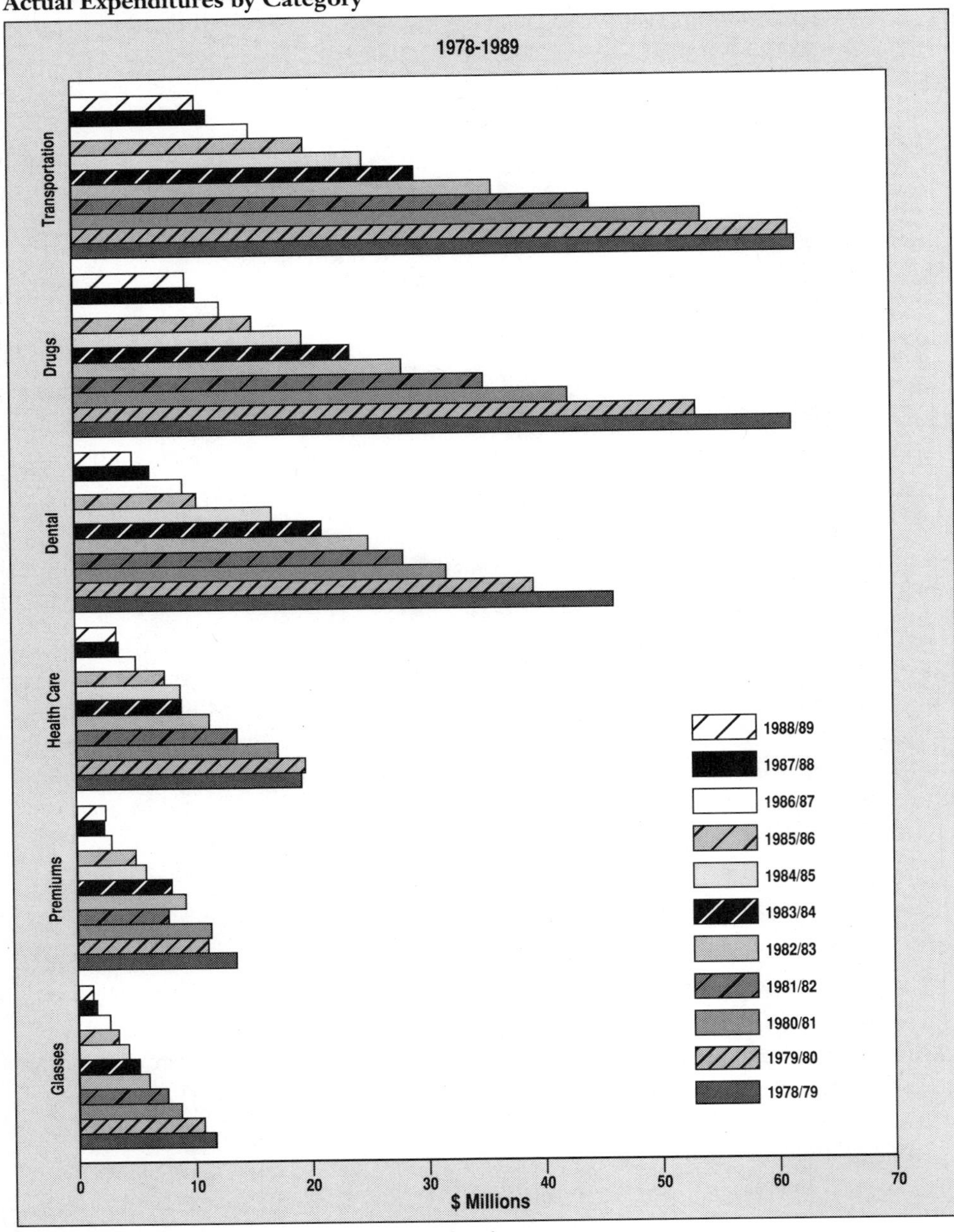

Source: Medical Services Branch, Health and Welfare Canada

Figure 2

Non-Insured Health Benefits
Actual and Forecast

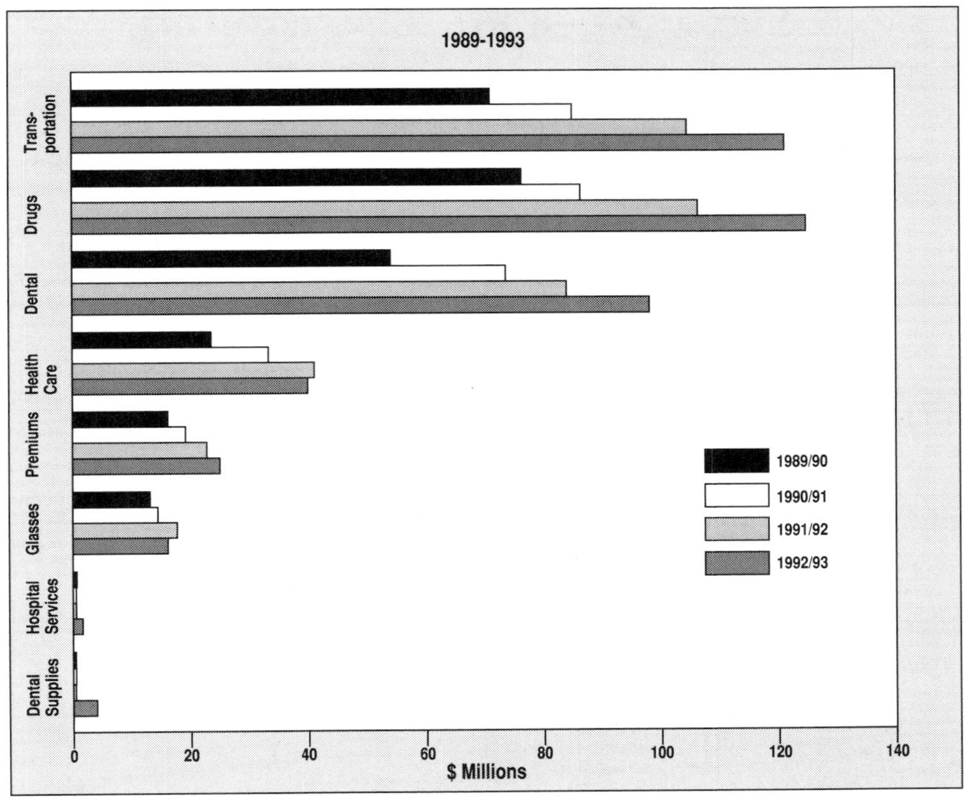

Source: Medical Services Branch, Health and Welfare Canada

References

Adrian Gibbons and Associates. *Short-Term Evaluation of Indian Health Transfer*. January 1992.

Barer, Morris L. and Greg. L. Stoddart. *Toward Integrated Medical Resource Policies for Canada*. Report prepared for the Federal/Provincial/Territorial Conference of Deputy Ministers of Health. June 1991.

Health and Welfare Canada. *Canada Assistance Plan Annual Report 1989-1990*. Cat. H75-8/1990, ISBN 0-662-59218-2. 1992.

Health and Welfare Canada, Program Transfer, Policy and Planning Directorate, Medical Services Branch. *Health Program Transfer Handbook*. Revised. September 1989.

Johnson, Judy. *A Review of Community-Administered Non-Insured Health Benefits*. June 1992.

Deficits, Foundation and Aspirations Signal Need for Restructuring

*W.J. (Bill) Mussell**

What Indigenous peoples do not have, as represented by programs and services made accessible to them, and what they want, seem to be far, far apart. What is required to satisfy essential needs and therefore to build a solid cultural foundation has not been seriously investigated. The deficits or challenges facing Indigenous peoples, given their aspirations, do call for restructuring within their communities and on the part of extra-community structures serving them and to which they are related.

Indigenous leaders of our country aspire to self-government. They want improvements in the lifestyles shared by their electors and a secure heritage for their future generations. Social, economic and political aspects of their lives indicate the need for radical change. Such successful changes will gradually enrich their collective abilities to take charge of their lives and to know social justice. Evidence of needs requiring attention reveal why social justice is a long-term goal.

Programs and services to combat addiction to alcohol and other substances, violence and sexual abuse, child neglect, youth suicide, and remedial kinds of education and training, for example, are reported by increasing numbers of community leaders as priority needs. Such needs clearly reflect serious problems and issues that began to receive some serious attention about a decade ago. These needs also reflect a strong deficiency orientation, which creates additional

* Researcher, author, community and curriculum development and trainer. Member of the Skwah Band, Sto:lo Culture, British Columbia

difficulties for all stakeholders committed to the processes necessary to create positive social, economic and political change.

Connecting a self-governing vision with these realities is a challenge facing this author, who is expected to share workable models that will promote what is necessary for collectives of people to become subjects of life. As strategic tools, models are most meaningful when posed after considering the historical context or the roots that give meaning to the whats and whys of present reality shared by most Indigenous communities. This discussion paper will be presented, therefore, in three major parts: the big picture that has a past and present, the future and restructuring necessary to get there, and discussion of favoured strategies together with recommendations for action. Questions pertinent to restructuring will be posed in this paper. The third part will be addressed in the presentation to be made at the Round Table.

Historical Context

In the late 1960s and early 1970s the late George Manuel and Harold Cardinal, two Indigenous leaders, spoke of justice as something not characterizing the lives of their people. Controlled by outsiders perceived as colonizers and oppressors, Indigenous societies began to think about 'the unjust society' and the meaning of the concept justice.

Three basic definitions of social justice can be related to the modern history of Indigenous peoples. By aspiring to self-government, their leaders may be perceived as not being satisfied with the status quo definition or the reformist one. The status quo definition, which emphasizes the rights of individuals, accepts that there is not enough justice for everyone. The reformist definition accepts that there is not enough justice for the poor and others deprived of it, so the government is expected to play a key role in protecting the rights of individuals. The Diefenbaker government's *Bill of Rights* was instrumental in making this definition real for many people in this country.

After three decades of this approach of protecting individual rights to promote greater equality among all Canadians, the Canadian government and its electors are being confronted now by Aboriginal leaders to change the laws in order to entrench the right to self-government and to consider the creation of new and different structures to promote social justice in Indigenous communities. What the Indigenous leaders are saying, it appears, is that society, as currently experienced, is unjust; therefore, new social, political and economic structures must be created to eliminate the root causes of injustice. This perception of social justice will be used here to make a case for radical restructuring.

Guiding Questions

1. What are some of the workable models that allow Aboriginal individuals/communities to take responsibility for health?
2. How can the movement toward self-management be facilitated, and what role should each health partner (communities, individuals, care systems and governments) play to facilitate self-management?

This paper should address the most effective ways to empower communities and individuals to take responsibility for health... Self-management must be clearly defined.

Two Dimensions of the Big Picture: Past and Present

Groups of people who have known continuous exploitation, domination and alienation share similar realities. According to Paulo Freire, a Brazilian educator, groups that have been oppressed are faced with the need to define clearly the effects of positive and negative forces in their lives. Knowing the myths or false beliefs that control their lives is a necessary part of the knowledge they require to plan for their future. How people empower themselves is the focus of Freire's work. By analyzing inequities in their lives, the people create the working knowledge necessary to restructure their lives. This process of empowerment is necessary to transform a lifestyle of dependence (living as objects of life) to one of self-control and self-determination (living as subjects of life). A subject of life is a person who acts and knows and by knowing is able to continue to create knowledge and make history. This perspective will be employed to discuss the substance of this paper. The spirit of process or the flow of energy over time and under certain conditions to make change, it is hoped, is conveyed in the graphic on page 4.

Vision

Let us assume that the best description of 'desired future lifestyle' or vision is self-government. What lifestyle is wanted? Values such as family, Mother Earth, natural resources, holistic health, co-operation, and sharing, for example, suggest that quality of life is very, very important. Its importance becomes apparent when we stop to consider evidence of its absence in significant numbers of communities. Many forces in the dynamics of life in these communities are dehumanizing. Paulo Freire's notion of a humanized society, therefore, may also be employed to convey the nature of the desired lifestyle.

Communities suffering from the effects of oppression, like individuals, seldom experience desired change and in fact often rally their energies to resist change. They are most comfortable with 'the way things are', and if they are unhappy with decisions made by others, they usually ask others to do something about them. Such people tend not to perceive themselves as having the personal and

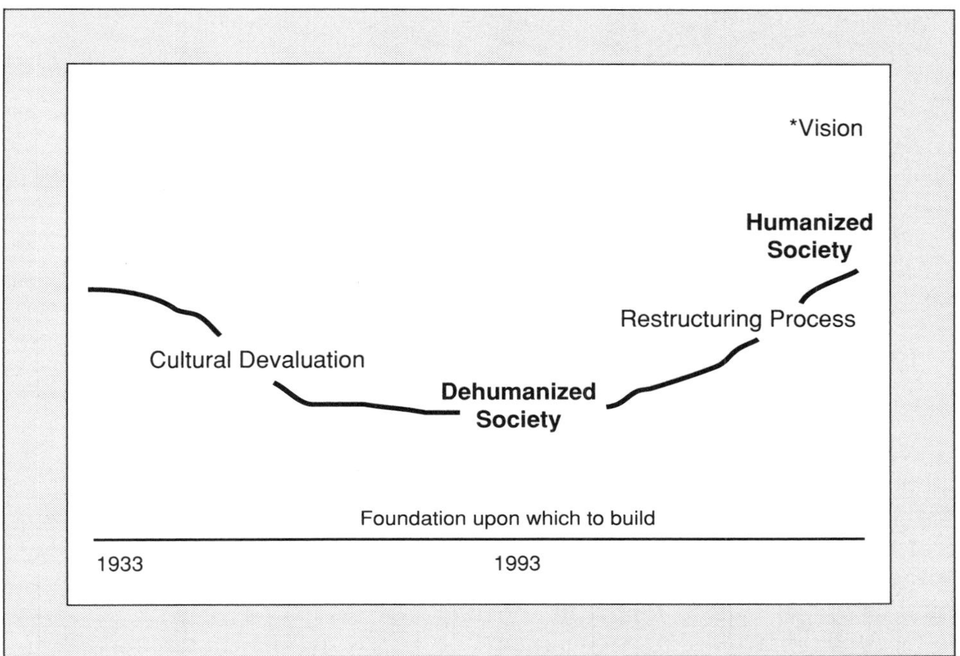

material resources to take constructive action themselves. In fact, they do not welcome responsibilities and frequently fear them. Over the past century, Aboriginal peoples have learned how to react to what others decide and only now are beginning to discover the significance of being proactive. Why are most Aboriginal groups crippled by inaction? A review of relations between Aboriginal groups and the settlers who assumed control over the country will suggest reasons for contemporary conditions in Indigenous societies.

Cultural Devaluation

The concept of cultural devaluation is used to convey the effects of negative forces in the lives of Indigenous peoples for over a century and much longer for other Indigenous groups in other parts of Canada. Culture is perceived as lifestyle, which changes over time as a result of both forces imposed from outside and forces generated from within the social entity.

During the earliest periods of settlement by immigrant populations in Canada, Indigenous peoples were perceived to be uncivilized, and various kinds of strategies were employed to change them. Reserves were created both to protect and to prepare them to become assimilated within the emerging Canadian society. Reserves were also created to severely restrict the use of their traditional land base; as a result, in time, most traditional economies disappeared. Thus, not making it possible for Aboriginal peoples to flourish as separate societies may be viewed as preferring to eliminate them as culturally unique and distinct peoples.

Children were removed from the influences of their families and communities to be trained. To promote this end, agents of the church and government housed them in residential schools where they were forced to learn English and to adopt new ways of dressing, thinking and behaving. Most of these children, generation after generation, lost their ability to communicate with their families, and many of them learned to reject their culture and identity. They were severely punished whenever they demonstrated behaviour that was identified with their culture and were rewarded for adapting successfully to the new way of life. Institutionalized ways, associated with custodial care, became a feature of their formative years and therefore of their lives.

Conformity was demanded in the residential schools. For many years, the curriculum used was to prepare consecutive generations of adults to become 'hired help' – not nurses, teachers, doctors, lawyers or entrepreneurs. Most young people met the expectations of the administrators and teachers and returned home without the social, academic, and life skills to manage their lives within their own societies or in the neighbouring ones. It can be concluded that they were not perceived to 'have what it takes' to become a professional in the western context. And if they were seen to have the abilities, no significant ways were found to prepare and equip them with the tools to become successful. First Nations and other Indigenous communities continue to live with this attitude.

Many people in these communities do not perceive themselves as having the ability to 'get a good education' or to compete effectively with other Canadians at school, in the workplace, or even to 'make it' in their own community. Many of them have internalized what they were trained to think about themselves by the administrators and teachers running the residences and the schools. As the first few generations of young people 'graduated' from these schools, married, and had children, they practised what they were taught. By doing this, they prepared their children for a life characterized by conformity and dependence upon others to do their thinking and acting for them.

As a result, families and individuals who are self-caring, self-sufficient, disciplined and socially confident and who exercise their ability to provide for others are often isolated and put down by neighbours. They are not usually perceived as a valued human resource, a resource whose lifestyle is anchored in strong traditions of their heritage and culture. They have had success as learners at home, in the community and at school. They think for themselves. They make their own decisions and can often express why they think and feel as they do. The negativity and the rejections they experience are often expressions of unhappiness, jealousy and other powerful negative feelings projected upon them by others. These individuals and families, who know some freedom, value their heritage and want a strong community, are being seen, however, by a gradually increasing number of other Indigenous people as desirable leaders. Among other major challenges, their personal, social and other resources are needed in order to overcome the 'power' of the status quo, which has come to represent the passive dependent population.

How and why First Nations and other Indigenous communities seldom experience planned change from within their own communities become clearer by knowing what the study of history can teach us and by knowing what people of a variety of other cultures have learned. If cycles of oppressive forces inside and outside Indigenous communities are not broken, the demeaning forces will continue to fuel their devaluation.

Dehumanized Society: Reality Today

The reality of dehumanized society in Indigenous communities today is apparent in their current social conditions.

1. Social dislocation occasioned by disruption of support networks such as extended family and clan through (a) institutionalization of school-age children to educate them for up to six generations in some parts of the country; (b) birth of children outside marriage; (c) separation and divorce; (d) child neglect or abuse, occasioning wardship; and (e) adoption of children outside their cultural milieu.
2. Incidence of family violence, youth suicide, elder abuse, and drug, alcohol and other kinds of addiction.
3. Aboriginal people are at greater risk than the general population regarding all physical ills, including respiratory, circulatory, gastrointestinal and infectious diseases, parasitic infections, accidental injuries and poisoning.
4. Inadequate housing and sanitary facilities.
5. Poor psychological and social environments and economic conditions.
6. Inadequate, inaccessible and culturally inappropriate health, social and educational services.
7. People are divided by fear, suspicion, jealousies and inability to interact reciprocally.
8. Powers of extra-community institutions are greater than those within the community.
9. Programs and services created to 'serve Aboriginal people' usually compensate for deficiencies rather than activate abilities to change.
10. Programs and services are highly fragmented. It is not unusual for families to have three, four, and sometimes more workers who do not collaborate or aim to co-ordinate their efforts and resources.
11. Network systems of the community are often treated with indifference.

12. Policies created tend to be the product of accidents and incidents, not viable and proactive kinds of planning.
13. Information, knowledge and skills produced in earlier decades and in foreign cultures are being applied with continuing poor outcomes.

Cultural invasion, as conceived by Paulo Freire, is a major feature of oppressed peoples' lifestyles. Each of these facets of a dehumanized society, in various ways, is related to or describes actual disruptions in Indigenous cultures. The collective abilities of Indigenous peoples to transmit the building blocks and tools of their respective cultures have been seriously damaged. When the people emulate the oppressor, the ways of the oppressor become the ways of the oppressed. Now that five, six and perhaps seven generations have been subjected to the powers of extra-community exploitation, domination and alienation, similar powers have taken root within their communities. Outsiders are no longer required for negative, demeaning and dehumanizing treatment to occur.

Cultural Foundation

The existing cultural foundation of Indigenous communities is another indication of the need for restructuring to bring lifestyles into greater congruence with cultural values.

1. The family is the primary institution of Indigenous 'communities'. It is not uncommon for individuals to value family over individual needs and wants, although there is evidence of movement toward increasing individualism.
2. The land base and associated natural resources are essential to sustain the integrity of the cultural ways of the people.
3. Traditions that have been brought into the present era have been sustained because they are working. They are valued for what they do to ensure survival and ability to meet challenges as the future unfolds.
4. New structures for making and implementing decisions with implications for all community members are being recreated, and sometimes strengthened, using the knowledge of elders who lived during times when they learned of traditional social, economic and political ways to ensure that safety, survival, developmental and other priority needs are satisfied.
5. Discovery and re-discovery of spiritual practices used in earlier times is stimulating a greater interest in Indigenous history and a strong sense of pride in increasing numbers of Indigenous individuals and families.
6. Discovery and re-discovery of the essence of teaching and learning, together with experiential and associated methods anchored in traditional ways, are taking place. The thrust of such discoveries is the creation of conditions and situations to activate the power to change or modify self.

7. Renewed and strengthened belief in the right to have a life in this land and to have their own communities and societies. The struggle for recognition and entrenchment of basic rights, which has resulted in decisions to co-manage fishery and forestry resources, for example, reflects a new ideology.

8. Belief in an optimistic future has prevailed over the years. That things will be better tomorrow is a strong attitude.

9. Holistic health, addressing wellness physically, emotionally, intellectually and spiritually, is a value anchored in strong Indigenous traditions that continues to be a shared goal among many, many families.

Reality as a Bridge to the Future

Integration of working knowledge – represented by vision, cultural devaluation, reality today and the cultural foundation – paints a picture that can be used (a) to discuss the strengths and weaknesses of programs and services being extended to Indigenous peoples and (b) to frame the presentation of strategies for change. Given the focus of this Round Table, health and related social areas will be given the most attention. Key features of the picture include the following:

1. Indigenous communities as places with a future.
2. Indigenous communities with an important history and cultural foundation.
3. Lack of working knowledge that makes it possible to define reality clearly and to do the planning necessary to restructure their societies.
4. Community leaders and workers want to strengthen the community's foundation, improve its quality of life, and have access to resources to make change.
5. Few individuals in the community have successfully completed high school.
6. More than half the families rely upon social assistance to survive.
7. Custodial care is the way of life for more than 60 per cent of families.
8. The nuclear and extended family are the primary social institutions.
9. Many individuals and families do not believe in their abilities to change themselves, their families or communities.
10. Many individuals and families believe that 'white is right'.
11. Healing is necessary, because traumas suffered during early childhood within families, in residential schools and in other settings seriously affect the lives of up to 80 per cent of the people.
12. About 20 per cent of the population from birth to 18 years is affected by either fetal alcohol syndrome or fetal alcohol effects.

13. Serious problems and issues consume the energies of leaders and workers.

14. Strategies used to solve problems have usually failed; for example, doing one-to-one counselling of a client whose life is controlled by alcohol without working through the family's strengths.

15. Extra-community institutions have greater powers than in-community ones; for example, the Department of Indian Affairs and Northern Development and the Medical Services Branch of Health and Welfare Canada.

New strategies are required to solve the problems that sap the energies and limited resources of Indigenous communities. These strategies must build upon the traditions and other cultural strengths of the people. The family, both nuclear and extended, is the key social institution. Instead of focusing upon serving or treating the individual, working through and with the strengths of the family, where possible, expands the opportunities to share and expand knowledge. First Nations and other Indigenous communities are here to stay. It is important, therefore, to employ community development practices that are necessary to strengthen the fabric of life that is shared by all families.

A re-ordering of other priorities is also essential. Community-based administration, starting with the elected council, was imposed from the outside. There is no significant evidence to show that this structure works; that is, it is inadequate to meet the need for local control (responsibility and accountability), inadequate to meet the challenges of managing its interests that are managed by extra-community organizations and agencies, and lacks the wherewithal for effective planning. Although there have been serious problems with elected councils, resources to support pertinent research and development work to investigate traditional means of governing and meeting mutual needs have not been made available or accessible to Indigenous groups. Research addressing questions such as healing, holistic health, childrearing practices and so on is similarly lacking.

It is accepted in most health, education and social fields of work that Indigenous peoples lack self-worth and tend not to believe in their ability to modify self. Only within the past year or so have some people in these same fields begun to discover that significant numbers of these people were traumatized in their earlier lives and could be assisted to take charge of their personal lives through healing (grieving of losses) and personal growth (learning the whats, hows and whys of holistic growth) before undertaking serious academic study or seeking employment, especially in the human services fields. Education and training that are tailored to building on the experience of the learner (to make the teaching/learning process culturally relevant) have not yet become reality in the classroom. Given education levels and histories of unhappiness in formal education systems, coupled with the need for competent professionals as managers, administrators, therapists, counsellors, teachers, lawyers and entrepreneurs, for example, new strategies and innovations must be found. This need has implications for research and education and training opportunities. Besides being guided by the stated conditions, such opportunities must also consider the serious dependence upon social welfare assistance, which is becoming an inter-generational phenomenon.

Vision and Restructuring

Individuals with a secure identity have the greatest ability to interact with others, to pose reasonable and thoughtful questions and to make time to listen to what others have to share; they are also individuals with a vision. Like the point on a map that shows the destination of a long journey, the vision can be seen to represent the purpose of one's life. Expressions of vision, in western Canadian Indigenous societies, began to become popular less than two decades ago. Such expressions made implicit the need to know where one has been or to know one's family and community history. Knowing the past provides knowledge to know the present and its continuity into the future. Most discussions about vision, in the author's experience, took place within meetings while exploring strategies to build a healthy and strong community of families.

Having a clear perception of realities makes it possible to categorize strengths and weaknesses. When the community is the subject being investigated, leaders, workers and volunteers doing the planning can identify what they wish to change, as an earlier stage in the process. This investigation can lead to a description of some characteristics of health and associated programs and services that are delivered to their community. Many of these traits will describe the parent of these programs and services, either the first or second orders of government in most instances.

1. Most services are designed and delivered in ways to compensate for deficiencies. Although needs may be satisfied in the short term, how they are satisfied does not usually involve creation of knowledge necessary for patients or clients to find their own solutions or to feel the satisfaction associated with knowing how to do something more for self or others. This approach perpetuates the status quo – more and more passive dependence!
2. Whatever is promoted for Indigenous communities duplicates 'dominant' cultural services, even though there is ample evidence that such approaches and methodologies bring questionable results. Risks of 'feeding' passive dependence are high!
3. That which is delivered is highly fragmented and not necessarily designed to address effectively the needs of a family, a whole person or community. Training tailored to promote co-operation, co-ordination and mutual aid among workers serving the same families has not been given serious attention by any stakeholder. Unless education and training to do this are undertaken, conditions will remain much as they are.

4. The focus is always on negatives or deficiencies. This has been the case for enough generations for today's Indigenous populations to perceive their deficiencies more clearly than their strengths. Most of them know that statistics that highlight their weaknesses are useful in making cases for funding. How does this perception impinge upon efforts to promote empowerment?

5. No significant attention is given to the community's strengths. Until recently, children in need of protection were normally placed in homes outside the community and culture. Even today, it is difficult to obtain resources to undertake community development initiatives designed to bring community-wide change. Has any serious commitment been made to date to promote change from within the existing structures of the Indigenous community?

6. No notable building up of internal structures, systems and pertinent manpower resources, which are required to assume duties and responsibilities being transferred by federal and provincial bureaucracies, has been done. Although plans for transfer have been known for some time, education and training of community-based personnel have not been a priority. The same may be said of research and development work necessary to describe and to create culturally cogent governing structures and associated systems. How does this reflect upon pertinent extra-community agencies involved in the devolution process?

7. When efforts are made to find mutually agreeable strategies or solutions, the process is more akin to anti-dialogue than dialogue. The outcome does not usually produce what the people thought they had expressed as wants or needs. This outcome affirms that the process did not result in the creation or recreation of knowledge which characterizes dialogue or reciprocal interaction between two or more parties committed to finding mutually satisfactory answers. Consultations between Indigenous leaders and government officials and Indigenous officials and community people often fail to satisfy the purpose of the quest.

Most of these descriptions apply to first- and second-order governments and those governing organizations created by Indigenous leaders themselves. This brings us to some of the issues pertaining to what is needed to restructure and therefore make it possible for Indigenous societies to know social justice as described early in this paper. The following questions are pertinent to the purpose of this Round Table:

1. Can it be agreed that First Nation and other Indigenous communities are acceptable as separate and unique parts of the country's mosaic?

2. Can it be agreed that First Nation and other Indigenous communities do have a legitimate history and culture?

3. How do First Nation and other Indigenous communities define themselves in relation to the outside society?

4. Can there be a common vision shared by all Indigenous communities? Can there be a common vision between bands of the various definable cultures in the twenty-first century?

5. Is it possible for extra-community institutions to prepare and to equip the full range of community-based cultural leadership required to manage the affairs of First Nation and other Indigenous communities?

6. The more that extra-community systems impinge on the life of the Indigenous community, the less ability it has to control its own affairs. Are systems that manage economic matters (production, distribution and consumption), socialization (schools, courts, policing), and mutual aid (family and child welfare), which are now delivered by an impersonal bureaucracy, willing to give up their control, even by sharing it as a partner?

7. Is true dialogue achievable when the backgrounds, traditions, ideologies, and languages of the parties in the process of consultation and/or negotiation are so different?

8. The role of the elected leader is changing in Aboriginal communities. It seems to be changing in Canadian society generally. The referendum experience taught and perhaps retaught a few lessons. How might it be possible for people to move in a unified way? Once something is determined as wanted, then what? Do we not need a way for leaders to make and implement policy changes?

9. Community gatherings, which are characterized by discussion, appear to be an acceptable forum for decision making in the Indigenous community. Participants, it seems, feel a sense of ownership for what is decided, as long as their spokespeople honour the intent of the decisions made. How can the needs of Indigenous communities be reconciled with conventional Canadian leadership practices?

10. The wage economy and the provision of social assistance changed the relationship of people with one another and with the land, it appears. Consequences of the resulting passive dependence are devastating to their quality of life. What can be done to promote self-care and mutual aid and to create healthy community environments?

The Treaty Right to Health

*Alma Favel-King**

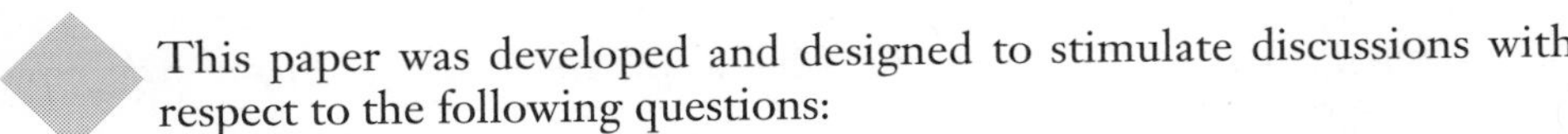

This paper was developed and designed to stimulate discussions with respect to the following questions:

- How will the federal government transfer process, enabling community control of health services and the recognition of treaty rights to health, affect the future health status of First Nations people?
- Will this process facilitate a holistic approach to health maintenance, and how will this be achieved?
- How will the role of provincial and federal health agencies change as a result?

In view of the complexity and nature of this subject, some background information is necessary to facilitate a comprehensive discussion of the issues. Because of the nature of the special relationship between the federal government and Treaty First Nations and the discussion parameters, this paper will address the issue only as it affects Treaty First Nations people.

Historical Review

It is a belief, held strongly and fervently by all First Nations, that accessibility to and availability of health benefits/services are based on a treaty right to health. Historical evidence indicates that the future well-being of First Nations was a

* Executive Director for the health and social development portfolio, Federation of Saskatchewan Indians.

major concern of Indian people during the negotiations of treaties. With the effects of the dwindling buffalo population and the introduction of European diseases already evident, our forefathers wanted to ensure the survival of future generations. Specific reference to the treaty right to health is contained in Treaty 6, in which the Queen's representatives promised that a "medicine chest" would be available for access by First Nations through the Indian Agent. How this clause has been interpreted by the federal government and by First Nations has been a point of contention for many years. In addition, their philosophical concepts of health and use of language are intrinsically different.

It is the federal government's view that clause refers to the equivalent of a first aid kit. However, it is the view of the First Nations that this means access and availability of a wide range of primary, secondary and tertiary health services.

Testimony from elders indicates that at the time of the negotiation of treaties, the Queen promised her subjects that she would look after them in the manner in which they had looked after themselves. First Nations' holistic concept and understanding of health led to a broad interpretation of this agreement.

Until the late 1940s, the department of Indian Affairs maintained responsibility for all aspects of programs and services to Indian people. While the intent behind the decision has not been researched in depth for this paper, responsibility for health services to First Nations people was transferred to Health and Welfare Canada, Medical Services Branch. It is evident Medical Services Branch (MSB) assumed responsibility for health services without regard to or acknowledgement of the perceived treaty right to health services. The design and delivery of health services by the federal government is based on the notion that their involvement in health services flows simply from humanitarian principles.

Although the Department of Indian Affairs and Northern Development (DIAND) transferred health services to MSB, it maintained responsibility for all other aspects of services and programs for First Nations. These include areas with a direct relation to health status, such as roads, housing, and water and sewer systems, as well as financial assistance to cover such basic needs as food, clothing, shelter and what the department refers to as "adult care". In addition, several other federal government departments have associated responsibilities. The complexity resulting from multiple federal departmental roles and responsibilities and the lack of integrated planning are demonstrated clearly with respect to water and sewage. With respect to the incidence of water-borne diseases, a problem common to many First Nation communities, the Environmental Health Officer of Health and Welfare Canada is responsible for recommending community infrastructure systems that will address the problem. DIAND is responsible for funding community systems, and MSB is responsible for ensuring that treatment and prevention activities occur. Funding by DIAND to the band does not take into consideration the water-borne disease rate of that community, nor is there an avenue for the recommendations of health care workers or band authorities to be considered by DIAND. The lack of co-ordinated planning results in some departments spending excessive funds to rectify problems that should not have occurred in the first place.

The working relationship between the two departments (DIAND and MSB) has not always been geared to meeting the needs of First Nations but rather carrying out their respective mandates as dictated by the legislators of the day. This has been particularly evident when First Nations want to address the issue of the treaty right to health. It has always been the position of Medical Services Branch that although they have responsibility for health services, this responsibility has been carried out on the basis of a moral obligation of the federal Crown and that DIAND has responsibility for dealing with treaty matters. The position of Medical Services Branch is that

> the responsibility for discussing treaties on behalf of the federal government resides with DIAND. Where DIAND has received a mandate to discuss treaty matters with First Nations, and if the treaty matters to be discussed include health, the Department of National Health and Welfare, through MSB, will participate in that substantive discussion. MSB participation will be subject to the overall DIAND mandate and framework for treaty discussions.

However, DIAND has indicated that because Medical Services Branch is responsible for health, the issue of a treaty right to health is an MSB responsibility. There has been no documented case where the two departments have ever agreed to a joint process to address the treaty right to health issue.

Transfer Policy and Potential Effects on the Treaty Right to Health

In 1979, the federal government announced the Indian Health Policy. This policy outlined, for the first time in its history, the principles by which Medical Services Branch would work toward improving the health status of First Nations people. The policy approach was to be built upon three pillars:

- Community development, both socio-economic and culturally appropriate to remove/reduce the conditions that limit the achievement of community wellness;
- Reaffirming the traditional trust relationship between First Nations and the federal government; and
- Integration with the existing Canadian health care system.

This period also saw a general rise in First Nations' aspirations with respect to constitutional entrenchment of the right to self-government and the recognition of any and all treaty rights. The passing of the *Constitution Act, 1982* focused the debate on self-government and the control of Indian services, including health.

During the period 1983-1986, Medical Services Branch funded a number of demonstration projects in First Nations communities across the country as an experiment in the administrative transfer of health services to First Nations governments. As a result of these projects and increased demands by First Nations for control of and involvement in the delivery of health services, the federal government announced the Health Transfer Initiative. The objectives of the initiative were

- to enable Indian bands to design health programs, establish services and allocate funds according to community health priorities;
- to strengthen and enhance the accountability of Indian bands to band members; and
- to ensure public health and safety are maintained through adherence to mandatory programs.

These objectives were acceptable to First Nations communities, many of which took advantage of this new funding initiative to conduct a community needs assessment and begin a process of planning strategies for the types of approaches and health services that were required to improve the health status of people and communities. This funding initiative has enabled First Nations to test their own ability to manage programs and to remove cultural and language barriers to health care services. The services controlled and delivered by First Nations are more acceptable to people and have in many instances resulted in an increase demand. The limited resources available through this initiative do not allow flexibility to meet this increased demand for services, however, particularly with respect to mental health programming. The federal government has consistently refused to consider funding activities they consider to be "program enrichments" through the Health Transfer Program. This has seriously hampered the ability of First Nations fully to address their specific health priorities within the confines of historical spending by the government and forced them to spend valuable resources to develop proposals and lobby for funding from other sources.

The Short-Term Evaluation of Indian Health Transfer, completed in 1992, evaluated eight communities that had signed transfer agreements and eighteen communities involved in pre-transfer planning and negotiations. The evaluation noted that "people involved with transfer repeatedly point out...the lack of recognition of Treaty Rights to Health." The question is, if First Nations are agreeing to transfer, are they in fact defining their treaty right to health in the future. In a recent ruling by the Supreme Court of Canada, the Bear Island Decision (*Temougami* v. *Ontario*), the court indicated that past conduct will assist in the present and future interpretation of treaties. If your 'walk' is different from your 'talk', the Supreme Court will use the past walk of First Nations to assist the court in reaching decisions. With respect to the health transfer program, if a band accepts delegated responsibility for health care delivery from Medical Services Branch and delegated authority for these services under the

Indian Act, will the treaty right to health be defined in light of the decisions First Nations have made in written agreements with the federal government?

It can be argued that the treaty right to health is being defined by various policies being instituted and enforced by bureaucrats within the federal government. Medical Services Branch has designed its non-insured health benefits program on the principle of being the agency of last resort. The recent contract between Medical Services Branch and Blue Cross to administer some of the responsibilities of the Non-Insured Health Benefits Unit within Medical Services Branch resulted in a serious reduction and limitation of drugs available to First Nations people. In addition, non-insured health benefits policies associated with eye examinations and the approval of prescriptions, dental care and requests for aids to independent living are being rewritten to reflect the changing and downsizing of provincial programs and services. This domino effect is a result of economic difficulties and realities. What is apparent, in fact, is that the treaty right to health is being defined by economic conditions of the national and regional government, not by an understanding of treaty obligations.

Legislation and Jurisdictional Issues

As the economic times result in both provincial and federal governments offloading responsibilities or downsizing the range of services they provide to citizens, First Nations people are being treated the same as other citizens in Canada. Provincial health care systems across Canada are being evaluated and reorganized, resulting in new legislation being passed. Provincial legislation is not recognizing First Nations jurisdiction, nor does it reflect understanding or recognition of the self-government process. In the absence of federal law or First Nations law, provincial law applies to First Nations lands. Once jurisdictional authority is assumed by provincial governments, it may be very difficult to regain authority. Again, if First Nations recognize and accept the application of provincial law, will this impinge on the development of self-government?

Federal Government and Reorganization Issues

Recently DIAND and MSB have undergone major restructuring processes to meet internal government downsizing objectives. In some instances these changes have not been responsive to the support requirements identified by First Nations to achieve their goals of infrastructure development for administrative control of programs and services and self-government. The restructuring of federal government systems has not resulted in improved communication and co-ordinated planning between the two federal departments but rather has left many key regional staff scrambling to identify what their roles and responsibilities are under the new structures. Again the needs and goals of First Nations do not seem to be reflected in these organizational changes.

First Nations' Definition of Health

Throughout the history of First Nations people, the definition of health evolved around the whole being of each person – the physical, emotional, mental and spiritual aspects of a person being in balance and harmony with each other as well with the environment and other beings. This has clashed with the western medical model which, until very recently, has perpetuated the concept of health as being 'the absence of disease'. The perception and understanding of health held by each group have prevented communication. The program delivery model designed and implemented by Medical Services Branch reflected the western European understanding of health. The current health and social conditions being experienced by most First Nations in this country clearly demonstrate the barriers this conceptual difference has created.

Present Conditions

The health and social conditions of First Nations have been well documented throughout the past few decades. In general, the health and welfare of First Nations people in Canada is a national and international disgrace. First Nations people have had consistently higher mortality and morbidity rates than the national average. Their life expectancy at birth is nearly a decade less than that of the general non-Aboriginal population. Fetal and infant death among First Nations babies was nearly twice the national average reported since 1987. First Nations youth have the highest suicide rates in the country. Substance abuse is a way of life in many First Nations communities. A First Nations youth is more likely to be incarcerated than to graduate from high school.

Despite these depressing conditions, many First Nations have begun a process to address the healing that is required. They face many challenges, however, both from their constituents and from present federal policies and guidelines. In spite of the growing recognition by the general population that the inherent right to self-government must be addressed, it appears that the two federal departments responsible for health and social development with respect to First Nations people continue to operate as they have in the past.

Requirement for Change

The present conditions in First Nations communities require steps to begin to address the problems. To compound the problem, the ping-pong approach being used by the federal government with respect to who has responsibility for the treaty right to health has created numerous problems for First Nations communities. Therefore the most desirable approach would be as follows:

First, recognition of the right to self-government;

Second, although the *Constitution Act, 1982* reaffirmed treaty and Aboriginal rights, the federal government has not provided the leadership necessary to put into practice what is contained in the Constitution. Steps have to be taken to ensure that treaty understandings become the basis of any programs, policies, and procedures adopted by the federal government.

Third, a reorganization of the federal government with respect to the responsibility of all programs and services for First Nations would be required.

Fourth, an office of a Federal Treaty Commissioner or Treaty Ombudsman should be established. This office would monitor and be a watchdog over how the federal government meets its treaty obligations to First Nations.

A more detailed description of these recommendations is presented below.

1. Recognition of the Inherent Right to Self-Government

First Nations' position has been consistently that despite the lack of formal recognition of their inherent right to self-government, the right to govern themselves existed prior to contact with Europeans and is an inherent right.

During the recent discussions concerning the proposed amendments to the *Constitution Act, 1982*, it appeared that there would finally be a solution to this longstanding impasse. Despite the rejection of the proposals by the Canadian public, it was evident that the inherent right to self-government would have been recognized and achieved if it had not been part of a package of other controversial proposals.

Upon the defeat of the constitutional amendments, many government leaders and politicians stated that the inherent right to self-government could be achieved by working closely with First Nations on the issue and that there were other means of achieving this goal outside the constitutional process.

Many First Nations have initiated activities with respect to the development of their own unique form of self-government.

Because of the vast differences among First Nations communities, it is impossible to describe fully what a self-government model would look like and how health would be incorporated. However, some common components would exist. First Nations would define their jurisdiction over a wide range of health services, policies, standards and enforcement. Implicit in this self-government model is the legislative power of First Nations. It is reasonable to expect that First Nations would pursue the development of a community-based First Nations Health Act. Depending on the circumstances, legislation could also be required at the provincial and national level.

The First Nations Health Act would describe

- the powers that will be the exclusive jurisdiction of the treaty First Nation;

- the powers that are/will be shared with or delegated to the provincial government and the federal government;
- the powers that are the exclusive jurisdiction of the federal government by virtue of treaty;
- the healing philosophy;
- the program principles;
- the health standards of the community; and
- how standards will be monitored and enforced.

As a result of First Nations health legislation, the role of both the federal government and provincial governments would be fundamentally affected. It is assumed that the federal government would provide the necessary resources to First Nations for the design, management and implementation of a First Nations health care system but would no longer have any responsibility for the direct delivery of health services. In addition, the federal government would facilitate discussions between present providers of service and First Nations and assist in the development of how these services would be assumed by First Nations. An example of this is Blue Cross administration of non-insured benefits.

It is expected that the federal government would provide the necessary resources to First Nations, similar to current arrangements for transfer payments to provincial governments, as well as resources for specific health services now provided by the federal government.

First Nations would have the ability to negotiate agreements with provincial and/or municipal governments for specific services such as hospital services and other health care services. This would ensure that service providers would be accountable to First Nations.

2. Application of the **Constitution Act, 1982**

As indicated previously, the *Constitution Act, 1982* reaffirms treaty and Aboriginal rights. Although this constitutional amendment was adopted twelve years ago, there has been no visible movement on the part of the federal government to address the treaty right to health. While differences exist with respect to the interpretation of a treaty right to health between the federal government and First Nations, it is critical that a joint understanding be developed between the two parties. How this will be achieved will depend on the First Nations in each of the various treaty areas.

There have been arguments presented for those First Nations that had negotiated treaties prior to the signing of Treaty 6 with its reference to the medicine chest. It could be argued that the right to health is an Aboriginal right as defined by the *Constitution Act*.

Lack of a common understanding of the treaty right to health will continue to perpetuate the confusion and disagreement that now exist. The federal government must begin a process that will finally acknowledge its responsibilities with respect to the treaty right to health.

3. *Reorganization of the Federal Government*

Once the federal government acknowledges its trust and fiduciary responsibility for health services for First Nations based upon a treaty obligation, a reorganization would be necessary to carry out this obligation.

In addition to DIAND and MSB, other federal departments have assumed various components of services that directly affect the lives of First Nations people. Examples include Employment and Immigration for training, Canada Mortgage and Housing Corporation for housing, Department of the Environment for the Greenplan, Secretary of State, Solicitor General, Health and Welfare Canada (Environmental Health), and Public Works (on-reserve health services buildings).

To meet the needs of First Nations effectively, all aspects of federal programming, funding and support services must be channelled through one federal department, with one minister having total responsibility. The positive effects of this would be as follows:

- Lower administrative costs for the operation of all programs and services. At present, each department has its own administrative and financial structures. Amalgamating all of these operations would free up administrative funds that could be used more effectively at the First Nations level. Regional branches of the proposed ministry should be established on the basis of provincial boundaries, not the 'super regions' currently being organized. Since Confederation, relationships among First Nations have been developed within provincial geographical boundaries. These relationships must be recognized, and the federal government should not, at its whim, change the working relationships of First Nations at this critical time of development with respect to self-government and the assumption of control over programs and services. This integrated ministry needs to delegate strong authorities to its regional bodies to enable timely and effective decision making.
- The integration and appropriate approaches to First Nations issues and priorities could be achieved under one central government department. The health needs of First Nations could be addressed effectively if First Nations had the resources to plan housing, water and sewer infrastructure, training and other priorities in a holistic manner, rather than having to go to a multitude of departments to resolve issues. First Nations recognize the importance of the development of multifaceted planning and implementation of integrated community infrastructure development in strategies to address family violence, addictions and in fact all issues with a direct impact on the health status of First Nations people.

4. Establishment of a Federal Treaty Commissioner/Ombudsman

To ensure that the both the federal government and First Nations abide by their respective responsibilities around a common understanding and the delivery of services to First Nations people, it is imperative that a monitoring system be implemented. The establishment of an Office of the Federal Treaty Commissioner or Treaty Ombudsman is necessary. It would be expected that First Nations would negotiate the terms of reference for this function. However, some of the responsibilities that could be considered might include monitoring and regulating of the federal government's performance with respect to the delivery of treaty obligations. This office would intervene and resolve breaches of treaty obligations.

Impact of Recommendations

Recognition of the treaty right to health, development of legislation and jurisdiction within a self-government framework, and co-ordination of federal government activities are essential if First Nations are to address health and social issues in a manner that is responsive, culturally appropriate and acceptable to First Nations consumers. Only if health and social approaches are integrated, community-based and multi-faceted, and only if they respect the inherent rights of First Nations, will health status improve and wellness be achieved.

Conclusion

This paper contains recommendations that are realistic and achievable only if the federal government is serious in addressing the health and social needs of First Nations.

Urgent changes are required if First Nations are to assume their rightful place in Canadian society. First Nations are prepared to meet the challenge of change, but this change must take place in partnership with Canada, both its people and its governments.

Aboriginal People Living in Remote and Northern Areas

*Iris Allen**

The Labrador Inuit Health Commission (LIHC) is very pleased to have this opportunity to participate in this process of discussion and problem solving. We have a great deal of information to share with you, as LIHC has developed a series of documents/reports on health issues pertinent to the Labrador Inuit. Since time is limited we will highlight certain key areas in an oral presentation and will provide you with a set of written reports. We will commence by telling you a little about our problems, then move on to what we currently do and where we are going from there. We will then outline some of the barriers that we believe are preventing us from moving in a positive direction. We will conclude by making some recommendations that we believe will help us solve some of our most serious problems with health care in Labrador Inuit communities.

Labrador Inuit: Health Status

Briefly, the health status of the Labrador Inuit is considerably worse than that of average Canadians. Our problems include low income, unemployment or underemployment, inadequate education, inadequate housing, alcohol abuse, tobacco use, inadequate water and sewer infrastructure, family violence, etc. These are the same problems surfacing in Aboriginal communities all across

* Executive Director, Labrador Inuit Health Commission.

Canada, which are certainly already well documented. The reports to be tabled will describe the incidence of disease, mortality rates, etc.

The health issue that is now taking precedence is that of mental health. We are deeply concerned about the violence in our families and between our people. We feel helpless, even though we know that some communities are beginning to pull together and develop strategies and plans. Child abuse, vandalism, gas sniffing, etc. all fall under mental health and are a major concern.

One of our communities, Nain, is now holding public meetings where these problems are being discussed with a view to the community making some real changes and accepting responsibility for the changes. The other community is Rigolet, which has just gone through a homicide/suicide and is now looking at ways to deal with such a crisis at the community level.

The Labrador Inuit Health Commission

The Labrador Inuit Health Commission (LIHC) is the affiliate created by the Labrador Inuit Association (LIA) to deal with health issues. It was formed in 1985 and reports to the LIA Board of Directors. Funding comes from Medical Services Branch of Health and Welfare Canada.

The philosophy, goals and objectives of LIHC are well documented in our Policy and Procedure Manual. Briefly, LIHC is very concerned with the issues of housing, meaningful employment, etc. and how they affect the health of the Labrador Inuit. The workings of the health care delivery system are also of concern, but are only a small part of health.

We have been fortunate to have an ongoing core of programs. The Community Health Representative (CHR) Program has been operating since 1985. CHRs in Labrador do not provide primary health care as they do in other parts of northern Canada. We are fortunate that our CHRs can devote their time to health education and promotion in their communities, with much emphasis on school involvement. We currently have a CHR in Nain, Hopedale, Makkovik, Postville and Rigolet. Despite considerable numbers of Labrador Inuit in Northwest River and Happy Valley/Goose Bay, we have been unsuccessful in convincing Medical Services Branch (MSB) that the program should extend to these communities.

Another core program is the Health Liaison Program. This involves helping Labrador Inuit through the health care system wherever they might be. The program is anchored by a referral clerk and an interpreter/translator, who both work out of the Melville Hospital in Happy Valley/Goose Bay. Other interpreters are hired on an as-needed basis to accompany a patient to hospital in St. Anthony. We depend on the Friendship Centre in St. John's to assist when patients are sent there.

The Non-Insured Health Benefits (NIHBs) operates from our head office in Northwest River with the help of the CHRs and the Health Liaison Team. LIHC is extremely proud of this program, as we are one of only two Aboriginal groups in the country to administer a comprehensive program ourselves rather than having MSB do it. MSB has recently commissioned a report on our program and that of Conne River with positive results.

One of our more recent programs is Dental Therapy. LIHC has recently hired a dental therapist for the community of Nain. In the past seven months, this program has already shown excellent results – especially with respect to the dental hygiene of our school-age children. LIHC hopes to extend dental therapy to other communities as we gain more experience from Nain.

LIHC is hoping to become more active in areas of family violence. A researcher was hired in 1992 to do a needs assessment on the extent of family violence in the Inuit communities of Labrador. This assessment encompassed the following: the level of need, services already available, problems or obstacles facing the present services, and statistical data. The assessment has been completed and a report submitted. The next step in this process would be to plan, co-ordinate and lobby for family violence services and programs according to the needs identified by the Labrador Inuit communities.

LIHC recently hired a family violence co-ordinator, who has commenced her advocacy role for family violence projects for the Labrador Inuit. LIHC will determine the missing links in the present service base and will begin to fill in the gaps. This will involve much co-ordination and communication at all levels – LIHC feels it can take a role in this area for the LIA membership. Both of these projects – the assessment and the co-ordination – have been funded by recent federal initiatives.

LIHC is responding to the demands for further mental health intervention for the Labrador Inuit communities. Under the Brighter Futures Initiative, LIHC has recently hired a mental health co-ordinator and a suicide intervention fieldworker. These staff members will be addressing the ongoing and escalating problem with suicides and its many repercussions. Suicide intervention and counselling services are the immediate priority for the two Labrador Inuit communities now in crisis – Nain and Rigolet.

Through the newly hired mental health staff, LIHC proposes to develop, in consultation with the Labrador Inuit Association, Labrador College, community leaders and other health care workers, a comprehensive training package for community health and services workers in all pertinent areas of mental health.

The mental health staff will also be directed to facilitate the development of a crisis response team in each community. This process will be completed in consultation with leaders, elders, professionals and all interested parties. The mental health workers will be directed to be part of this team and include other local field personnel – CHRs, LIADAP fieldworkers, LIA fieldworkers – in the process. In this way, the supports for the clients remain in the community and are not removed when the visiting professional leaves.

LIHC also proposes to set up counselling programs in communities. These programs will include a crisis line for Nain in the initial stages, which will then be extended to the entire Labrador Inuit region. This crisis line will include support and debriefing services for clients as well as local caregivers.

LIHC is also looking to obtain the services of a psychologist for an extended period of time. The professional would be working with the mental health team – to provide training so staff can begin to acquire counselling skills, to conduct workshops, to work one-to-one with clients, and generally to help staff gain expertise in all areas of community mental health supports and networks.

LIHC is able to use existing resources to get involved in many other aspects of health care. We work with LIA's education adviser to promote health careers through individual counselling, tours of health facilities and educational settings, and through advocacy.

LIHC and LIA have been instrumental in getting the Nursing Access Program at Labrador College off the ground. We take great pride in the four members of the Labrador Inuit Association now enroled in the Nursing Access Program in Goose Bay. There are also a number of members completing degrees in nursing at Memorial University of Newfoundland. The graduation of these health care professionals will do much to begin to meet the need for Aboriginal personnel.

To help promote awareness of the Inuit culture among health care professionals, LIHC and Torngasok (the Cultural Institute of LIA) undertook a workshop at the Melville Hospital in Goose Bay. This undertaking was very well received and has prompted requests for others at the Grenfell Regional Health Services Hospital in St. Anthony and at the Western Memorial Regional Hospital in Corner Brook. This request will help the nursing access students when they move to Corner Brook to complete their nursing training.

LIHC is also active in many aspects of Aboriginal health issues and research at the national level. We have conducted our own research in many areas and are involved in monitoring all health research in Labrador. LIA has established a Health Committee within its Board of Directors; this committee has a mandate to monitor all health-related research conducted in conjunction with the Labrador Inuit.

Future Plans

LIA and LIHC have just completed a process of community consultation to plan for the next five years. It began with a health conference in the fall of 1991 at which community delegates stated the current problems and looked at various organizational structures that would best serve the needs of the Labrador Inuit. This process continued at the annual general meeting in the spring of 1992, where the membership directed LIA, LIHC and the Labrador Inuit Alcohol and Drug Abuse Program (LIADAP) to proceed with a gradual staged process that will result in the amalgamation of all health programs for the Labrador Inuit under a Community Health Department of LIA. This will include the activities of LIHC and LIADAP as well as public health services now provided by the province of Newfoundland through Grenfell Regional Health Services. Community health committees will be set up as part of this new Community Health Department. The transition stages between program acquisition and takeover will involve constant and ongoing education for present staff and newly acquired staff. This education and knowledge in the realm of health care must then be translated to the membership of LIA – so they can take on the roles and accountabilities that come with takeover and transfer. Employees and members alike must be well prepared for the expectations and duties that will come their way. It is the responsibility of LIHC to see that everyone begins to undertake these roles in a responsible fashion. Once this is operational, the next stage will be to take over the operation of the nursing stations in our communities.

In keeping with this plan, LIHC is beginning to develop a Community Health Plan to deal with the specifics of this undertaking. While this sounds like an ambitious agenda, it is a natural progression along a path that has seen us take on a new program once the previous one is running smoothly. And while it essentially means the end of LIHC as it now exists, the larger more comprehensive Community Health Department is more in line with the holistic picture of health perceived by the membership.

LIA's Community Health Department – The Barriers

Several barriers must be overcome for the Labrador Inuit to move ahead in the area of health care. For a more detailed discussion we refer you to the Review of Labrador Inuit Health and Health Services.

1. Jurisdictional issues and eligibility still create everyday problems in our dealings with various levels of government. Each time access is requested to a new program or a new government initiative, the question of whether we are eligible surfaces and delays movement for several months. Non-Insured Health Benefits is a good example. It took MSB three years to deliberate on our eligibility. We obtained this program only in 1989. The Family Violence Initiative is another example. It was not automatically extended to us, as it was to other Aboriginal groups, until we requested and lobbied for it, and even then we were given only some parts of the program and not others.

2. The product of the jurisdictional confusion is that there are currently four different groups that define health policy for the Labrador Inuit: (1) the

federal government through Indian and Inuit Health Services, Medical Services Branch, Health and Welfare Canada; (2) the provincial government of Newfoundland through the Department of Health; (3) Regional Health Services – Grenfell Regional Health Services (which operates the nursing stations and the public health program); and (4) the Labrador Inuit Association membership through the Labrador Inuit Health Commission. These groups do not work well together, despite efforts on everyone's part. All groups have different priorities and different understandings of the needs and how they should be met.

To illustrate this point, and keeping in mind that the Labrador Inuit are our prime concern, here is one example:

> A mother whose child has a serious ear problem attempting to fit into the confused health care system can often find getting appropriate medical care difficult and frustrating. The referral policy of GRHS is such that the child must be sent to their secondary care facility in St. Anthony. The parent is not given the right to choose where the child could be seen – i.e., a specialist in St. John's. The Non-Insured Program is a program of last resort. Therefore, we must use services provided within the Grenfell region. The MSB Program does not allow for individual choices.
>
> The whole process could then lead to a waiting list and possibly one trip to St. Anthony, only to be referred on to St. John's. This is a confusing health care delivery system to our membership.

3. The CHR program has not reached its full potential. While we are fortunate in that our CHRs have received basic training and there is a very low turnover of CHRs in our communities, we have been unable to get ongoing refresher training programs for them. This is very important for a group of health workers who are operating alone in isolated communities. We have also had to be very creative in finding ways to provide adequate supervision and co-ordination so that each CHR does not always have to develop their own resource material from scratch.

   Our CHRs have not been recognized as full, participating members of the health care team by health professionals. This situation is improving, but we have to continue to promote our CHRs as key community health workers who have local knowledge that many of the health professionals lack. An introduction to the CHR program could also be incorporated in the training of health care professionals before they work in northern communities.

4. The Labrador Inuit are the only Inuit group in the Atlantic region. The organizational structure of MSB is oriented north to south, so that we have little

opportunity to network with Inuit in Quebec. Since the Northwest Territories have undergone transfer, we also have virtually no opportunity to meet with the Inuit in the N.W.T. We do not feel that regional and national MSB personnel are sensitive to the differences between Inuit and Indians. We are constantly sent documents that refer only to status Indians, to chief and council, to tribal councils, etc. At meetings we always have to remind people that we do not live on reserves, that our circumstances are different. There is also a lack of understanding about how isolated our communities are. We are not an urban Aboriginal group – our communities are isolated and rugged, the climate is harsh, economic opportunities are limited, and transportation to obtain services and basic necessities is difficult. One document written by MSB and presented to us at a national meeting actually said that there were no isolated communities in the Atlantic region.

5. Services for people with disabilities are very limited in communities in northern Labrador. Labrador Inuit with disabilities were always the responsibility of the provincial department of social services. In the recent past, LIHC had only the services of the community health representatives to offer these clients. CHRs visit people with disabilities on a regular basis, act on their individual and collective requests, and refer to appropriate service agencies when possible. These duties are carried out in conjunction with many other responsibilities.

   Recent funding received from DIAND and MSB is being used to hire a researcher and carry out a needs assessment for people with disabilities in all Labrador Inuit communities.

   Some of the problems facing people with disabilities in their communities are as follows:

   - very few buildings are wheelchair-accessible;
   - the only mode of transport in the winter is ski-doo and komatik – a very uncomfortable mode of travel when one already has some affliction;
   - in summer and fall the gravel roads are poorly maintained, and once again a truck or all-terrain vehicle ride is very uncomfortable;
   - employment opportunities and training programs are limited;
   - homes are poorly designed, restricting movement in a wheelchair;
   - home support programs – respite and homecare – are limited and often nonexistent; and
   - knowledge of services available through various agencies is often lacking; if special services are required and available only outside the community, travel is by air, and that brings its own problems.

Much is needed to begin to meet the needs of the Labrador Inuit with disabilities.

6. LIHC is hoping to begin to take on more responsibility for public health nurses and nursing stations. Negotiations for public health nurses are already under way. We realize it will be a long process; however, we believe that with co-operation and a good honest working relationship with all parties, it does not have to be a long dragged out process.

   With regard to northern nurses and nursing stations, it is of great concern to the Labrador Inuit that in some communities there is just one nurse in a nursing station. The nurse is put in a difficult and stressful situation. He/she must work five days a week and be on call twenty-four hours a day, seven days a week, three hundred and sixty-five days a year. We hope to resolve this situation in our own community health plan and are communicating these concerns to the appropriate agencies.

   In regard to speciality services such as cardiology, gynaecology, etc., patients must travel outside their communities as far away as St. John's, Newfoundland or Halifax, Nova Scotia. This means a long time away from home and could be a traumatic experience in itself – feeling unwell, alone and far from home.

Possible Solutions or Recommendations

1. The federal government, in consultation with the provincial government, should make some sort of interim decision on the eligibility of Labrador Inuit for health and social programs while awaiting the results of the land claims process, which may take several more years.
2. MSB should commit funds to provide continuing training programs for CHRs, NNADAP and all mental health workers.
3. All levels of government that deliver health care to the Labrador Inuit must work together. Only then will the membership receive the same health care standards enjoyed by the average Canadian.
4. Increased financial and professional assistance should be made available to Labrador Inuit communities as we work toward solutions to our problems, especially in the area of mental health.
5. Inuit communities must be given the opportunity to have a say in health care programs and to take control of our lives and the future of our children.
6. The Labrador Inuit must be given the authority to set up Labrador Inuit health boards and committees in order to plan, implement and control all health services for their communities. We must be given the opportunity to have ownership of and responsibility for our own health care.
7. More effort has to be placed on bringing services to the communities rather than having people go elsewhere for speciality services.

8. More emphasis has to be placed on promoting health careers in order to have more Inuit nurses, doctors and allied health professionals.

9. There need to be working water and sewer systems, adequate housing and meaningful employment in all isolated communities.

10. Emergency resources must be made available to communities in crisis – these resources should be well developed and easily mobilized.

11. For people with disabilities:

    - funds should be made available to build ramps, etc. to all public buildings and to private homes when necessary;
    - all people with disabilities should be given every opportunity to have meaningful employment and to take part in all community events or activities, etc.;
    - more effort must be placed on providing suitable transportation in northern communities such as modification to snowmobiles, wheelchairs, etc.;
    - ongoing homecare and respite programs should be available in all communities; and
    - the needs of people with disabilities must be taken into consideration when planning and designing new homes and modifying present homes for northern communities.

    Labrador Inuit, through LIHC, should be given adequate funding and authority to be responsible for all health care services for people with disabilities.

12. There should be at least two nurses in each northern community, with adequate support at the community and regional level.

13. Health care delivery agencies should be directed to have specialists travel to Labrador Inuit communities on a regular basis.

14. The Labrador Inuit Health Commission should be recognized for its ever increasing expertise in health care delivery.

Health and Social Issues of Aboriginal People with Disabilities: An Alberta Perspective

*Brenda J. Sinclair**

This discussion paper looks specifically at the current status of Aboriginal people with disabilities, the health and social conditions that affect their lives, and possible recommendations that can be developed on a nation-wide basis. To simplify the paper and to devote the entire document to the needs of Aboriginal people with disabilities, a list of relevant studies is provided as source of further information.

For purposes of this paper, health care includes both health care services and traditional healing. In addition, one section on barriers to independent living includes the following service areas:

- personal supports,
- accessibility (community/housing), and
- transportation.

The service areas not covered in this report are financial supports, cultural activities and recreation, information, education and training.

Also for purposes of the paper, Aboriginal people includes treaty Indians and band members on and off reserve, those whose status has been reinstated under Bill C-31, non-status Indians, and Métis on and off settlements.

The information in this report is based on a research project the author conducted in 1991-93 on Alberta Aboriginal people with disabilities.

---

* Consultant, Alberta Indian Health Care Commission.

Current Status of Aboriginal People with Disabilities

> The special problems and needs of Indian people with disabilities are complex, defy simplistic solutions and require special considerations.
>
> *A Study of the Special Problems and Needs of North American Indians with handicaps both on and off the reservation*, Native American Research and Training Centre, 1987

This statement is as true for Canada today at it was for the United States in 1987. Health care issues of Aboriginal people living with disabilities often result from the mix of responsibilities for Aboriginal people on the part of various governments and the lack of programs and services that reflect Aboriginal cultures and traditions.

Health Care and Traditional Healing

Health Care as a Treaty Right

Aboriginal people with treaty status consider health a treaty right. However, Aboriginal people registered under the *Indian Act* – particularly those living on reserves or in isolated areas – do not have access to the full range of health services that are available to urban Aboriginal people or non-Aboriginal Canadians. Furthermore, the services they do have are not community-based or Aboriginal-controlled, nor have they been developed in consultation with Aboriginal people.

Non-Insured Benefits Program

Aboriginal people who are registered under the *Indian Act* or those whose status has been reinstated under Bill C-31 are eligible through the Medical Services Branch (MSB) of Health and Welfare Canada. The benefits they receive fall under the Non-Insured Health Benefits Program and include dental treatment, vision care, prescription drugs, drugs for therapeutic purposes, various supplies and equipment required for medical treatment, and medical transportation. Whether or not they are prescribed by a physician, special items are covered only if they fall under MSB guidelines.

Coverage for Métis and Non-Status Indians

Métis and non-status Aboriginal people are covered under provincial insurance plans. This means that although they have access to such programs as respite care, home nursing care and rehabilitative programs, none of which are covered through MSB, they do not have coverage for dental and optometric services or costs related to special needs.

Coverage for Traditional Healing

Status Indians have one advantage in that traditional healing is covered by MSB. A person wishing the services of a traditional healer must apply in writing to the MSB director in his or her zone. The expenses involved in travelling to the traditional healer are covered. Traditional healing is not covered under provincial programs.

The People Speak

The section consists of the statements and comments of Aboriginal people living with disabilities.

Difficulties Obtaining Necessary Health Care

> There is no hospital here so when we get really sick we are sent away from our home and families – we lie in the hospital and worry about them.
>
> – *Band Member on Reserve*

> No medical care on settlement – must leave community.
>
> – *Métis on Settlement*

Specific Health Care Problems and Solutions
A major problem faced by Aboriginal people with disabilities, whether they live on or off reserve, on or off settlements, is isolation. On reserves and settlements this problem is compounded by the lack of a specific authority responsible for the health care needs of Aboriginal people living with disabilities.

Isolation and Lack of Home Care Visits. What Aboriginal persons with disabilities want:

- An Aboriginal health care worker to work with them on reserves, in settlements and in rural communities.
- Regular home visits to persons with disabilities.
- A worker to assist with forms.
- A worker to help gain access to services and programs.
- A worker to do health needs assessment.
- Train workers for better understanding of the needs of people with disabilities, as well as services and programs available.
- Regular home visits: a nurse once a week; homemaker once a week; spring and fall clean-up program; summer yard work and painting; home winterization program.

Lack of Programs and Appropriate Policies. What Aboriginal people with disabilities want:

- Culturally based health care programs available in the community, including a program for persons with mental disabilities.

- A disabled support group from the community to promote the needs of persons with disabilities to the chief and council, settlement leaders and community leaders.
- Change health care services 'upon request' policy, to become more aggressive health care service providers.

Improved Health Care Services at the Community Level. What Aboriginal people with disabilities want:

- A doctor in the community once a week.
- An accessible doctor's office.
- A hospital unit with full-time doctor.
- A health clinic in the community.
- Community health centre, occupational therapists, doctors, nurses, CHRs.
- Funding available for a community-based mental health worker.
- More funding to upgrade services and facilities.

Difficulties in Obtaining Traditional Healing

> All our lives we use our ways, when we need it most they don't allow it.
>
> *– Band Member on Reserve*

> Hospitals will not allow our medicine men and women to look after our people when they are in the hospital.
>
> *– Band Member on Reserve*

> There has to be a place to send him to be with the elders, away from the society that hinders him…to receive healing…the caring, love, honesty that he needs to heal.
>
> *– Band Member off Reserve*

Clash of Cultures

Access to traditional healing is difficult for many Aboriginal people with disabilities, particularly those who are in hospital or living in urban centres. Because many doctors practising under the western medical model are sceptical of traditional healing, especially with regard to the ethical and legal implications in the use of natural medicines, their attitude makes it difficult for Aboriginal people to seek out traditional healers. Hospitals too are often reluctant to accommodate traditional healers because of the possibility of liability, the problems of mixing western and traditional medications, hospital codes and ventilation concerns.

In addition to not having access to traditional healing, Aboriginal people with disabilities are most likely to be cared for by health are professionals who are neither trained in nor familiar with Aboriginal cultures or traditions, and this can lead to discomfort for the person being treated.

Difficulties in Access to Traditional Healing. What Aboriginal people with disabilities want:

- Restore our culture.
- People who have cultural training to come into our area.
- Outside help from people who are trained in our culture.
- Travelling monies to visit healers in other communities.
- Traditional healing should be allowed in hospitals.
- A special meeting with hospital administration to co-ordinate a special room for traditional healing practices.
- Monies for intensive traditional healing, to cover travel, meals, accommodation for a week or more.
- Hospitals to allow our medicine men and women to look after our people when they are in the hospital.

In summary, the following health care and traditional healing issues were identified:

1. Doctors and medical services are not available on most reserves or settlements; some communities are visited by doctors weekly.
2. Specialized medical services (speech therapy, physical therapy) are available only in large centres.
3. Health care professionals are not usually Aboriginal and often not trained in Aboriginal cultures.
4. Doctors' clinics are sometimes inaccessible; the waiting time for treatment is lengthy.
5. Funds for travel and some medical expenses are not covered by provincial insurance plans (e.g., dental bills, eye glasses, special dietary needs).
6. Preventive health and well-being are not being promoted.
7. Traditional healing is not always available locally, so travel and funding become issues.
8. Hospital policies prohibit the practice of traditional healing.
9. There is no specific authority locally or provincially to advocate for Aboriginal people living with disabilities.

Possible Recommendations

- Review and revision of MSB Non-Insured Health Benefits Program to ensure that the needs of people living with disabilities are identified through consultation and that these needs are considered when policies are established.
- Band chiefs and councils and Métis leaders to set as a priority increasing the awareness of Aboriginal cultures and traditions among health care professionals.
- Band chiefs and councils and Métis leaders to focus on preventive health for Aboriginal people on their reserves and settlements by introducing and encouraging programs.

- Aboriginal leaders to support the establishment of local and provincial organizations to represent the interests of Aboriginal people with disabilities.

Barriers to Independent Living: Personal Supports

Difficulties in Obtaining Personal Supports

> The agencies do what they want, not what we want. They give services but only the way they want it.
>
> – *Band Member on Reserve*

> Social services says it's Indian Affairs, Indian Affairs says it's MSB, MSB says no...so no one helps me.
>
> – *Band Member on Reserve*

> Nothing established in the community yet for personal supports.
>
> – *Métis on Settlement*

> The equipment gets brought into the community, but no one installs it...so it is useless.
>
> – *Métis on Settlement*

Access to Personal Supports

Personal supports for people with disabilities include technical aids or equipment and human services that assist the individual at home, at work or in the community. Supports and services can be obtained through various government departments, special interest agencies, educational institutions or voluntary organizations. A person's access to the supports needed often depends on the nature of that person's disability, his or her knowledge of what is available and how to obtain it, as well as where he or she lives. Aboriginal people with disabilities who live in rural areas, who are not strong advocates or do not have an advocate working for them, and who have a disability (or disabilities) that do not fall within the mandate of available service providers are most at risk in trying to obtain personal supports.

Federal Government Programs

Status Aboriginal people with disabilities living on or off reserves are eligible for personal support in the form of programs and equipment through either the Department of Indian Affairs and Northern Development (DIAND) or the Medical Services Branch (MSB). With regard to equipment, MSB is responsible for anything that moves (prosthetics, wheelchairs, hearing aids), while DIAND covers anything that is bolted down. Both departments fund adult care programs designed to "address the health, social and personal care needs of individuals who have not had or have lost some capacity for self-care". MSB provides services under community health programs, and DIAND funds social services under their Adult Care Program.

In-Home Care Services

The in-home care services provided under DIAND's Adult Care Program are primarily homemaker services intended to assist individuals with housekeeping, meals and social support. In-home care is usually administered by bands or social development workers. Services are funded on an individual basis. The availability of services is inconsistent, as are standards related to assessment, supervision, case management and training requirements. The provision of personal care, such as assistance with bathing, is not funded, nor are services to families such as respite care. Bands have the option of being given funds to provide their own services, but very few take on this responsibility.

Provincial Programs

All non-status and Métis people with disabilities qualify for the same programs that serve other provincial citizens. Aids to Daily Living provides Aboriginal people with disabilities with equipment such as wheelchairs and supports other organizations that help meet the needs of people with disabilities such as the CNIB.

The People Speak

The section consists of the statements and comments of Aboriginal people living with disabilities.

Lack of Support Services

What Aboriginal People with disabilities want:

- Support programs in the community to help achieve independent living.
- Support services that meet the needs of the disabled individual, not the needs of the agency.
- Métis Nation to start having support services available.
- Workers, especially social workers, more sensitive to and respectful of traditional ways.
- A health care program with home care/health care workers; Indian Affairs and MSB should be more responsive to our needs.
- More services and resources to help gain access to services.
- Program for health care workers and nurses to work with persons with disabilities on settlements.

Lack of Trained Personnel/Resources/Information

What Aboriginal people with disabilities want:

- Good qualified workers delivering services.
- A life skills/living skills program, informational workshops, trained personnel, and resource people.
- Educate the people as to what living with a disability means.
- Chiefs and councils and Métis leaders to recognize that the lifestyle of people with disabilities needs improving.
- Leaders to start requesting money for programs in their communities.

Lack of Home Care, Adult Care and Medical Home Visits

What Aboriginal people with disabilities want:

- A reliable homemaker service in the community.
- Home care services to look after daughter, give caregiver a break.
- A home care service to look after people with disabilities in the winter. The band should have a program for people with disabilities and a way to supply them with wild meat and fish.
- Payment for the caregivers who are looking after and keeping the disabled clean and well.
- Adult care for people with disabilities on reserve.
- Home visits from medical staff.
- More specific, regular therapy/counselling sessions.
- More home visits from CHRs and more respect of confidentiality.

Lack of Aboriginal Health Care Personnel.

What Aboriginal people with disabilities want:

- More Aboriginal health care workers.
- Service organizations to recruit Aboriginal personnel in order to provide much needed services to Aboriginal people with disabilities.
- CNIB should have an Aboriginal person working with sight-impaired Aboriginal people.
- Committee from the community to identify needs and acquire services of Aboriginal home care worker for people with disabilities.
- Expand health care assistance by obtaining services of Aboriginal workers: nurses, home care workers, counsellors for people with disabilities.

Lack of Independent Living Program

What Aboriginal people with disabilities want:

- A supervised home setting for people with mental/emotional disabilities that is based on Aboriginal culture.
- A program for independent living in home community.

In summary, the issues raised with respect to the need for personal supports were as follows:

1. Aboriginal people with disabilities feel that agencies are inflexible or bureaucratic and slow. On reserves, the fragmentation of responsibility between federal departments leads to confusion about which department provides which service.
2. Information about services is lacking or difficult to understand.
3. There are not enough service/care providers to supply the support needed, and definitely not enough Aboriginal service/care providers.
4. Few special needs services or programs exist for Aboriginal people with disabilities or their families (e.g., respite care, special equipment). Support services for persons with mental disabilities are particularly inadequate.
5. Home care visits are scarce. Few workers are trained to deal specifically with disabled people or are familiar with Aboriginal ways.

Possible Recommendations

- Priority to be given to the needs of Aboriginal people with disabilities:
  - address the issues of fragmentation of responsibilities and service delivery by consolidating services relating to health, social services and education.
  - act immediately to address the lack of services for Aboriginal people with disabilities living on reserves and settlements.
  - undertake extensive consultation with Aboriginal governments on the issues, principles and preferred methods of delivering services to Aboriginal persons with disabilities.
- Band chiefs and councils and Métis leaders to introduce programs on reserves and settlements designed to train Aboriginal People as health care professionals.
- Band chiefs and councils to request all health care professionals working on reserve to acquire training in understanding Aboriginal culture and traditions.

Barriers to Independent Living: Accessibility

Problems with Accessibility

Housing

> All homes are two-storey with the front door on the top level. There are no ramps in any of the buildings on the reserve. Isolation! Ramps come from Housing Authority – not a priority!
>
> – *Band Member on Reserve*

House has ramps, but doorways are not big enough for wheelchair.

– Band Member on Reserve

My home has no furnace, no running water; without my husband I would have a hard time, I could not live alone.

– Métis Person in Rural Area

The council are not recognizing the specialness of mental illness, the need for special housing units.

– Métis on Settlement

There are three families living in the house with the disabled.

– Band Member on Reserve

Community

All ramps are on the side doors, not main doors, like we are second-class citizens.

– Métis on Settlement

There is no escort service or transportation for the blind so all community buildings are inaccessible without help.

– Non-Status Person in Rural Area

Disabled people and their needs are not a priority for Council.

– Métis on Settlement

The builders never think of accessibility. This limits the disabled in numerous programs and projects.

– Band Member on Reserve

Community is not paved for people in wheelchairs and walkers, not enough attention is paid to services – snow and ice removal.

– Band Member on Reserve

The accessibility to most services – education, therapy, training – means having to leave home and community to access, leaving behind support structures, family.

– Band Member on Reserve

Accessibility in Rural Areas

While access to public buildings and facilities is a problem for most people with disabilities, for Aboriginal people, the problem is heightened because so many live in rural locations where buildings and their surroundings have not been modified. Although the federal government has included barrier-free design standards in the national building code, the standards apply only to buildings over which it has jurisdiction. This includes buildings owned by the federal government and leased to other tenants. Accessibility to these buildings has typically been defined as meaning wheelchair-accessible. People with other disabilities – such as hearing or visual impairments – are not necessarily accommodated.

Neither the national nor any provincial building code addresses sufficiently the issues of compliance and enforcement. There are no penalties for non-compliance. A disabled person who cannot gain access to a public building can complain under the Canadian Human Rights Act, but to do so involves a long and often complicated process.

Lack of Awareness

This is often the greatest barrier to accessibility. Many building adaptations that would improve accessibility cost very little money (ramps, handrails, improved lighting, signage), but owners or occupiers of the buildings often fail to consider such modifications because they are unaware of the needs of people with disabilities. This lack of awareness extends to business people and professionals alike. Aboriginal people with disabilities find their local churches, medical centres, band offices, settlement offices, educational facilities, recreational facilities and their own community halls inaccessible. Aboriginal people with disabilities living in urban centres have the same level of access as do non-Aboriginals with disabilities. The issue of accessibility has not been addressed for all people with disabilities living on reserves or settlements.

Federal Incentives

These are available for building owners who want to improve accessibility for disabled Aboriginal persons. For example, DIAND makes a one-time grant available to bands wishing to retrofit a public building on reserve. Similarly, under the Canadian Jobs Strategy, Employment and Immigration Canada makes up to $10,000 available to employers wishing to upgrade their work sites to a barrier-free design.

Federal tax exemptions are available to owners wishing to renovate old or existing buildings. On reserves, these incentives are not being used, either because band leaders are not aware of them or they are not sensitive to meeting the needs of their members who have disabilities.

The People Speak

Lack of Suitable Homes

What Aboriginal people with disabilities want:

- Homes built to national standards of accessibility.
- Recognition of the needs of people with all types of disabilities before a building is constructed.

- Change type of homes built on reserve for disabled people to ground-floor dwellings.
- People specialized in building barrier-free homes/renovations to train people to build ramps, handrails, doorways, shower supports.
- Low-cost housing with heat and running water for people with disabilities.
- Housing should be a priority because of the potential for emotional, physical and mental distress when needs go unmet.
- Push for completing renovation requests.
- More accessible funding for renovations.
- MSB and Indian Affairs and housing should co-ordinate and pay for renovations and services. Improve information!
- Indian Affairs and CMHC should look into how housing monies are being spent.

Lack of Supervised Housing

What Aboriginal people with disabilities want:

- A supervised housing unit should be built for the mentally disabled. This housing needs to be run by Aboriginal people, with Aboriginal values, just like the values in their own parents' home.
- There should be apartments/houses with qualified supervision to look after the disabled and help with medication.
- Safety! Elders and people with disabilities are fearful of people coming to their home and hurting them or stealing from them.

Inaccessible Community Buildings

What Aboriginal people with disabilities want:

- A community task force to help in the construction and renovation of buildings for the disabled.
- Disabled people and their needs must become a priority for band councils.
- An action group to help solve problems, build awareness.
- Change of attitude of council and politicians.
- Workshops for housing departments on reserve for total accessibility of buildings and homes.
- Public buildings to be accessible to the physically disabled. Uphold national/provincial building codes.
- An escort service and transportation for the blind. All buildings are inaccessible without help.
- Community should pave at least a 2-mile stretch of road.

In summary, the issues raised with respect to accessibility in communities were as follows:

Housing

1. Existing housing is substandard and not equipped to accommodate special needs (no ramps, hard-to-reach faucets and knobs; no inside plumbing, inadequate heating).
2. Disabled people lack funds or ability to make the necessary renovations to their homes.
3. People do not know where to go for help. Information is lacking or difficult to understand. Government agencies seem inflexible or bureaucratic.
4. Aboriginal leaders appear not to understand the needs of disabled persons, and their needs tend to be low priority when houses are being designed and allocated.
5. New homes are too expensive for disabled people and not necessarily suited to their physical needs.
6. Overcrowding is common.

Community

1. Fragmentation of responsibility leads to confusion in the minds of Aboriginal people with disabilities about whether DIAND or MSB is responsible for addressing accessibility-related issues.
2. Many public buildings have not been adapted for people with mobility or sight-related disabilities (no ramps, no sliding doors, no safety railings, poor lighting, steep stairs).
3. The lack of paved roads, sidewalks and snow and ice removal restricts mobility.

Possible Recommendations

- National Aboriginal leaders to draw up a policy statement identifying the provision of suitable housing for Aboriginal people with disabilities as a priority.
- Canada Mortgage and Housing Corporation to modify its policies to make housing for disabled Aboriginal people a priority.
- Band chiefs and councils and Métis leaders to set as a priority the collection and dissemination of information relating to the provision of suitable housing and necessary services to disabled people in their communities.
- Band chief and councils and Métis leaders to set barrier-free access as a priority.
- Individuals with disabilities and groups representing Aboriginal persons with disabilities be encouraged to challenge restrictions on their access to public buildings using either federal or provincial human rights legislation.
- Band chiefs and councils to recommend to DIAND and MSB that the issue of fragmentation of responsibility for federally funded public buildings on reserves be addressed and resolved.

- Band chief and councils to ensure that any programs or special activities (education, training, culture and recreation) offered on reserves are accessible to persons with disabilities.

Barriers to Independent Living: Transportation

> People today don't give free rides because of the high cost of gas and living.
>
> – *Band Member on Reserve*

> No services here, taxi to town is $45.00 one way.
>
> – *Métis on Settlement*

> No medical van or such that could accommodate a wheelchair.
>
> – *Métis on Settlement*

> No means. No sidewalks for wheelchairs. No handivan for community use.
>
> – *Band Member off Reserve*

> I have my own vehicle, however no money for gas, plates and insurance. The store is 55 kilometres away.
>
> – *Band Member on Reserve*

Inadequate Transportation Limits Activity

Transportation is one of the major problems for Aboriginal people with disabilities, many of whom live in rural communities or isolated areas. Transportation is so inadequate and the opportunity to make even a short trip so infrequent, that some disabled people have difficulty meeting their basic needs, such as shopping or attending medical appointments.

For many there is almost no opportunity to pursue educational, recreation, social, cultural or employment-related activities. This lack of transportation has serious implications for children, whose access to education and recreation can be restricted as a result.

Funding for Transportation is Inadequate

Transportation coverage under MSB is inadequate for people with special needs, particularly those living in urban centres, since MSB does not provide medical transportation for status Aboriginal people living off reserve. If an individual living on a reserve requires an extended visit to a health centre for medical treatment, his or her costs for accommodation and meals while travelling, as well as transportation costs, are covered. The program covers an escort's expenses only if the escort is essential for medical reasons; compassionate travel is not covered. This is significant, because MSB does not provide home nursing or nurse-supervised home care except on an emergency basis when no other assistance is available. As a result, Aboriginal people with disabilities who require medical care but would prefer to remain at home in the company of family and friends cannot necessarily receive adequate care if they do so. At the same time, if they travel off the reserve to receive care, the travel costs of a friend or family member accompanying them are not covered.

Medical Transportation

Transportation for medical purposes is a problem for most disabled Aboriginal people regardless of where they live or whether they qualify under the *Indian Act*. Doctors and medical services are generally not available on reserves and settlements, and the specialized medical services that disabled people may require are available only in urban centres. Public transportation for Aboriginal disabled people is either not available at all or is inadequate, and few reserves or settlements have vehicles equipped to carry people in a wheelchair.

Transportation to School

Under a federal government program, funding is available for Aboriginal disabled children who are between the ages of 6 and 19 and attending school, or for band members attending a post-secondary program. Seasonal transportation is one of the costs covered. This applies whether the person attends a local school or has had to move away to attend school. Individuals must apply through their band or tribal council for this funding. Provincial education provides transportation to elementary or secondary school for all disabled Aboriginal children and is reimbursed by the federal government for the costs of transporting status children.

Children's activities are limited, however, because those with disabilities do not necessarily have transportation to extracurricular or social activities and, depending on the nature of their disability, Aboriginal children may be forced to leave home and move to an urban centre for special education or training.

No Public Transportation

Public transportation from reserves and settlements to other reserves or urban centres is inadequate for most Aboriginal people, but virtually non-existent for Aboriginal people with disabilities. Although capital funding is available to assist Aboriginal leaders to purchase a vehicle suitable to provide a transportation service, local bands and councils usually find they cannot afford to run such a service, and funding for operating costs is not available. In cases where bands have been able to afford to buy and run an equipped vehicle, it has not necessarily been used exclusively to transport people with disabilities and is often unavailable. Individual owners have not been inclined to adapt their vehicles for several reasons: vehicles are expensive to adapt, and at present there is no government assistance for private owners. In addition, drivers of adapted vehicles must complete a special training program, which involves additional expense. Because of the lack of financial incentives and the high costs of operation, private companies have not become involved in transport for disabled people. The net result is a lack of transportation for disabled Aboriginal people living in rural/isolated areas.

The People Speak

Transportation People with Severe Disabilities

What Aboriginal people with disabilities want:

- Qualified medical transportation personnel to transport the severely disabled.
- A service like DATS should be developed in rural communities.
- Transportation for disabled to get medical attention without having to pay cash.
- A wheelchair-accessible handivan.

Lack of Non-Medical Transportation

- Band van for disabled for basic needs: shopping, employment, daily living.
- Community-owned handivan for social and recreation purposes.
- Handivan and a combination of services that allow for transportation of disabled on/off reserve/settlement.
- Voucher system for taxi service through social services.

Lack of Programs/Transportation

- A program to help disabled get out of the house.
- A referral unit plus a handicap bus.
- A service agency to help people with disabilities to do things – recreational, social, cultural, personal – under supervision.
- More information regarding transportation services, programs available.

In summary, the difficulties identified with respect to transportation were as follows:

1. Accessible transportation is difficult to obtain and often expensive. Only a few communities have a wheelchair-equipped van.
2. There is almost a complete absence of public transportation to reserves, settlements and rural areas, and virtually no transportation available for people with disabilities for social, recreational or daily living purposes.
3. Private transportation is scarce, costly, and often not safe or comfortable for people with disabilities.
4. Aboriginal people living with disabilities in rural areas or on reserves and settlements are without transportation and are therefore unable to fulfil their educational, health, employment, recreational and cultural needs.

5. Although capital funding is available for the purchase of adapted vehicles, there is no government assistance for operating costs. The operating costs deter most bands from investing in transportation for people with disabilities.

Possible Recommendations

- MSB be requested to include as a benefit, under the Non-Insured Health Benefits Program, transportation expenses for compassionate travel for an escort.
- The federal and provincial governments jointly develop and fund a program supporting the purchase and/or modification of private vehicles to meet the transportation needs of disabled Aboriginal people.
- The federal and provincial governments to provide Aboriginal communities with a special transportation grant covering capital and operating costs.
- Aboriginal community leaders to set the transportation needs of people with disabilities as a priority.

Conclusion

In 1988, a Disabled Native Persons Think Tank was held in Cornwall, Ontario. The purpose was to provide a forum to allow Aboriginal persons with disabilities and their supporters to discuss the situation facing Aboriginal people with disabilities. As a result a number of issues were identified.

1. The attitudes of communities, band chiefs, councils, government and health professionals toward people with disabilities.
2. Physical barriers in private homes, recreational facilities, and public transportation.
3. Lack of information on services that provide financial support, counselling, medical care, etc.
4. Lack of growth opportunities in vocational and educational areas.
5. The poor co-ordination of services and unclear jurisdiction.

It is now 1993, and the same issues are still manifest in the lives of Aboriginal people living with disabilities.

In 1990 the National Aboriginal Network on Disability was founded. Its goals are to

- restrict Aboriginal people with disabilities; and
- create opportunities for Aboriginal people with disabilities to improve their quality of life and to contribute meaningfully to the development of their community, their region, and Canada.

At this time the National Aboriginal Network on Disability is the only voice speaking out for all Aboriginal people living with disabilities across Canada.

In June of 1992 a First Nations People with Disabilities Conference was held in Alberta. The following recommendation resulted:

- That a provincial organization for the disabled be formed with representation from all Aboriginal people with disabilities.

Action is being taken in Alberta to organize local support groups, to give voice to the individual needs and concerns of Aboriginal people with disabilities, and to establish a provincial organization to look after the interests of all Aboriginal people living with disabilities in Alberta.

As stated by the people, the interests of Aboriginal people with disabilities have not been understood or given primacy by either their leaders or government departments. Decisions that affect them are made without their involvement, often by non-Aboriginal government representatives in distant cities.

The problems of multiple jurisdiction and isolation by distance, disability and economic circumstances create often insurmountable barriers to Aboriginal people with disabilities who wish to participate fully in all aspects of community life in Canada.

Their needs are not being met in terms of accessibility, housing, education, transportation, health care, cultural and recreational opportunities, and financial and personal supports. Even when there are programs or government assistance available to help them, they do not know about this help or have access to it. Consequently, Aboriginal people with disabilities feel passive and alienated and believe that no one is listening to them.

However, Aboriginal people with disabilities in Alberta are now organizing themselves, and soon their voice will be heard not only at the national level through the National Aboriginal Network on Disabilities, but at provincial, regional and local levels.

The author now wishes to put forth one last recommendation for discussion:

- That the Royal Commission on Aboriginal Peoples encourage all Aboriginal people with disabilities to participate actively in the establishment of local and provincial organizations to represent the interests of Aboriginal people living with disabilities.

References

Obstacles, the Report of the Special Committee on the Disabled and the Handicapped, Follow-up Report, Native Population, 1980-81.

Proceedings of the Disabled Native Persons' Think Tank, Cornwall, Ontario, 1988.

National Aboriginal Network on Disability, *Information Kit; Literacy and Aboriginal People with Disabilities*, 1990; *Management Training and Aboriginal Persons with Disabilities*, 1990.

A Needs Assessment: Aboriginal People and Disability, National Aboriginal Network on Disability, September 1990.

Beyond the Caregivers: Health and Social Services Policy for the 1990s

*Sharon Helin**

The World Health Organization defines health as a state of complete physical, mental and social well-being, and not merely the absence of disease or infirmity. It is in this context that the term health is used in this paper. For many years now, First Nations people have journeyed in search of wellness, acceptable health care and culturally appropriate standards for social services delivery. This journey has at times proved fruitful and at times been fraught with difficulty. Along the way there have been some notable improvements in health status that parallel those of the mainstream population in areas such as infectious diseases. Along the way we have seen the development and successful implementation of social service programs such as the Nuu-chah-nulth Family Child Services program. Countless stories have been told and re-told by First Nations people over the years extolling the need for improved health care delivery and, in some cases, the need even for the presence of health care personnel. Countless stories have been told by First Nations people about the apprehension of First Nations children by government agencies, stories of child sexual abuse and the residential school experience. Each of these stories recounts individual and collective suffering. Countless studies have been commissioned and completed. Yet the health status of First Nations people remains deficient relative to the general population, a fact that has been well documented in the literature. Further, in a comparative study of First Nations health in the

* B.A., M.P.H., President, Sharon Helin and Associates.

United States and Canada, indications are that the health status of First Nations people here in Canada also lags behind that of our American counterparts. It would be erroneous to assume that the current state of health and social services delivery for First Nations is a result of inadequate consideration of the issues. It appears the opposite may be true, since there must now exist sufficiently detailed studies to demand innovative attempts to synthesize emerging recommendations and themes with policy development and service delivery.

Health care is perceived as a fundamental necessity for First Nations people, and the grassroots movement across this country has been successful from coast to coast, from Puktawagan, to Kahnawake, Nuu-chah-nulth, and the Nass Valley and back to the Atikamekw Health and Social Services Project. The blueprint for change lies out there in First Nations communities. To effect change and continue with this successful trend, change must occur at both the micro and macro levels of institutions.

Health Service Delivery

There are many contemporary health care issues in Indian country today. Among these are home care for the elderly, child health, mental health, solvent abuse, injury prevention, healthy babies, parenting, cancer screening, cancer research, arthritis, service to people with disabilities, adolescent health, HIV/AIDS, preventable diseases and associated risk-factor behaviour. In addition to program issues, there are also concerns about jurisdictional issues, the non-insured health benefits program currently administered by Medical Services Branch, comparable wage scales for employees of health care programs transferred to First Nations control, development of health by-laws and a deep-rooted commitment by First Nations to ensuring that all First Nations people have access to quality health care service. It is paramount that health care systems be culturally appropriate.

Social Services

During 1992 at least three impressive reports were published in British Columbia alone; it would be safe to assume that similar reports were also completed in other provinces across the country. The British Columbia reports were entitled *Liberating Our Children – Liberating Our Nations* (Report of the Aboriginal Committee, Family and Children's Services, Legislative Review in British Columbia, October 1992); *Protecting Our Children – Supporting Our Families* (A Review of Child Protection Issues in British Columbia, January 1992); and *Indian Child and Family Services Standards Project* (Final Report, First Nations Congress, July 1992).

An overview of recommendations and comments from *Liberating Our Children – Liberating Our Nations* speaks clearly to the issues and a selection of them is provided here:

> Provincial legislation must explicitly acknowledge the jurisdiction and responsibility of Aboriginal nations to make decisions, and resolve problems with respect to Aboriginal families and children; there must be formation of Aboriginal child and family service agencies, definition of Aboriginal and Aboriginal family; development of legislation that would compel provincial governments to recognize the right of an Aboriginal Nation or community to assume decision-making authority for all, or any part of, the administration of the *Family and Child Services Act* through an agency that is mandated by an Aboriginal Nation or community to undertake that responsibility.
>
> Family and child services to the Aboriginal community are characterized by their absence, inadequacy and fragmentation. Behind these characteristics is the failure of both the federal and provincial governments to recognize their obligations to Aboriginal people. If we are to achieve any change in this pattern, then clearly we must heed the voices of First Nations people with regard to service delivery.
>
> If we are to see a reduction in the number of Native children in care in British Columbia, then the responsibility for the welfare of our children must be turned back over to Native communities. In addition to giving recognition to this reality we cannot emphasize enough the need for government to also recognize that there are real and substantial costs involved.
>
> *Ktunaxa/Kinbasket Tribal Council*

> What must be achieved is a system of child care and healing of our families where our traditions and cultures become the primary guideline.
>
> *Louis Riel Metis Association*

> It is imperative that the community membership becomes so pro-active in the planning/resolution and decision-making within the child welfare process.
>
> *Heiltsuk Band Council*

> We are talking about so much more than child welfare, we are talking about services to children, social services, social development, child welfare, development of legislation, the re-building

of family values, unity and how we live together. Not only how we live together as individuals, but how we live together as families and communities.

USMA Family & Child Services

Culturally appropriate resources for children and families specifically addressing child physical, sexual, emotional abuse, child neglect and family development should be established in Aboriginal communities.

Squamish Nation Council

First Nations people are the ones who can make the best decisions for the well-being of our children. Not by outside standards, but by our own standards.

Northwest Band Social Workers Association

Aboriginal nations and communities must have ongoing financial resources to implement a wide range of preventative services that are holistic and unfragmented. The services must be available in a culturally appropriate manner, as determined by the specific Aboriginal Nation or community, and delivered by people from that community.

We recommend that governments must make resources available to Aboriginal Nations and communities to develop methods of replacing non-Aboriginal standards with culturally appropriate methods for sharing knowledge and providing care.

There is no doubt in my mind that the system has to change completely.

Indian Homemakers Association of B.C.

The responsibility for development and delivery of family and child services must be turned over to Native communities.

Ktunaxa/Kinbasket Tribal Council

There is something inherently wrong in a system that will pay 'strangers' more money to look after our children than they would allot to an Aboriginal family.

Louis Riel Metis Association

It is painfully obvious that the provincial government has failed dismally in previous attempts to fulfil its child protection role, especially in regard to Native children.

Ktunaxa/Kinbasket Tribal Council

> Your methods of removing children from their families has created a lot of sorrow in communities, sorrows which will take generations to mend.
>
> *Metis Council of Port Alberni*

We must harmonize man-made laws, legislation, policies and regulations with the Laws of Nature to meet our obligations to our children, our families and our communities.

So What's The Problem?

A historical perspective on the health and social services issues that have long plagued First Nations people is well documented, yet to this day we have not been able to achieve a health status for Indian people that is anywhere near that of the general population. Without a doubt, First Nations have clearly stated that the source of hinderance has been the imposition of the dominant society's standards and solutions for all Aboriginal issues. The provincial report of the Aboriginal Committee states:

> The prevalent feature of cultural chauvinism is the dominating culture's assumption that its cultural values are in fact the only reflection of human nature. From this perspective, the values of any other culture are not only ignored, but are seen to be abnormal and in need of correction.

From ICFS Standards Report:

> It does not take a great leap of faith to realize that the development of First Nations based service delivery does not imply a rejection of Euro-Canadian standards but rather a simple acknowledgement that different cultures may have different priorities and that there is more than one way to ensure the health, safety and general well-being of children.

In a 1991 publication entitled *What is the Indian Problem*, Noel Dyck, an associate professor at Simon Fraser University, critically examines past and present relations between Indian people and governments in Canada, demonstrating the manner in which the Indian 'problem' was created, and how it has been maintained and exacerbated by the policies and administrative practices designed to solve the problem in the first place. He says that discussions of the Indian problem revolve around a deep-rooted belief that perceived differences between Indians and other Canadians constitute a regrettable situation that needs to be remedied.

Paradoxically, the phrase 'what is the Indian problem' is not so much a question as an assertion that a problem exists. This belief is so widespread that discussions of the Indian problem may proceed without even having to state the question explicitly. The assumption that there is an Indian problem is taken for granted.

Dyck says that we should deal with the Indian question as a question rather than simply a call for solutions. How often have we entered into substantive discussion with preconceived solutions in hand?

> To develop culturally appropriate programs, we must learn to see the world through more than one cultural window. Unfortunately, in mainstream education systems, Indian children have long been urged by educators to see things and to name them in terms of the cultural package of white people, though such training divests them of their unique grasp of reality, of their own dissimilar cultural package....While...children of the dominant society are rarely given the opportunity to know the world as others know it. Therefore they come to believe that there is only one world, one reality, one truth – the one they personally know; and they are inclined to dismiss all others...

Clearly, this way of doing business has not worked. If we are to have any impact on health and social services delivery in the '90s, we must define a new direction, a new way of coming together and working together that is inclusive of both cultures. Given the statistics and current state of our communities, we must advocate for change and believe that because it is necessary, it is also possible. If we can accept the paradox that the real humanity of people is understood through cultural differences and are ready to accept the notion that "it is possible that there is not one truth, but many; not only one experience, but many realities; not one history, but many different and valid ways of looking...at the resolution of issues and development of programs."

Adjustments to Service Delivery

Before proceeding with a discussion on adjustments to service delivery, it is essential to examine the thread of continuity that runs through the literature, since health and social services issues should not be considered as isolated entities. Rather, we must look at the entire socio-economic and political picture as we begin to review recommendations and develop policy that is flexible enough to meet local community needs. Some have said that it is better to move in the right direction, however slow and awkward, than not to move at all. The questions becomes, what is the right direction? What are the elements required to transform recommendations into reality?

The First Nations population is very young, with a high birth rate, educational levels are lower than the general population, high unemployment contributes to a depressed economy and subsequent detrimental health and social effects, many people live in rural/isolated communities not of their own choosing, transportation in and out of these communities in often difficult and expensive, and the culture and lifestyle of First Nations people are different from that of the dominant Canadian culture. Generally there are limited opportunities for First Nations people to achieve their full potential as individuals, families and healthy communities. Finally, although the effects of colonization are well known, we must give credence to the continuing effects of colonization – a fact that is often forgotten and underrated.

From an institutional perspective, there is a tremendous discrepancy between the government's recognition of who is 'First Nations' and who is identified as 'First Nations' by communities. This issue of citizenship again is best defined by First Nations communities.

It appears that bureaucracies have simply not been organized enough to develop a co-ordinated approach to the provision of care when requested or necessary. On a regular basis, First Nations communities are shuffled between departments, and between provincial and federal jurisdiction. To address this, First Nations need to heard at the very highest level of decision making if we are to see notable improvements in service delivery for the '90s.

First Nations have long stated the need to incorporate traditional ways and cultural perspectives into the planning and implementation of community programs. When it has been possible to achieve this, the outcome of program implementation has been for the most part very successful. A holistic approach to caregiving is what is required, yet most government bureaucracies work within a framework that is hierarchical by nature, with decisions coming from the top down. In the arena of health and social services, individuals often are caught in the middle between provision of services by Indian Affairs and by Medical Services Branch. One way to address this continuing dilemma would be to have an effective interdepartmental committee that works closely with First Nations people across the country. Another possibility would be to use the model used by Program Transfer before the program actually became a reality; a First Nations committee was established to examine the issues around program transfer and provide direction to the process. Representation on this committee was geographically selected from across the country, and the process seemed to be a beneficial one for all parties. While I am not a huge fan of committee work, an interactive committee, with membership from both First Nations and government, may be one way to start working on new policy directions.

A commitment must be made by governments to listen to the voices of First Nations people and to take action immediately if we are to be a part of Health for All by the year 2000.

If real change is to occur, we must look beyond the caregivers at how decisions are made, when they are made and by whom they are made. We must initiate change at both micro and macro levels of organizations. We must examine the impact of community-based studies on program design and implementation and be cognizant of both successes and failures. For example, First Nations people have lobbied successfully to demand a transfer of health services from Medical Services Branch and, for some, the transfer of family and children's services from provincial institutions to local control. It should be noted that neither of these transferred programs was intended as a panacea for all ills in health care or social services. Indeed, these transfers should be considered only a portion of the overall picture. Indeed, throughout the years there have been many concerns raised about funding levels, growing populations and the ability to provide quality care to communities on an ongoing basis. From the Ktunaxa/Kinbasket Tribal Council, 1992:

> If we are to see a reduction in the number of children in care in British Columbia, then the responsibility for the welfare of our children must be turned back over to Native communities. In addition to giving recognition to this reality, we cannot emphasize enough the need for government to also recognize that there are real and substantial costs involved.

Further, the cost of health care operations, funding, facilities, and the non-insured health benefits program have been a major issue identified by the Assembly of First Nations during the two National Conferences on Health Transfer.

The hierarchy of health and social services includes communities, individuals, family, caregivers, mid-managers, policy development officers, community-based consultation committees, departmental committees, assistant deputy ministers, deputy ministers, ministers, a prime minister, premiers, judges, lawyers, courts and law enforcement. Somewhere amidst the multitude, decisions are made on a regular basis that affect the daily lives of First Nations people and their communities. In short, we have large bureaucracies whose work is directed in part to alleviating or eliminating what Dyck has termed the 'Indian problem':

> The fact that government departments are still dealing with the Indian problem today, in spite of extraordinary policies and actions that have been...approved in the past...stands not only as a condemnation of past governments and policies, but also as evidence of the amazing...resiliency and determination of...First Nations communities...to retain their integrity...as First Nations ...people.

The work of our grandfathers and grandmothers has had a substantial impact on the dissolution of inappropriate policy for First Nations people, an example of this being the response of First Nations people to the 1969 White Paper. Since then there have been many accomplishments. Today, the work of First Nations people across the country has already had an impact on the way governments do business. There is much work that remains.

In addition to the caregivers and agencies, there are contributing factors that must be considered, such as differing values, cultural concepts, jurisdictional issues, and the perceptions of the power brokers and the powerless. A primary example of a decision in action is how the dominant culture and the First Nations culture perceive and implement programs for the elderly.

Eldership has always been a moving force through First Nations communities, it has been and will always be the elders in our midst who hold individuals, families and communities together. They go about their work softly and quietly, leaving footsteps for us brave enough to follow. When I was an infant, my grandparents gave me roots; as a young adult they gave me wings as I bounded off in search of worldly treasures. With the passing of my grandfather in 1984, my grandmother and I once again chose to live together, albeit with resistance and tears from me. In retrospect, the tears were for naught and the years we have shared together are worth more than any worldly treasures. Once again she gave me roots, and in July of 1992, when she needed someone home on a full-time basis, I quit a full-time job to be with her. In doing so, I have once again experienced an exhilarating sense of freedom. Thank you, Grandmother.

The world of health care and medicine does not see my grandmother with the same eyes. They see an elderly non-person who has lived a relatively long life, with deformed platelets, low haemoglobin, malfunctioning kidneys, cardiac dysfunction, cataract formation in both eyes and a stumble in her walk. Sadly, she is only one of many elderly people, First Nations and mainstream alike, that fall between the bureaucratic cracks of government programs and services. Direct caregivers and providers of care at the community level are caught in a jurisdictional debate over who is responsible for care. At times, even when the caregiver knows what needs to be done and how to do it, she/he is unable to do so because of liability issues and jurisdictional issues. Coupled with the attitudes of the medical profession toward the elderly, the battle for service is turbulent even at the best of times. People who have survived great hardships, served us so well and continue to teach us deserve so much more than we can now offer. Policy development for the elderly must necessarily look at the ethics of medical care. At what age is it deemed appropriate for people to die? Who decides? At the very least, we must strive to maintain the dignity of individuals and find a way to develop policy that respects the individual and collective worth of our First Nations elderly population in a world that appears to believe that people decrease in value as they grow older. Into those same bureaucratic cracks fall women, children and communities; despite the 'trickle-down' theory of the 1980s, very few benefits are trickling down to those individuals who fall between the perennial cracks.

Caregivers stand along with individuals, families and communities. To effect change we must step beyond the caregivers and examine the decision-making process. Stepping beyond the caregivers does not imply that communities and caregivers are left behind, rather that they become part of the decision-making process to facilitate a co-ordinated approach to policy development and implementation. This has to occur if people are to have a sense of ownership about programs and communities and if we are to survive as a nation.

Optimism Should Not Be Considered in Poor Taste

There are many issues to be addressed in health and social services, and thus many points of intervention. If intervention occurs in accordance with a holistic approach to care, it will likely have a greater effect than the current federal policies, which attempt to solve the Indian problem on a piecemeal basis.

In recent years we have witnessed the successful transition of some services for health, families and children from government institutions to local control. This transition has occurred without any detrimental effects on the mainstream institutions; they remain intact and ever-present. The success of these community-based programs provides testimony to the fact that not only are First Nations people capable of operating programs, but in many ways they are operating programs much more effectively than any government agency ever has. There are two schools of thought about transfers to First Nations; one school subscribes to the belief that the initiatives are simply another way for federal and provincial governments to expunge themselves of principal and fiscal responsibility for the poor health of First Nations people. The second school of thought is one rooted in self-government and self-determination: "At this point in time, transfer may not offer everything we want, but it provides us with certain elements of control, and we'll take control anyway we can." This control, of course, must be in keeping with traditions and culture.

Policy development could build upon the framework of success already established in some First Nations communities. Although progress has not always been at the pace most would prefer, still there has been progress. Before 1945, responsibility for Indian health rested with the Department of Mines and Surveys; today that responsibility is with Health and Welfare Canada, Medical Services Branch. The mission of Medical Services Branch is "to provide and/or co-ordinate the provision of health care to the client groups for whom it has responsibility...to increase community participation in all aspects of the health program." Let us hold them to this commitment and ensure that the co-ordination of health services is in the hands of First Nations people. Let us work together to develop health and social services systems that are culturally appropriate. Let us hold them ever responsible when the logical outcome of culturally appropriate service delivery results in an increased use of services.

Ideally, to facilitate further change, greater emphasis needs to be placed on the training and education of First Nations people to assume key roles in all areas of health and social services. This is being addressed in part by health careers initiatives such as the First Nations Health Care Professions Program at the University of British Columbia, the Special Premedical Studies Program at the University of Manitoba, and other such programs at the universities of Alberta, Toronto and Saskatchewan. However, the time has long since passed to examine funding for these programs. At present, they are funded as three-year demonstration projects and are encouraged to seek funding at other levels of governments. To some extent, there has been some success in securing funds from sources other than the federal government; in some cases, however, this has just not been possible. To increase the number of Aboriginal health professionals in First Nations communities will require the ongoing commitment of the federal government, as continuity in program delivery is critical. Health care professionals will be required at all levels of caregiving, in both rural and urban settings, at both the administrative/policy levels and in direct services.

The challenge before us is great, and how we rise to accept this challenge will determine the future for our children, our families and our communities. How will we facilitate the development of policy in respect of and adherence to culture? How will we facilitate the change within service delivery systems at both micro and macro levels? How will we transform the recommendations of many into reality ?

"We cannot wait for the world to turn," said the philosopher Beatrice Bruteau, "for times to change that we might change with them, for the revolution to come and carry us around in its new course. We ourselves are the future. We are the revolution." The stories, the studies, the journeys reflect our history; the decisions we make today will define our future. How will we develop policy for our communities that is reflective of culture and community?

The Current Environment

We live in a world of shifting paradigms, hospital closures, bed closures, user fees, hospital personnel lay-offs, a growing list of what physicians will cover, what non-insured benefits will cover, physicians are moving south of the border and oftentimes in health care, we discover that there is more we have to pay for. The province of British Columbia is in the midst of reorganizing regional districts and hospital boards. What used to be hospital boards will now become community health councils, and for those First Nations that have worked so hard to get representation on those boards, the work now begins to get representation on the health councils. Medical Services Branch is in the process of re-structuring, the non-insured health benefits study has yet to be tabled, and the federal government is facing an election in the fall. It is in this context that we must place the discussion of culturally appropriate health and social service delivery.

Ideally, there should not be any outside institutions providing direction over the daily lives of First Nations people, but for now we must work within existing structures and institutions. To facilitate institutional change, we need dialogue and exchanges of information between the western and traditional ways. With reciprocal consultation, it is possible to find solutions together.

In a world of re-structuring, reorganization, devolution, transfer, and shifting paradigms, it is still possible to alter the direction of policy for First Nations communities. Throughout the years, there has been one constant approach to health care that has not altered through the years, an approach that has proved successful time and time again. One paradigm has had a profound impact on the way health care services are provided to First Nations people – and that is the traditional approach to health care. This reality is reflected in the voices of community people, in the countless studies, in the stories, in the literature and in the many successful programs being implemented across this country; programs are most successful when people have ownership in the development of policy and program implementation. The task before is to develop a well co-ordinated disciplinary approach to care with sufficient resources to implement change.

References

Indian Conditions – A Survey, Minister of Indian Affairs and Northern Development (Ottawa: 1990).

Agenda for First Nations and Inuit Mental Health, Report of the Steering Committee, Medical Services Branch (June 1991).

Statement of the Government of Canada on Indian Policy, Minister of Indian Affairs and Northern Development (Ottawa: 1969).

The Aboriginal Peoples of British Columbia: A Profile, Province of British Columbia, Ministry of Native Affairs (1990).

First Nations Health Transfer Forum, Union of Ontario Indians and the Assembly of First Nations (November 1985).

Special Report: The National Indian Health Transfer Conference, Assembly of First Nations (Ottawa: 1987).

Sally M. Weaver, "Indian Policy in the New Conservative Government, Part I: The Nielson Task Force of 1985" in *Native Studies Review* (1986).

Indian Child & Family Services Standards Project: Final Report, First Nations Congress (July 1992).

Liberating Our Children – Liberating Our Nations, Report of the Aboriginal Committee, Community Panel, Family and Children's Services, Legislative Review in B.C. (October 1992).

Protecting Our Children, Supporting Our Families: A Review of Child Protection Issues in B.C., British Columbia Ministry of Social Services (January 1992).

Noel Dyck, *What is The Indian 'Problem': Tutelage and Resistance in Canadian Indian Administration*, Institute of Social and Economic Research, Memorial University of Newfoundland (St. John's: 1991).

Marilyn Ferguson, *The Aquarian Conspiracy: Personal and Social Transformation in the 1980s* (Los Angeles: J.P.Tarcher, Inc., 1980).

Jamake Highwater, *The Primal Mind: Vision and Reality in Indian America* New York: Harper & Row, 1981).

Pathways to a Dream: Professional Education in the Health Sciences

*Dianne Longboat**

Professional degrees, licences or certification in the health care field granted by universities to Aboriginal candidates have long been an elusive goal, achieved by few over the past generations.

A study by Health and Welfare Canada in 1983 noted only 200 Aboriginal health care professionals out of 325,000 surveyed across Canada. Of this number, there were only sixteen Aboriginal physicians, four dentists, one pharmacist, and one physical therapist. The remaining number were nurses (with no breakdown between BScNs and RNs provided). Thus, in 1983, less than one per cent of health professionals were of Aboriginal ancestry. No data were provided on the location of these people, or whether they were serving Aboriginal populations.

By 1993, there were 51 self-identified Aboriginal physicians in Canada, an additional physical therapist, one occupational therapist and one speech pathologist (MHSc). Current statistics are shown in Table 1, Appendix 2. The numbers exhibit minimal growth and are still inadequate to meet the health care demands of an Aboriginal population of approximately 1 million people in more than 600 communities, a population growing faster than the national average.

The goal of professional health education must be to educate Aboriginal students to have knowledge of both traditional Aboriginal healing practices and current health issues, as well as modern medical practices.

* B.A., B.Ed., M.Ed., First Nations House, Office of Aboriginal Student Services and Programs, University of Toronto. This paper was produced with the assistance of Ms. A.M. Hodes, University of Alberta, and Dr. Gene Degen, University of Manitoba.

First Nations citizens and all our relatives of Aboriginal ancestry have the right to expect medical services from Aboriginal health care professionals located in our communities, in our cultural milieu, and who can offer services in our languages. In order for these goals to be met, thousands of Aboriginal health care professionals must be trained over the coming generation. It is a monumental task. It demands strategy, policy, legislation and accompanying financial commitments by the partners:

- federal and provincial governments
- universities
- First Nations and Aboriginal associations

Institutional change in policy and funding is not easily achieved without legislation. First Nations and Aboriginal leadership must immediately set the goals and, with other governments and the universities as partners, develop strategy, policy, time lines, financial support and legislation to effect the changes needed to dissolve the barriers to access to professional health education.

We must be cognizant of the Indigenous reality in which these changes are proposed. Our population is extremely at risk. The scars of colonization have affected each generation of our people. We now have the highest rate of suicide in the country in the youngest age group, an estimated 60 to 80 per cent dropout rate from schools, the highest mortality and morbidity rates and the lowest educational attainment levels of any ethnic or racial group in Canada. In the United States, the graduation rate of Native Americans from university is roughly 10 per cent. In Canada, the same rate is around 6 per cent. The young men have a better chance of going to jail than graduating from university. Extreme poverty is a direct result of colonization. Forcible removal from traditional lands, a welfare economy, limitations on hunting and fishing rights – all are elements of the physical and cultural dislocation of traditional communities.

Inadequate and overcrowded housing, and poor sewage and water facilities contribute to poor general health conditions and the rise of communicable diseases and epidemics once thought to have been eliminated, such as tuberculosis. Alcoholism, substance abuse, and the physical and sexual abuse of women and children are pervasive and generational in their impact on virtually all Aboriginal peoples. The pain, the bitterness and the powerlessness have turned inward to cause hostility in families and personal relationships. Dysfunctional behaviours to some degree exist in all of us. Identity development, self-esteem, and self-respect are real issues to be confronted in the healing process. The Indigenous population has suffered from the genocidal actions of colonial governments. Though these actions are no longer blatant, the long-range effects remain. The spirit of the people has been affected by colonization, but not destroyed. The answers for us lie in recognition that we are the survivors of generations of our people who have endured that we might live today. Our survival as peoples depends on a healing process that, through traditional teachings and ceremony, can restore the spirit of the people. This is the only Aboriginal reality that has proven to be effective.

Every Aboriginal community, rural or urban, needs a healing lodge. Every activist, front-line Aboriginal association serving Indigenous people requires the help of elders, traditional teachers and healing circles to augment its function. Spirituality gives the people the strength to understand their purpose in life and be proud of themselves, and to tackle the issues that confront them with confidence, pride and the knowledge that future generations will benefit from the healing that occurs today.

Barriers to Professional Health Education

Academic Barriers to University Entrance

Most Aboriginal students seeking admission to university-level studies come from First Nations communities. They have emerged from a reserve-based elementary system that is seriously underfunded by the Department of Indian Affairs and Northern Development (DIAND). Rapid teacher turnover, lack of emphasis on science and mathematics in the curriculum, and the absence of laboratories contribute to producing a student who may not be adequately prepared academically for secondary-level studies in mathematics and science.

At the secondary level, most Aboriginal students from First Nations leave their communities to attend provincial high schools. By this time teachers and counsellors in Ontario have streamed students into basic (two-year occupational), general (four-year college-track) or advanced (five-year university track) level studies. A large percentage of Aboriginal students are ghettoized in the two-year and four-year programs as a result of the negative attitudes of individuals in decision-making positions. Anti-racist education is required to begin close examinations of the concept of 'privilege' among teaching and counselling staff.

The majority of Aboriginal students drop science and mathematics at about the Grade 10 level. The attitude that these courses are too difficult or too boring is pervasive. There is significant peer pressure to get out of school as quickly and as easily as possible. In Ontario, students can graduate from Grade 12 without a program of study that includes mathematics and science. This impedes university entrance into BSc programs in the health sciences.

The dropout rate can vary from 60 per cent to 80 per cent, depending on the school. Students say they cannot relate to the curriculum. There is peer pressure against excelling.

Many secondary schools in the North do not offer advanced-level courses leading to the Ontario Academic Credits necessary to meet admission requirements to university-level studies. Students in northern schools do not have the same opportunity for access to university as do their southern counterparts.

Counselling and career planning are inadequate. Students rarely know of their career and educational options. Counsellors hand out forms for applying to college or university without an in-depth understanding of student attributes or academic strengths. In most cases, counsellors do not have current university admissions policies at their fingertips. This causes delays in applications and poor student access to admissions information. Counsellors usually do not work with students on career planning from the time they enter high school with a long-term view to placing students in the most appropriate program. Students usually find themselves alone in deciding which program to enter at which university. The choices a student makes can be a gamble: time and money are lost when students then drop out, change programs or use summer courses to make up lost time.

As a result of all these academic barriers, a large proportion – approximately 30 per cent of all students – fall into the mature student category. They are over 25 years old, often with two or more children, primarily single mothers, who require upgrading before university entrance can become a reality. The extra years added to their schooling create financial hardship. They set up a catch-up attitude that affects self-esteem.

At university, a different set of academic barriers comes into play. Aboriginal students often have trouble wading through the admissions process. With thousands of applications annually (20,000 to the University of Toronto alone), it is common for the computerized system to establish a minimum grade level (e.g., 78 per cent) for admissions and automatically reject all applications below that level, regardless of the student's academic promise or capabilities. Aboriginal students often become discouraged if they are not accepted in the first round of applications. They may be often reluctant to discuss how to correct academic deficiencies and strengthen their applications the second time around. Students are often unwilling to ask for assistance regrading course planning to raise their marks. When no one offers to help the Aboriginal student make sense of the letter of rejection, the student will often take the rejection as permanent. Faculty advisers or counsellors need to be part of the admissions process to help deal with rejections and strengthen a second application.

Counsellors need to be as much a part of the rejection process as the admissions process. It is the responsibility of the university to make culturally appropriate counselling part of its student services.

Currently in Ontario, unlike some of the western provinces, there is no way to identify Aboriginal students admitted into programs of study. On application forms, there is no section where information can be provided voluntarily by Aboriginal applicants. It is virtually impossible to identify the Aboriginal client group attending university unless they choose to identify themselves. Universities need to examine a process of obtaining an exemption from human rights codes that would allow for the collection of information supplied voluntarily by the Aboriginal student. Aboriginal student service organizations must be able to identify their client group to plan effectively for enrichment of their educational experience.

Many students may need advocacy, tutoring or counselling services yet not know that these exist for their benefit. In some instances, use of these services may mean the difference between increasing the grade point average and leaving school.

A university may be virtually oblivious to its Aboriginal student population, preferring to rely on its equality of access admission provisions and the notion of academic freedom to teach what it pleases. It may be content to believe that whatever Aboriginal students are in attendance are quite integrated into the norms and values of university life. In these environments, it is quite likely that no Aboriginal studies programs exist. Aboriginal content may be found in some history or anthropology courses and in few other places. The Aboriginal student in mainstream courses may feel like a marginal participant, since little or none of the content relates to Aboriginal issues or development needs. The lack of cultural components or Aboriginal health issues in the health science courses prevents students from relating the material to real life.

If the institution does not recognize the special needs of Aboriginal students, there may be no culturally appropriate student services, such as

- recruitment
- admissions advocacy
- counselling
- tutoring
- academic advice
- scholarships and bursaries
- housing
- daycare referrals
- Aboriginal student associations
- cultural programming

These services provide a safety net for students, many of whom build a family away from home with friends they make through this network of services. Personal support offered by people of the same culture helps make the foreign environment of the university a more comfortable place.

The university itself needs to work on its public image. Many First Nations see institutions as self-serving and not at all interested in Aboriginal issues. With this image, the university will continue to be viewed as an agent of colonization by First Nations. When the Aboriginal associations require consultants or specialists, they rarely approach universities. This means that a serious evaluation needs to be done by university senior management in conjunction with Aboriginal representatives to discuss how to work effectively with Aboriginal peoples, particularly in health transfer. University policies in the conduct of research need to be clear and fully cognizant of the cultural imperatives and participatory nature of the style of research to be done.

Institutional Barriers

Relatively few institutions in eastern Canada and certainly more in the west have articulated institution-wide policies to increase access of Aboriginal people to all sectors of the university's programs, staffing and committee structures. Aboriginal people need access not only to admission as students but also to employment and participation on key decision-making committees in the university.

To date, in Ontario, there seems to be an isolation of employment equity policies. They are not directly linked to a university-wide Aboriginal policy or strategy which includes recruitment and retention in employment and admissions.

There is also a tendency in institutions to place Aboriginal student needs and programs in a multicultural context, where the uniqueness of Indigenous programming is diluted by the aggressively stated needs of the other groups. This is particularly true on the east coast, where Aboriginal programs are grouped with black programs, and in Ontario, where Aboriginal groups are listed with women and people with disabilities or as part of the multicultural fabric of the city of Toronto.

Financial Barriers

DIAND/First Nations Financial Guidelines

Of all the factors affecting a student's academic success, the lack of adequate finances is the most crucial and most common reason for dropping out of school.

DIAND rates for student living expenses are grossly inadequate for city living, given the expenses that all students incur. On the average, single students work part-time to meet their debt load. Their marks suffer for it. There are few incentives for graduate students. In fact, support for graduate-level studies and professional licensing becomes less likely as the demand increases among a growing population that wishes to enter university for a first degree. Graduate degrees or second entry programs, such as dentistry, medicine or speech pathology, may not be supported as legitimate student months receiving DIAND or First Nation financial support. A priority system has now been set up to fund secondary school graduates moving forward for a first degree as the priority group to receive funding.

Post-secondary funding was stabilized and capped by DIAND years ago. A growing population now competes for funding that has not increased to meet demand. An inordinate amount of stress is created in the students when funding is not assured beyond one-year commitments from the First Nations or DIAND.

Allegedly in order to curb abuses, the government of Canada set a limit on the number of months that a student could receive federal funding. The idea was to prevent people from becoming permanent students, making a living on student living allowances.

Medical school years are often longer than the academic year in other faculties. Medical studies are continuous through years 3 and 4 with clinical placements. Federal funding guidelines do not take this into account for student financing. By the time medical students reach the residency period, all of their allotted student months have been used up. Funding guidelines must be adjusted to take into account length of academic program.

Students often incur debts for eyeglasses, health insurance, hearing aids, learning disability study aids, dental bills or expensive prescriptions which are not covered through federal grants. This adds to the pressure on these students to find paid work in addition to their school work.

There are also difficulties with funding bodies such as First Nations administrations and DIAND, who often require transcripts as proof of attendance or success. Most institutions does not produce them half-way through the year. January funding is often late for the student as a result. Students borrow funds or run lines of credit, which they cannot repay until late summer.

Ontario Student Assistance Program

There is a critical lack of funding for Métis and non-status students. The Ontario Student Assistance Program (OSAP) is one avenue of aid, though only loans (not grants) are now available. Aboriginal people are generally reluctant to take loans and may walk away from schooling if loans are the only option.

Outstanding Needs

Most Aboriginal students are the first generation of their families to attend university. In this situation there may likely be younger children at home requiring parental support. Students receive little or no financial help from their families. Older students often have two or more children to support. Federal or First Nations funds do not meet family expenses, and students in this dilemma run up debts throughout the year, hoping to find work in the summer and rarely being able to catch up financially. The allowance of $675 per month for single students falls about $200 short and needs to be revised. Current book allowances cover only about one-third of actual costs. A realistic revision of this category would place actual costs at $600 per year.

Government policy on Aboriginal post-secondary education needs review and change to recognize

- student demand for assistance
- student needs
- program supports at universities
- First Nations targets in employing graduates
- long-term strategy to increase the number of graduates
- long-term funding commitments

In some institutions, the universities have accorded very minimal base budget funding for Aboriginal education. The prevailing expectation seems to be that Aboriginal people are responsible for raising funds for Aboriginal programming. Many First Nations view this attitude as one of paying lip service to the needs of Aboriginal students. A university-wide policy placing Aboriginal educational needs as an emerging priority needs to be established with consistent base budget support for counselling, bursaries, academic advice, curriculum revision and the hiring of Aboriginal faculty.

Geographical Barriers

First Nations communities and Métis communities are rural in location for the most part. There is a growing segment of the Aboriginal population (51 per cent) now living in towns or urban centres. For those nations in rural or northern areas, access to current information on admissions policies to universities, in-service workshops for counsellors, and summer jobs for students is slow in arriving. The participation of northern students or their counsellors in summer enrichment courses or in-service workshops is sometimes avoided because of the high cost of travel, which limits their access to services.

Students attending university whose families are left behind, sometimes hundreds or thousands of kilometres away, experience periods of extreme loneliness, homesickness and depression. This is often manifested in the student's inability to detach from the family and concentrate on studying. Community events and family gatherings also affect the students, drawing their attention from work. Multiple deaths in the family have caused some students to interrupt their studies to seek the healing of spirit they require.

Aboriginal students have a strong connection to family and community. They come from communal cultures where there are community expectations of their behaviour, participation and responsibilities. Aboriginal students in the health sciences are in some of the most demanding programs at the university. They require money to allow for breaks to visit family, renew relationships with Elders, and attend ceremonies. This is an integral part of maintaining a cultural identity, a balance of mind, body and spirit, and a strong connection to one's people. Consideration should be given to establishing a category of federal funding for travel to fulfil family and community obligations.

Education counsellors require in-service training at the university to enable them to experience the university environment and understand current admissions policies, meet their university counterparts and have an opportunity to experience the range of services available to support the Aboriginal students. Funds should be provided by DIAND to cover counsellor travel costs. The long-term impacts of such a course of action would be better informed front-line student service workers who have current and accurate knowledge about

- professional certification requirements
- course planning
- choices of universities to attend
- the range of employment possibilities

Summer job placements with mentors is particularly useful in the health care field. Students who live in remote or northern areas usually have little access to this type of enrichment because of the travel costs and living expenses involved in supporting the student away from home.

Travel expenses and geographic distances are also critical factors in planning summer science and mathematics enrichment-type courses. Sometimes publications that advertise these events don't reach the counsellors and students in time. In some cases, students who do hear about the programs are reluctant to leave home, worried about travelling alone, particularly by air, or they may have the chance of obtaining a summer job to earn self-support money for the academic year. Community-based courses will meet the students' need in this case.

Health care professions are not always preferred careers among Aboriginal students. The negative image of health care professionals needs to be re-focused. The high turnover of non-Aboriginal health professionals in First Nations and Aboriginal communities has caused problems in continuity of care, leading to mistrust in the physician/patient relationship.

Seriously ill patients are flown out of remote communities, to facilities staffed by non-Aboriginals, and are perceived by the patients and their families as remote and unfriendly. The impressions created by this experience make health care professions not the most desirable of fields to devote one's energies to. A new generation of Aboriginal health professionals could change the negative image.

Personal and Social Barriers

The lingering scars of colonization and latent racism have seriously affected the self-esteem of Aboriginal students. Some students have a lack of confidence in dealing effectively with the institution on admissions matters, academic difficulties or personal issues. The years of schooling for health science education (4 to 10 years) cause some Aboriginal students with low confidence levels to avoid taking up the challenge, regardless of their ability to succeed.

Many Aboriginal students have not been encouraged to work consistently to achieve high grades. They have not been challenged by parents, teachers or counsellors to excel in school. The attitude that mathematics and science are too difficult is common: at the first opportunity, these courses are often dropped. This closes the door to entrance to university health science programs.

For the minority of high achievers, these students of the 1980s and '90s have had to deal with the high expectations set for them by their communities. For a large percentage of them, they are the first members of their families to gain university entrance. As much as education is valued, there are re-entry problems after graduation as students re-adjust to community values and norms. Sometimes there is peer pressure not to leave the community for university. There may be concerns about losing one's culture, or criticism from traditional people with respect to certain procedures in school (for example, dissection in anatomy class).

When students reach university, there are times when they will feel the racial stereotyping by fellow students and faculty. Specialized counselling by Aboriginal counsellors helps in the short run, but an Aboriginal studies program in the long term provides an academic foundation for affirming Aboriginal issues and providing the anti-racist education for all students. Courses in health science faculties on traditional healing or Aboriginal health issues are essential.

Aboriginal students can feel a backlash from other students against funding from DIAND or from First Nations and against scholarships targeted for Aboriginal health sciences students only. Affirmative action or equity measures are sometimes seen as reverse discrimination; these attitudes can create an uncomfortable atmosphere for the Aboriginal students and can polarize the student body. Aboriginal students may feel additional pressure by being placed in the public eye and watched constantly to see how they achieve academically. Role-modelling is an important imaging process that is very weak in the health sciences. The lack of Aboriginal health professionals to act as mentors or as guest lecturers at high schools and universities has a direct impact on the effectiveness of recruitment of students into health care fields. Members of the National Aboriginal Physicians Association (NAPA, whose membership includes the allied health professions) do lecture at a few Ontario universities, but the full impact of their work is not yet felt at the high school level by Aboriginal students.

Although First Nations and Aboriginal associations have stated that their priority is community health, it must be emphasized here that professional education is the key to effective leadership at the community level. Professional health care providers move easily into management and policy positions. Along with community health, professional education has a key role to play in developing role models and conducting public education regarding Aboriginal health issues. The members of NAPA are important activists in this regard. Their presence is a clear signal that professional health education is attainable. As an organization, their input into resolving barriers and developing strategies to increase their members is central to the rethinking of policy and legislation.

Strategies to Increase the Number of Health Care Practitioners

Aboriginal Leadership Establishes Goals

The leadership of First Nations and national Aboriginal associations needs to establish the political will with federal and provincial governments and the financial investment necessary to ensure that Aboriginal post-secondary education is a high priority in preparation for self-government and health transfer. Federal legislation for college and university education, along with annual Treasury Board allocations, is required.

First Nations must take the initiative to work more closely with universities for more relevant programming in health sciences that accommodates Aboriginal health needs and ways of healing. Culturally appropriate student services should be placed at all universities in Canada.

Universities must develop a partnership with First Nations to understand the professional training needs and numbers of graduates required to prepare for self- government. There are many graduates of health science programs who are not readily known by First Nations. Universities need a forum, such as a graduation ceremony and pow wow, to feature their graduates of Aboriginal ancestry. These social events raise consciousness about the importance of university education and clearly establish role models for younger students.

Focus on Secondary School Improvements

Aboriginal students are at risk for streaming or for dropping mathematics and sciences at about the Grade 7 to 10 level. Puberty, peer pressure and employment complicate the retention issue. Not enough emphasis has been placed on this age group. Regardless of how effective university-based recruitment and student support services seem to be, there are simply not the numbers of Aboriginal secondary school graduates with Ontario academic credits or Grade 12 mathematics and science that there should be. The number of Aboriginal students entering university health science programs is minuscule and indicative of the high dropout rates in Grades 10 and 11.

The focus for the 1990s should be on secondary learners and Grades 7 to 10. Summer programs in science and mathematics enrichment, which are accredited by boards of education or the provincial government, need to be offered to students and their parents or guardians at the community level or in residence at universities. Currently, the First Nations House at the University of Toronto has such a program in the planning stage but has yet to find adequate funding (First Nations Summer Science Programs for Grades 7-OAC level).

In order to promote retention of students, science and mathematics curriculum at the Grade 7 to 10 level should be redesigned to accommodate Aboriginal content, teaching style and methods of evaluation. The content should be tied to the applicability to real-life situations with experiential learning situations and environmental relevance. The Aboriginal Science and Mathematics Pilot Project at the Mohawk community of Akwesasne is testimony to the effectiveness of this strategy.

Accommodating University Environments

At the university a different set of strategies needs to be set in place. In Appendix 1, there is a discussion of the success of the applications of these strategies. This section identifies the needs and strategies.

The university must create an environment where it is obvious to First Nations and to Aboriginal students that there is an institutional commitment to meeting Aboriginal education needs. The commitment includes

- increased interaction between First Nations and the university to place Aboriginal committees in decision-making capacities within the university to guide the development of Aboriginal education policy, academic programs, and student services;
- support expressed by the president of the university and the deans of the health science faculties;
- favourable admissions policies for health sciences programs until discrepancies in numbers are rectified (i.e., ratio of Aboriginal physicians to Aboriginal people is 1:33,333 whereas in the general Canadian population it is 1:575);
- recruitment strategy with Aboriginal-specific recruitment brochures and posters; travel funds for recruiters to reach First Nations and Aboriginal students on reserves and in cities; outreach by Aboriginal students to Aboriginal communities;
- culturally appropriate student services and support structures in professional and pre-professional years, staffed by Aboriginal people;
- admissions assistance and advice;
- academic planning;
- counselling – personal, financial and academic;
- elder in residence and cultural seminars;
- culturally and clinically relevant summer employment;
- adequate financial support for single students and students with families;
- Aboriginal-specific scholarships and bursaries;
- Aboriginal residences;
- daycare referrals;
- Aboriginal health issues integrated into the curriculum;
- new courses on Aboriginal health issues relevant to Aboriginal community needs;
- clinical placements in Aboriginal communities, enabling the students to work with Aboriginal patients;

- culturally based pre-university preparation courses with credits;
- hiring of Aboriginal faculty, guest lecturers, elders and healers to work with health science faculties;
- Aboriginal seats on hiring committees at the university;
- provision of university base budget support;
- linkages with other universities as a network to provide the most efficient and best quality of service to the Aboriginal students;
- staff development funds for liaison with other universities, attendance at conferences, and the development of networks of resource people; and
- interaction among traditional healers, faculty, students, Medical Services Branch personnel, Aboriginal professionals, and Aboriginal health organizations.

Barriers to the Support of Health Science Advocacy Programs

Long-Term Nature of Programs

The strategies outlined earlier are long-term initiatives reaching into the elementary and secondary schools and also providing mature students with pre-university preparation courses. The programs of study for medical school usually require a four-year Bsc degree, a four-year MD degree, and two years of residency for a licence. Ten years of training face a student who likely will not receive DIAND/band financial support for all of that time. Successful education strategies require a long-term commitment in policy and funding, understanding that graduates will not be forthcoming until some years down the road. The long-term nature of advocacy programs is a barrier to the development of such programs at universities.

Funding

> In the past, universities have had difficulties with finding money to support these types of programs because they are facing financial difficulties themselves and therefore do not have the money to fund programs which are perceived to be directed at special interest groups or perceived to be non-cost-effective due to the small numbers of students involved.
>
> As a result all Indian and Inuit Health Careers Programs were initially funded through the federal government, in Manitoba through a joint federal-provincial initiative and the others through the Medical Services Branch Indian and Inuit Health Careers Program.
>
> Medical Services Branch, Health and Welfare Canada has a time limit on developmental funding. Initially funding for a

> program is given for a three year term with an opportunity for an extension for another three years based on the fact that no student can graduate from a four year degree program (standard for most professional health careers) in three years.
>
> It is obvious then that the present government policy is geared to funding programs to recruit students into health careers. The University of Alberta has demonstrated that it is possible to recruit successfully and consistently. Yet after six years the bigger task – retention – lies ahead. In six years the University of Alberta will have graduated three physicians. But if funding is withdrawn the bulk of the students (8 plus a minimum of 4 projected entering students) will be left in limbo, their support systems withdrawn....
>
> Many private foundations have policies similar to those of the federal government. They are willing to provide short-term developmental funding with a stated time limit. In some cases they are willing to fund program components – the University of Alberta has been able to obtain bursary money for students, for example, from a foundation and money for student outreach travel from a professional organization. However, these foundations are not prepared to give operating dollars to continue programs started by developmental money from elsewhere.
>
> *A.M. Hodes, University of Alberta, 1993*

Foundations are more likely to fund projects of a developmental nature with measurable outputs. At the University of Toronto, foundation funds have assisted in financing the Aboriginal Science and Mathematics Pilot Project at Akwesasne and the First Nations Summer Sciences Program for students in Grades 7 to OAC level. Long-term funding must be found to continue these projects. No educational programs are completely self-supporting financially.

> Funding difficulties are compounded for programs designed to produce health professionals by accusations that such programs are elitist because health professions, especially medicine, are perceived as elitist. There is resistance at the government level to the idea that money should be concentrated on a relatively small number of elitist students when it could be spent on a larger group.
>
> This attitude is held by some First Nations groups who also resist the idea that the money should go to an institution when it could be spent at the community level. Political pressure from these groups puts pressure on Medical Services Branch who then consider cutting successful programs.

> If these attitudes prevail, nothing will change at the community level. Support and aide positions in health centres on reserves and adjacent hospitals will continue to be filled by First Nations staff but the professional and managerial positions will continue to be staffed by non-native people with no stake in the betterment of Aboriginal health. As a result First Nations will continue to have no control over their own health at the professional level.
>
> The danger at the institutional level – and this has been demonstrated in numerous U.S. programs – is twofold. Once larger numbers of under-represented students are admitted, the university feels it has done enough. Programs are cut because it is felt with larger numbers enroled there is no longer a problem with representation. No thought is given to retention. When problems develop with students and there is no program to address these, a strain is put on the system. The university then draws back its support and cuts back on admissions because it has no facilities to deal with what it now perceives to be a group of 'problem' students. The very success of the program creates its demise.
>
> *A.M. Hodes, University of Alberta, 1993*

Strategies for Change

Recognition of Needs

The programs that are most successful at producing Aboriginal health sciences graduates are cognizant of the needs of First Nations and Aboriginal associations regarding the move toward self-government. The programs are tied closely to Aboriginal communities and are supported by these communities through strong decision-making Aboriginal committees placed appropriately in the structure of the university.

The transfer of health services from federal government to First Nations control has provided the impetus or the *raison d'être* of health science advocacy programs. The licensed Aboriginal health professionals will be leaders in policy formulation and primary care services, able to offer care in the cultural milieu (and language) of the population they are serving.

It is this group who will begin to establish the co-operative relationship between modern medical practitioners and traditional healers. As alternative medicine becomes part of the medical school curriculum, there will be increased opportunities to work together at all levels.

Students have expressed the need to retain their culture, language and traditional values while studying. The best advocacy programs build culture into the curriculum and into the student service component, recognizing the need for self-actualization. Native science, healing practices and current health issues find affirmation as to their efficacy in this environment.

Aboriginal educators need to work closely with universities to continue

- to present the health professions as a realistic and attainable goal;
- to revise K-10 science, English and mathematics programs to add Aboriginal knowledge and adapt to Aboriginal teaching styles;
- to work with university-level programs designed to encourage Aboriginal students to gain access to professional health careers;
- to revise funding guidelines to accommodate student expenses in the long years of demanding study in the health sciences where student costs are higher; and
- to demand that the Medical Services Branch support successful programs to enable these programs to be fully integrated into the university system.

An Aboriginal educational foundation or endowment fund is urgently required with a mandate similar to the Native American College Fund. Student educational expenses, a curriculum design fund, and institutional student support core funding could be part of the funding mandate for such an organization.

As Aboriginal nations move toward control of their own institutions under self-government, the likelihood of Aboriginal-controlled universities or colleges forming within the next ten years becomes more of a reality. As these developments move ahead, plans should include an assessment of partnerships to enable universities to do what they do best and allow Aboriginal institutions the freedom to develop in their strongest program areas.

Recommendations

First Nations

The Aboriginal leadership must set the pace for change by establishing a partnership with governments and universities to agree on goals for post-secondary education, adequate funding levels, and support for institutions that are striving to open clear pathways to the health sciences. Legislation is required to protect Aboriginal post-secondary education from a continuing slump in financing.

First Nations leadership must lead the way to articulate strategies for the educational advancement of their people. Aboriginal decision-making bodies should be established at the highest level of the university structure to influence policy, programming and student services.

Aboriginal policy development should include

- an assessment of student needs, community needs in preparation for self-government;
- a review of existing university/college programs as to recruitment and retention;
- revision of government funding guidelines for students and student service programs;
- development of Aboriginal professional training targets over a five-year period;
- estimation of the number of graduates needed in each profession; support for student service programs at universities; support for new program development, including distance education models; and
- looking to the future for Aboriginal-controlled university/college structure.

The Government of Canada

Enabling legislation must be devised to enable the government of Canada to relate to First Nations and Aboriginal governments on the issue of post-secondary education provision, policy and funding based on need. Aboriginal governments should control post-secondary funds that flow from annual Treasury Board allocations. Financial support is required for

- student tuition, books, living expenses, travel, daycare;
- student support services at institutions (co-funding);
- new program development on curriculum, research;
- planning and development funds to establish Aboriginal post-secondary institutions;
- long-term (10-year) developmental funding to health careers programs at universities in order to graduate and license physicians and others in the allied health professions; and
- raising the level of funding for the IIHC bursary and scholarship program of the Medical Services Branch to enable students to be supported financially until they graduate.

Universities

Universities are more likely to respond to Aboriginal education needs when First Nations and Aboriginal associations make their needs clearly known and when there is initial developmental funding to help establish student services, curriculum innovation and research.

Universities need to engage in policy development to establish

- admissions policies; goals/targets for increasing access to all faculties and programs in the health sciences and others;
- culturally appropriate student services;
- financial incentives for students;
- appropriate clinical placements in Aboriginal communities;

- university-wide policies on Aboriginal access to education and to employment;
- curriculum renewal across all disciplines to integrate Indigenous knowledge into existing curriculum and develop new courses on traditional healing, Aboriginal health issues and Aboriginal science;
- admissions policy must recognize Aboriginal people as a special needs group representing an under-represented population in the health care field; student applicants should be examined in a separate pool;
- pre-university health science preparation programs are a necessity (like the SPSP at the University of Manitoba – see Appendix 1) to prepare mature students for university entrance;
- culturally appropriate student services are a requirement at every college and university;
- Aboriginal studies programs are also required; new full-credit courses should be developed to enhance identity, language and cultural knowledge; Aboriginal faculty are important to present the Aboriginal viewpoint and act as role models;
- provincial and national planning is required to co-ordinate programs to best meet student needs and ensure that duplication does not occur;
- there should be high visibility of support for Aboriginal issues at the university; for example, a graduation pow-wow, Aboriginal scholarships, Aboriginal residences;
- there should be provision for voluntary identification of Aboriginal students on admission forms; and
- there should be a permanent health sciences advocacy co-ordinator in every university.

There are successful health science advocacy programs for Aboriginal students that have contributed to this paper.

- University of Manitoba: Special Pre-Medical Studies Program
- University of Alberta: Native Health Careers Program
- University of Toronto: Office of Aboriginal Student Services and Programs and the Aboriginal Health Professions Program

A full description of their goals, services and impacts can be found in Appendix 1.

Appendix 1

Health Science Advocacy Programs for Aboriginal Students at Four Canadian Universities

Preparing Aboriginal People For Health Studies: Special Premedical Studies Program At The University of Manitoba

M.C. Stephens, MD, PhD, G. Degen, MEd, C. Hoy, MD, S. Matusik, MEd
Departments of Community Health Sciences & Continuing Education, University of Manitoba

Overview

Since 1979, the Special Premedical Studies Program at the University of Manitoba has had solid success in preparing Aboriginal students admitted through to graduation as professionals.

This unique program actively recruits students to premedical study, and assists those selected with comprehensive supports including academic, financial and personal support, plus ongoing enrichment through the Faculty of Medicine.

Graduates of the programs (including five doctors, three dentists, one pharmacist and one physiotherapist) make their practice largely with Aboriginal people throughout the province. In addition, they are increasingly involved at many other levels to improve health care for the Aboriginal population.

Introduction

Ten years ago, in Manitoba, one known Aboriginal physician had graduated in medicine at the University. Today there are six additional known Aboriginal physicians in the province, five of whom graduated from the Special Premedical Studies Program (SPSP). In addition, three dentists, one physiotherapist, and one pharmacist have graduated from this program, and the program presently has three students in medicine, one in dentistry, and two in medical rehabilitation, all of Aboriginal ancestry. Other SPSP students have graduated in degree nursing, and three more are currently studying nursing.

What is the SPSP?

It is a program established in 1979 in Manitoba with the goal of preparing Aboriginal students, mainly mature students, for admission to one of the health faculties. It was established to address the under representation of this group in those health careers.

SPSP was modeled after other ACCESS programs at the University of Manitoba, at Brandon University and at community colleges, as well as after INMED, of the University of North Dakota.

Some numbers and results:

As of January 1991:	
Total SPSP enrolment	146
Current students in SPSP	28
Potential Graduates	118
Graduates other than health careers	28/118
Graduates in health careers	13/118
present professional health faculty students (from SPSP only)	9/118
Success Rates	
Total	43%
into professional health faculties	19%
from professional health faculties	100%

Program

The SPSP is located at the centre of the main campus in the Continuing Education Division. The program can be viewed as having five main components: recruitment, selection, personal support, financial support, and academic support and enrichment.

Recruitment

Staff, and occasionally students, make trips throughout the year to communities to present information about the program and identify prospective applicants. Recruitment packets are also sent out to schools, organizations and social service agencies and other contacts. In recent years, media has been utilized; newspaper and radio ads are purchased, and a short video has been developed and widely distributed to ensure that the maximum number of potential applicants hear about the program.

Selection

Applications to the program are accepted up to April 1 each year. The selection of students takes place in two phases. First, an initial screening process is conducted to select applicants for interviews. Second, those screened in applicants are then brought to the University for a four day process. This process includes an orientation to the program and the University for their own information, and then their interviews. Candidates are chosen on the basis of their motivation and ability to pursue health care training as well as their academic, financial and social need for the program supports.

Types of Support

There are three areas of support which characterize SPSP:

1. Financial support for the premedical years as well as for the further professional schools, including relocation costs, tuition, books, tutors, living allowance, etc;
2. Personal support – to meet needs in the areas of adaptation to the city and to the University, of financial and time management, help with relocation, with baby-sitting, and with counselling in personal issues, there is a counsellor on permanent staff. Personal support continues for premedical years and further into professional studies, as needed; in general, by the time students enter the professional schools, those needs are much less or non existent. Others arise, such as those consequent to the overwhelming amount of reading necessary. However, like all other students, adaptation occurs, after some encouragement from many of the faculty members who know about the program and who come into contact repeatedly with these students;
3. Academic support and enrichment – many academic supports are vital to student success. Course planning, advising, and monitoring are basic. Remember that students who have been outside the mainstream of academic life must in four years be able to compete for entrance to highly competitive professional health faculties. Once there, they must survive. Therefore, all academic supports must emphasize student' developmental concerns. Advising is seen as a teaching function, helping students to learn to direct their own learning within a realistic framework of possibilities. Tutors are also made available in all subjects.

One of the most important characteristics of SPSP is the first year/second year 'bridging' in chemistry and physics for those students with a weak science background. Classes meet 6 hours a week minimally for chemistry and for physics, instead of the usual three, plus the courses are extended over an extra year. Initially it was thought that only chemistry and physics needed to be addressed with academic enrichment. However, it was soon realized that there was a great need, for the majority of students, of developing skills and knowledge in mathematics, of reading more efficiently and studying efficiently as well. Fora ll these activities, instructors are hired.

Students, however, do not spend all their time in separate classes, and by the third year all classes are regular. Counselling continues to be available as needed. Over the years, more flexibility has been added to the program, depending on the different academic and personal needs of each student. Someone might just need the program for some counselling and financial help. Others might need the total and intensive support system.

The Health Sciences Component is an important part of this extended program. In order to stimulate and maintain the interest in the long term goal, students regularly attend courses and participate in other activities at the Health Sciences campus. These activities are coordinated by an SPSP member, out of the Northern Medical Unit, Department of Community Health Sciences.

During the first year, on a weekly basis a seminar course in medical/dental/ medical rehabilitation lecture on topics of their specialties in a very informal atmosphere, so as to encourage free discussion. Students also visit clinics and hospitals all over the city. Whenever possible aboriginal speakers in health related professions also lecture, as well as ex-SPSP students who now are in the professional health faculties.

There are also six week summer field placement in medical settings arranged for the first and second year students. The settings include rural and urban hospitals, northern nursing stations, community clinics, drug and alcohol addiction treatment and education centres, health clinics, dental clinics, medical rehabilitation services, pharmacies, and so on.

During the second year, the seminar series continues, but now in more basic sciences topics – physiology – and here the instructors are graduate students. Demonstrations and visits to laboratories are held, and some clinical specialists are also invited.

For third year, we hold "MCAT/DAT preparation" classes on a weekly basis. This consists more in the repetition of exercises, reviewing, taking tests, and reading emphasis. The objective is mainly to ensure that, as far as it is possible, students understand what is involved in these types of exams, and possibly to stimulate their studies and review of the necessary materials. Another more intense, continuous six week session has been added for the summer before last year of SPSP, before the final MCAT/DAT.

Yet another regular component of the program is preparation for interviews for admission to the health faculties. One must keep in mind that practically all the students in the program are the first members of their families who attend university, let alone medical or dental schools. Mainstream students in general have relatives or close family friends who are university educated and/or physicians, dentists or therapists and can therefore become familiarized informally with the process of interview for admissions. In the case of SPSP, we provide that familiarization through the volunteer help of mentors in the various faculties and now our graduates as well. It is interesting to note that what we must really emphasize with out students are the many, many achievements they had in their pre-university years, which are undervalued by the students themselves, but highly valued by admissions committees.

Professional Health Program

As previously mentioned, once students graduate from SPSP, and if they successfully compete for a place in the health faculties, they become Professional Health Program (PHP) students.

PHP students continue contact established earlier on with staff of the J A Hildes Northern Medical Unit. In this respect Manitoba is fortunate because the very idea of this program arose from Dr. J A Hildes and his associates at what is now the Northern Medical Unit. Now twenty years old, the Northern Medical Unit provides physician services and is committed to the development of health care services, education and preventive measures to about 25,000 people living in rural and remote Manitoba and the Keewatin district of the Northwest Territories.

Because of this very long period of contact with indigenous communities, there are at the NMU many individuals who can provide all sorts of mentorship to the PHP students. For the PHP students, this is a special relationship, a "home base", which can be used for such things as actual teaching help, tutoring, advice on professional choices, advice on personal matters, and use of the facility at all hours. But, in addition, mentorship and support are provided by taking these students up north with one of the consultants for a short period of time, or by promoting interest in Aboriginal health issues and solutions. This is done either through regular students' programs at the Northern Medical Unit, or through other special mechanisms developed here.

Regular students' programs have always been present at the NMU, since its inception. Their purpose is to foster understanding by the medical or dental students of the health conditions in remote communities, and what are the factors which lead to those conditions, to familiarize students with a different culture and to promote understanding of that culture.

This is a summer northern program for first and second year medical students, of 10 weeks duration. There are also electives and family medicine rotations of 6 weeks duration. Finally, there is also the B.Sc. Med program in which research is done on a topic in Aboriginal health. In all these programs students will go up to the communities and work and learn. There are very few such programs in other health faculties in Canada. As far as the PHP students are concerned, we are always especially attentive to their desire to try these programs. In fact, all that have passed through medical school have taken the opportunity of going up north with one of the programs.

Other activities have also been a regular feature of the PHP program through the NMU contacts. For example, when we had the first class of PHP students going through the clinical training years (medicine, dentistry, and medical rehabilitation) we started contacts with the American Association of Indian Physicians and started sending all PHP students to their annual meetings. This continues to be a regular feature of the program, and grants are sought and often provided by medical Services Branch. The main purpose is exposure of students to professional role models of Aboriginal ancestry. It has resulted finally in a close relationship between the American and Canadian students and physicians, and had stimulated new ideas from our graduates, such as their pivotal role in the formation of a professional association of Aboriginal physicians in Canada, among other initiatives.

Also, since members of the Northern Medical Unit and its department, Community Health Sciences, have been very active in the circumpolar Health Organization, our students have been sent to the international meetings of this society, and presented papers.

Locally, we always try to inform students of activities such as health related conferences for Aboriginal peoples or others, educational conferences, workshops, etc. There is always a person at NMU trying to negotiate free admission to such meetings for our SPSP and PHP students. We try to foster the interest in Aboriginal issues and try, through all these activities, to enhance leadership characteristics in both SPSP and PHP students.

Program Funding

The program is funded entirely by the Province of Manitoba, through Manitoba Education and Training. All status students' living allowances, books and tuition are paid through agreements with the Manitoba Indian Bands, and the Department of Indian Affairs.

Conclusion

Notwithstanding the improvements that can still be made in SPSP and PHP, the general overview after twelve years is that in terms of effectiveness it has accomplished its goal of providing health professionals of Aboriginal ancestry to Manitoba. There is also a special contract with the Northwest Territorial Government whereby their students can participate in the program and indeed we have one such student at present.

Most graduates are working with Aboriginal communities in Northern Manitoba. There are physicians and dentists working in the Island Lake region, on the east side of Lake Winnipeg, in Churchill, in Cross Lake, and in Pukatawagan.

It would be an unreasonable goal to achieve a graduation rate into professional careers at university of 100%. That is not remotely possible in the mainstream population of premedical students who begin university with the intention of going into these health careers do end up in them? It is not known, but is thought to be quite small. In light of this, the program's success rate is encouraging.

It is important to note that students who do not end up in specific health careers continue university and obtain a degree at close to the same rate as the mainstream population. This is an important point of consideration, because these people will be university qualified and enter the labour force as such. This is also a very important side result.

As mentioned in an editorial of the Canadian Medical Association Journal, this is the grandfather of all such programs in Canada.[1] Finally, more recently, other provinces have begun programs at the professional schools level. That is very important, but more thought, effort and money must be put into preparation for admission into these professional faculties, because there are very few qualified students ready to be admissible. Even more important, all provincial and the federal governments should somehow direct their attention to the fact that approximately 80% of aboriginal students do not complete high school, compared to the 70% of all other Canadians who do! Until this is overcome, there is no good alternative to continuing these special ACCESS programs.

Another important consideration is the financial support needed to maintain students in universities. If they are mature students, and the majority in SPSP and other ACCESS programs are indeed older students, often with families, the financial support throughout is crucial. Besides this however, money alone is not enough.

It is generally known that Aboriginal students supported only financially have a much lower success rate in completing a first degree in Canada (around 5 to 6%)[2] Other supports such as significant academic and personal supports will still be necessary until there is a whole generation of Aboriginal university graduates who will supply these supports to subsequent generations.

Notes

1. A. Gilmore, Educating native MDs – always go back and serve your people in some larger way, *Can Med Assoc J* 1990 142, 160-162.
2. J. Hull, An overview of the education characteristics of registered Indians in Canada 1986, Working Margins Consulting Group, Winnipeg, for Indian and Northern Affairs Canada.

First Nations House, University of Toronto

Leadership, Spiritual Growth and Academic Excellence

From the time of the inception of the Aboriginal Health Professions Program in April of 1986 to the present day evolution of the Office of Aboriginal Student Services and Programs, the University of Toronto has demonstrated its commitment to providing Aboriginal students with the highest quality of academic programming and culturally appropriate student services. The self-identified student population has risen each year by 20 per cent since 1986, a factor that shows that students make their academic choices based on program excellence, especially so since this university has no Aboriginal studies program yet.

Very early on, the barriers to the attainment of post-secondary education were articulated clearly by First Nations students, counsellors, teachers, and leaders. Together, the Aboriginal communities and the university developed a profile of the successful Aboriginal student possessing a strong identity and the academic qualifications to provide leadership in one's chosen field.

Based on the needs of the student, programs and services were designed to afford the Aboriginal student every opportunity for success in university-level studies. The present retention rate of students is 95 per cent. We feel this high figure is clearly due to the cultural programming and support we have been able to offer the students. However, we recognize that, while impressive, this is an historical figure only, and if we are unable to be proactive with appropriate future programming and services we will soon see a downward trend. The needs of the community are changing, and if we hope to see our success continue, we must meet those needs as well in the future as we have in the past. It is with this goal in mind that we have designed the services and programs outlined in this proposal.

At present, we have 140 students who have self-identified as being of Aboriginal ancestry, although we know that the actual number of students is higher. Most of these 140 are pursuing professional qualifications or preparing for graduate programs. We have a very successful pre-university program which is preparing mature, adult learners for university-level study. Many of our graduates are the first Aboriginal professionals in their fields in Canada:

- speech pathology
- occupational therapy
- medical research

and, in Ontario,

- pharmacy

- physical therapy
- medicine (female physician)

We are educating the leadership of the next generation which will make self-government a reality in the First Nations communities of Ontario. First Nations leaders have specified to us that they require accomplished graduates with the highest quality of credentials, those who have a strong affiliation with their people, a respect for traditional values and spiritual traditions. From only 25 students in 1986 to over 140 today, we are now seeing graduates in law, social work, education, medicine, physical therapy, speech and language pathology, occupational therapy, community health, business administration, history and, very soon, in engineering, psychology, mathematics and pharmacy.

The accompanying table shows enrolment by faculty and graduates. Throughout the life of the OASSP and the AHPP we have done our best to honour the integrity of the directions given to us by First Nations leaders:

- educate to the highest standards,
- honour traditional teachings, and
- prepare for self-government.

Student Enrolment Statistics 1992-93

Faculty	No. of Students	Year of Study
Arts & Sciences (includes TYP)	98	Years 1 – 4
Community Health	2	PhD
Education	2	Year 1
Engineering	3	Years 1 and 2
English	1	PhD
Law	16	Years 1 – 3
Management (MBA)	1	MBA
Mathematics	1	PhD
Medicine	2	Year 2
Nursing	1	Year 3
OISE	6	MA and PhD
Pharmacy	2	Years 1 and 2
Rehabilitation Medicine (Physical Therapy)	3	Years 2 – 4
Social Work (MSW)	2	Year 1
Divinity (Theology)	1	MA

Note: Current admissions cannot be officially confirmed until late November.

Graduates (26)

Social Work (MSW)	4	Mathematics (MA)	1
History (MA)	1	Community Health (MA)	1
Speech Pathology (MA)	1	Law	1
Education (BEd)	4	Physical Therapy	1
Medicine	4	Occupational Therapy	1
Transitional Year Program	7		

Culturally Appropriate Student Services

These services are designed to increase Aboriginal student access to the University and to promote student retention.

The Office of Aboriginal Student Services and Programs of First Nations House offers:

- Recruitment
- Admissions Advocacy
- Personal Counselling
- Academic Tutoring
- Native Student Housing
- Day Care Referrals
- Library Resource Centre
- Scholarships and Bursaries
- Financial Planning
- Cultural Seminar Series
- Elder-In-Residence
- Native Students Association
- Aboriginal Health Professions Program:
    - Health Experience Workshop
    - First Nations Summer Science Program
    - Aboriginal Science and Mathematics Pilot Project

Recruitment

The Recruitment Officer conducts career fairs, workshops and conferences on educational planning for professional careers. The Officer travels to First Nations communities, and to urban secondary schools where there are large numbers of native students in attendance.

- A video production is available on health career options.
- Information kits on careers in many disciplines at the University are also available.

- A Native Student Handbook is available outlining admission standards, programs of study, and student services can be obtained from First Nations House, the OASSP.

To date, the Recruitment Officer has spoken to over 3,000 native students and visited approximately 75 communities in Ontario.

Admissions Advocacy

The Admissions and Academic Advisor assists students in gaining admission into the University of Toronto. Students are advised to contact the Advisor first to map out strategies and options. Information is also available on programs at other universities in Canada and the United States. Students are requested to complete the OASSP student advocacy form to enable staff to advocate on the student's behalf. Students who are changing courses or programs of study are also encouraged to see the Academic and Admissions Advisor. The Advisor is the bridge between Aboriginal student needs and the University administration to ensure that the student meets the academic criteria for passing and graduation. "Special consideration" admission status, and in some faculties, "reserved seats" are held for Aboriginal applicants.

Personal Counselling

Personal and spiritual counselling as well as career and financial planning are available to students both prior to enrolment and throughout their studies at the University. The Counsellor will see students by appointment and is also available to visit other schools. The role of the Counsellor is to ensure the emotional well-being of the student as well as their financial stability while they study at the University. The Counsellor also assists the students in the transition from rural to urban lifestyles, high school to university-level studies, and cross-cultural changes. The Counsellor manages the bursary fund for Aboriginal students. The Counsellor will also assist students in developing financial plans to meet the high cost of city living on a fixed budget.

Academic Tutoring

There are presently two tutors employed during the academic year for the benefit of all Aboriginal students attending the University of Toronto. The courses covered are:

- English, study skills, essay and exam preparation
- science and mathematics

In addition to the regular office hours of the tutors, students can arrange to set up individual appointments at mutually convenient times. Specialized workshops are offered by the tutors to meet student needs, particularly in essay writing, research skills, exam preparation, and multiple choice testing.

Financial Assistance, Scholarships and Bursaries

Financial assistance is available for those with status from the Department of Indian Affairs or through the students' Band Administration Office. Status students, as well as non-Status and Métis and those persons may apply for assistance from the O.A.S.S.P.

- Scholarship: In 1988-89, the O.A.S.S.P. established specific scholarships for First Nations students registered in full-time degree programs at the University
- Bursaries are available to full time, undergraduate students of Aboriginal ancestry.
- A bursary fund of $20,000 has been established by the University and is managed by the O.A.S.S.P. for the benefit of Aboriginal students.

Métis and non-status Native students may approach the Student Awards Office for information on the Ontario Student Assistance Program (O.S.A.P.)

Aboriginal Student Housing

O.A.S.S.P. has a house especially for Aboriginal students on 43 Sussex Avenue. It has five fully furnished rooms for rent at reasonable rates. The house is within walking distance of the campus, and it is available for summer accommodation.

In addition, the University has a number of general residences. The Counsellor will assist students in finding suitable accommodation either at the University or in private accommodations through the Housing Services.

Daycare Referrals

The counsellors refer students requiring daycare to a number of appropriate services throughout the city. A Native daycare agency is available in Toronto.

Library/Resource Centre

A study centre with the necessary facilities such as computers and a small but ever growing Native resource library is available for student use.

Cultural Programs

O.A.S.S.P. within First Nations House is more than just an administrative office. Both staff and students organize cultural workshops, retreats and ceremonies intended to expand our understanding about the importance of identity and traditional values in a modern world.

Elder-In-Residence

The Elder-In-Residence program offers a role-model of traditional teachings, counselling from a traditional spiritual perspective and a link to First Nations issues and community events. The Elders rotate their visits, thereby offering students a complementary understanding of indigenous knowledge and personal development from the Aboriginal viewpoint.

Native Students Association

The Native Students Association (N.S.A.) has an office and lounge at First Nations House where students can relax, socialize, enjoy a cup of coffee, and develop new friendships. It is a place where students can meet and provide support to one another. The N.S.A. organizes social gettogethers and various cultural and recreational events. Special events and Native Studies Week are part of the N.S.A.'s mandate. A purification lodge (sweat lodge) is also part of the NSA's mandate for cultural teachings.

Academic Planning and Development

Increase the Sensitivity and Awareness of the Institution to Aboriginal Cultures and Issues

The role of the OASSP is to establish an academic environment for Aboriginal students which is responsive to their intellectual, spiritual, and emotional needs.

The students have identified the need for a Program of Aboriginal Studies within the Faculty of Arts and Science. The core of 12 to 15 courses should be cross-referenced to professional faculties so that all students begin to have an understanding of Aboriginal issues. For example, a course in the Faculty of Pharmacy on traditional Aboriginal healing practices could also be offered to first year medical students and be housed in the Program of Aboriginal Studies. Discussions are under way at the Governing Council level on the question of establishing an Institute for Aboriginal Culture and Research.

The following faculties have initiated plans for curriculum change:

- Faculty of Arts and Science: preliminary discussions for an Aboriginal Studies Program, Linguistics, Drama Centre, Canadian Studies, Fine Arts, Women's Studies Program
- OISE: Indigenous Education Program
- Faculty of Social Work: Curriculum Review, Recruitment of Aboriginal Faculty, Library Resources, Recruitment Strategies
- Transitional Year Program: Curriculum Review, Tutoring
- Faculty of Law: Curriculum Design, Faculty Appointments, Native Student Advisor, Academic Support Program, Workshops on the Royal Commission
- Faculty of Education: Native Teacher Education Program
- Faculty of Nursing: Curriculum Review
- Faculty of Music: Ethnic Music Course

- Scarborough College: new courses – "Canada and Multi-Culturalism", "First Nations Cultures in North America", and "Canadian Native Peoples" (under design)
- Faculty of Forestry: Aboriginal Forestry Symposium, new course – Canada's Aboriginal Communities and Their Forestry Environments
- Faculty of Engineering: AMIK Program
- Faculty of Dentistry: Special award over 4 years of study
- Faculty of Pharmacy: New Course – "First Nations Healing Practices", Mentors, Scholarship, Recruitment
- Faculty of Medicine: Elective – "Traditional Aboriginal Healing Practices"
- Speech and Language Pathology Division: Mentor Program, new seminar
- Community Health: Visiting Lectureship in Native Health

Other faculties/divisions within the health sciences have had a long-standing commitment to the admission, retention and graduation of Aboriginal people in their programs of study:

- medicine
- dentistry
- pharmacy
- nursing
- physical therapy
- speech and language pathology
- occupational therapy
- physical and health education.

Research on Aboriginal Issues

The OASSP through its extensive contacts with Aboriginal associations and its membership on the President's and Provost's Aboriginal committees will be in a strong position to act as an advocate for the research priorities identified by the Management Committee. The OASSP's role in advising divisions and departments on such issues would lead to a better use of scarce resource dollars for research by spending it in areas identified by the Aboriginal community as being of importance.

The OASSP in addition should examine the feasibility of establishing a centre at the University of Toronto for research issues of self-government, economic self-reliance, environmental sustainability and community development.

Such a centre, in conjunction with other interested universities could develop knowledge and expertise in those areas identified by First Nations and Aboriginal associations as crucial to their growth, including sustainable agriculture, forestry management, human resource management, architectural studies, education, health sciences, natural resources management, law, cultural development and engineering. Contracts, assignments, and placements of students and faculty in Aboriginal environments as part of the research effort promotes more credible and usable research results but also produces experts with realistic world views of Aboriginal goals and development issues.

In the short-term, the OASSP through the decisions of the Management Committee is in a position to advise on research policy, priorities and process in those research projects where Aboriginal concerns are part of the research. The Office will continue to be a resource to the University community with regard to native concerns.

Aboriginal Health Professions Program

In 1986 the Aboriginal Health Professions Program (A.H.P.P.) was established at the University of Toronto. Its mandate is to increase the number of Aboriginal health care professionals having a knowledge of both traditional and modern medical practices so that they can better serve First Nations people whether in urban centres or First Nations communities.

Health Experience

This program is designed to encourage interest in careers in the health care field. Health Experience is a week-long workshop which brings Aboriginal students in grades 9 to OAC to the University of Toronto where they participate in hands-on health-oriented learning activities, both traditional and modern, and visit on-site with health care professionals.

First Nations Summer Science Program

The program will provide Aboriginal students with science and mathematics courses leading to intermediate and senior advanced-level and OAC credits. Grades 7 and 8 students are invited to apply for the entry-level courses. A student progresses through the program over a period of six summers, taking enriched science and mathematics courses the first two summers, and gaining credits in grades 10, 11, 12 and OAC science in the following four summers.

Classes and labs for the five-week course term are held on the University of Toronto campus. Elders/traditional teachers; Aboriginal teachers and counsellors; parents; and staff and counsellors of the University of Toronto Schools work together to create an environment which will enable students to strengthen their understanding of Aboriginal science and gain the tools necessary for future academic advancement in the sciences.

Aboriginal Science and Mathematics Pilot Project

The A.S.M.P.P. is a four year curriculum development project designed to revise and implement Aboriginal science, mathematics and pedagogy into grades 7 - 10 level studies. The project is a joint venture of the Stormont, Dundas, Glengarry Board of Education, the Akwesasne Mohawk Board of Education and the O.A.S.S.P.

Native Health Care Careers Program University of Alberta, Faculty of Medicine

Historical Background

The inequities in the health status of Canada's Aboriginal peoples are well known. These include shorter life expectancy, higher infant mortality rates and higher morbidity rates than in the general population. Aboriginal people who need and want access to physicians from their own culture are further disadvantaged. The ratio of Aboriginal physicians to the total Aboriginal population in 1993 stands at 1:33,333 compared to the overall ratio of physicians to the general population in Canada which is 1:515.

In Alberta where treaty Indians account for 2 per cent of the population, 3 of the approximately 4,000 physicians are of Aboriginal ancestry. The Faculty of Medicine at the University of Alberta will graduate its first Aboriginal physician in 1993. To achieve parity in number, at least 80 more physicians of treaty Indian ancestry are needed, and at least double that number is Metis and non-status Indians are taken into account.

Mandate of Native Health Care Careers Program

The mandate of the program is to encourage more Aboriginal students to consider a career in medicine and to facilitate their admission into the MD program in order to correct the under-representation of Aboriginal physicians in Canada.

It is the belief of the Faculty that Aboriginal students with a commitment to their cultural identity and traditions will serve as role models for Aboriginal youth, become leaders in effecting improvements in Aboriginal health standards, and enrich the life of the Faculty as a whole.

In order to fulfil this mandate the Faculty has instituted special status admission to the MD program for Aboriginal participants and an aggressive pro-active recruitment policy nationally.

In 1988, two positions per year were added in each entering class of the MD program for students of Aboriginal ancestry within the meaning of the Constitutional Act of 1982, Section 35, Part 2. These positions are limited to Aboriginal students. If none apply, they cannot be filled from the general applicant pool. All Aboriginal students must meet the prerequisites as outlined in the calendar. However, students who identify as being of Aboriginal ancestry will have their applications considered separately from those in the general applicant pool.

In order to implement this new admissions policy the Office of the Native Health Care Careers Program was opened within the Faculty staffed by a Coordinator funded by Medical Services Branch, Health and Welfare Canada. Since that time the number of Aboriginal MD students has grown to 11, exceeding the total number of students of Aboriginal ancestry enroled in Faculties of Medicine in all other Canadian universities combined. These students come from across Canada and represent Abenaki, Blackfoot, Cree, Delaware, Inuit, Metis, Mohawk, Ojibwa, Odawa, and Saulteaux nations.

Program Services

The Program offers the following:

Student Services

- academic counselling in admission procedures and pre-admission program planning
- remediation and tutorial services
- personal and financial counselling
- access to bursaries and scholarships
- assistance in obtaining summer employment with relevant clinical and cultural components
- referral to other professional health care faculties, all of which have special positions reserved for Aboriginal students.

Projects and Resources

- Annual Faculty of Medicine Aboriginal Health Day with prominent Aboriginal speakers from the Health field: both western trained physicians and traditional healers.
- Visiting speakers on various aspects of Aboriginal Health and Traditional Healing during the year.
- Darcy Tailfeathers Awards: Two $1,000 scholarships are offered and presented to Aboriginal MD students at an annual Darcy Tailfeathers Luncheon.
- Core curriculum courses in Aboriginal Health for all MD students in the Faculty.
- Participation in the SIHA Native Health Issues Committee including students retreats and traditional sweats with Aboriginal Elders.
- Outreach visits to schools with high Aboriginal enrolments; career workshops on reserves, and northern communities.

- Opportunities to visit reserve based clinics with contract physicians.
- Electives in culturally specific settings.
- Opportunities to interact socially with a broad spectrum of professionals involved in Aboriginal health.
- Opportunities to attend culturally and clinically relevant conferences and workshops.

Entrance Requirements to the MD Program

1. Applicants to the MD Program must complete a minimum of two years of university studies carrying a course load consisting of five full course equivalents prior to admission. An undergraduate degree is strongly recommended.
2. Applicants must achieve a minimum GPA of 7 on a 9 point scale.
3. All applicants must complete the following prerequisites: full course equivalents in Organic and Inorganic Chemistry, Biology, Physics and English and one half course in Statistics.
4. All applicants must write the Medical College Admissions Test (MCAT) at the latest the autumn prior to the year of entry.
5. All applicants must provide an autobiography, 2 letters of recommendation and undergo an interview.
6. All applicants must provide proof of Aboriginal ancestry.

University of British Columbia The First Nations Health Care Professions Program

Background

The First Nations Health Care Professions Program (FNHCPP), established in 1988, is essentially an access and support service program. Its primary mandates are 1) to increase the number of First Nations health care students at the University of B.C., and 2) to provide support services for students currently in the health sciences faculties, schools and programs.

From 1988 to 1991, full funding was provided by the Indian and Inuit Health Careers Program, Medical Services Branch, Health and Welfare Canada. Since 1991, the Medical Services Branch has partially funded the program along with assistance from the Province of British Columbia Ministry of Health and the

Ministry of Advanced Education. The Ministry of Aboriginal Affairs (B.C.) has provided valuable lobbying support.

At the University, governance of the program falls under the Vice-President, Academic and Provost's office. In 1990, the Faculty of Medicine agreed to form a partnership with the First Nations House of Learning to seek funds for the continuation of the program. Program direction and guidance is provided by an Advisory Committee which consists of faculty members, First Nations community members and UBC First Nations House of Learning staff. The program is currently located in space provided by the Office of the Health Sciences Coordinator's Office in the Woodward Instructional Resources Centre.

Program Objectives

As stated in the program brochure, the goals and objectives of the FNHCPP are:

- to increase accessibility and provide support services to First Nations students in health care studies at the University of B.C.
- to consult with First Nations communities to identify those health care issues which should be addressed.
- to collaborate with Faculty of Medicine and other health sciences faculties and schools in developing courses and seminars relevant to First Nations' health care needs.
- to liaise with First Nations communities in the development of community-based program initiatives or research activities pertinent to local health care.
- to encourage interest in health science careers at the high school level through a Summer Science Program.

Activities

To carry out the program objectives, the FNHCPP has been involved in the following activities:

- recruitment of students through participation in career fairs, First Nations community meetings, interaction with colleges and schools
- providing program and admissions information through mailouts, information booths and direct academic counselling
- networking with First Nations health training programs in Canada and the United States
- providing programs which heighten interest in health careers such as the Summer Science Program, the Synala Program and the Scientists in the Schools Program
- planning and implementing courses and seminars on native health issues
- providing support services to health sciences' students on campus

- establishing a resource centre for students, faculty and First Nations communities

Accomplishments of the Program

1. Student Enrolment

The number of First Nations students enrolled at UBC increased from three in 1988 to 22 in the current (1992/93) academic year. The first Native medical student will graduate this May, and a second Native medical student is now in year 1. Currently, students are enrolled in Medicine, Nursing, Graduate Studies (Science and Counselling Psychology), Social Work, pre-Medicine and pre-Dentistry.

2. Support Services

Support services on campus consist of the following:

- academic counselling in admissions procedures and course selection
- personal and financial counselling
- remediation and tutorial assistance
- placement in a mentoring program (where applicable)
- a resident Elder
- reinforcement of cultural identity
- limited financial assistance for relevant conferences and professional workshops

3. Networking

The program has established a strong network with health training programs, organizations and colleagues in Canada and the United States. Strong links were made with other Canadian programs at the 1991 National Symposium, "Preparing Health Care Professionals: First Nations Action Agenda for the Nineties", which was hosted by the First Nations Health Care Professions Program.

4. Liaison

The program has established firm ties with all health sciences faculties, schools and programs at U.B.C. As well, there is ongoing liaison with schools, colleges, health organizations, native communities and government ministries.

5. Promotion

To promote the program, the FNHCPP has developed and widely circulated a brochure and a poster. In addition, regular press releases are used to promote new programs. FNHCPP activities and programs have been featured in several newspapers and radio broadcasts. The unique Summer Science Program has been acknowledged in a national magazine.

6. Courses and Seminars

Native Health Awareness Days have been held annually to educate health students and faculty at the University. The two-day event generally features displays and speakers. For the past two years, Biology 448 has been offered through the Faculty of Science. This course focuses on native health issues. In addition, the Coordinator of the FNHCPP is regularly asked to speak to students in the health sciences.

7. Research

With funds received from the B.C. Ministry of Health, the program was able to gather data on research done for and by native communities on numerous health issues. This information is currently being entered into a database and will soon be available to native communities, academics and students.

8. Projects

To promote interest in health careers, the program has embarked on a number of programs which are designed to heighten student interest in health sciences and post-secondary education. These projects include:

Summer Science Program

This highly successful annual residential program has been offered at the University of B.C. for five summers. Two groups of 20 students experience a week of labs and lectures with University professors.

Scientists in the Schools Program

The FNHCPP utilizes this provincial program implemented by the Ministry of Education to promote general science and technology awareness. The coordinator has facilitated tours involving UBC scientists to schools with substantial native populations. The groups consist of health scientists as well as basic scientists.

Synala Honours Program

This program, based on the Rural Alaska Honours Program, was piloted at U.B.C. in the summer of 1992. This bridging program was designed to encourage Aboriginal students already on an academic track to continue on to an institute of higher education after graduation. Students and staff were unanimous in their recommendations for the continuation of the program.

AISES

The FNHCPP office was instrumental in the development of the first Canadian Chapter of the American Indian Science and Engineering Society (AISES) at U.B.C. The Society currently has a membership of 40 students. It is active in the recruitment of Native high school students to post-secondary training.

Appendix 2

Table 1: Native Physicians Association of Canada, 1992-1993, Current Statistics

Physicians in Practice

51 self-identified Aboriginal physicians.
34 in active membership with the Association.

University	Number In-Course	Graduates
Medical Students		
University of British Columbia	1*	
University of Alberta	10	1*
University of Manitoba	4	1
University of Western Ontario	1	
McMaster University	2	2
University of Toronto	3	4 (not self identified)
University of Montreal	1	1
TOTAL	**21**	**10**

*These will graduate in May-June 1993.

Source: Native Physicians Association of Canada.

Table 2: Allied Health Professions

University	Number In-Course	Graduates
Dental Students		
University of Alberta	1*	*(also 2 in Dental Hygiene and 1 graduate)
University of Manitoba	1	
Pharmacy Students		
University of Manitoba	1	
University of Toronto	2	
University of Alberta	2	
Rehabilitation Medicine Students (Occupational Therapy, Physical Therapy, Speech & Language Pathology)		
University of Manitoba	1 (p.t.)	
University of Toronto	3 (p.t.)	1 (s.p.)
		1 (o.t.)
		1 (p.t.)
University of Alberta	1	1
Nursing Students		
No information available from Aboriginal Nurses Association of Canada or Health and Welfare Canada, Nursing Division.		

Note: There is also one student in the Medical Laboratory Science Program in the Faculty of Medicine at the University of Alberta.

Source: Native Physicians Association of Canada

Table 3: University of Manitoba, Current Statistics, SPSP

- 15 students/year interested in medicine, dentistry, pharmacy, rehabilitation medicine.
- students successfully completing the program can apply to the faculty of their choice, where they will receive the support of the Professional Health Program.

Graduates		Applicants
Medicine – 7	3 in course	3
Dentistry – 3	1 in course	
Pharmacy – 1	1 in course	1
Rehab. Medicine – 1	5 in course	3

Almost all grads work with Aboriginal communities as clinicians, and some have recently risen to the policy management level.

Source: Dr. Gene Degen, University of Manitoba.

Table 4: University of Alberta, Current Statistics

Faculty of Medicine: Current Enrolment 1992-93

(a) MD Program: 11 students

Academic Year	Applicants	Admitted	Registered	Withdrew
1988	2	2	1	1
1989	3	3	1	0
1990	11	4	4	0
1991	4	3	3	0
1992	8	4	3	0
1993	8	1 (Deferred from 1993)		

(b) Medical Laboratory Science
Student registered in year 3

Faculty of Medicine: Graduates

(a) One student graduated in 1988 with a diploma in Health Services Administration.
(b) One student is expected to graduate with an MD in June 1993.

Faculty of Rehabilitation Medicine

(a) One student graduated in physical therapy in 1991.
(b) One student is expected to graduate with a degree in physical therapy in 1993.

Faculty of Pharmacy

(a) One student is expected to graduate in pharmacy in 1993.
(b) One student is registered in year one of pharmacy.

Faculty of Dentistry

(a) One student is registered in the first year of the DDS program.
(b) One student graduate in Dental Hygiene in 1992.
(c) One student is registered in Year 1 and one student is expected to graduate in Dental Hygiene in 1993.

Faculty of Nursing

In 1991-92 there were 10 registered native nursing students and one student graduated in 1992. The Faculty has not kept statistics on previous graduates.

All professional health faculties at the University of Alberta offer special positions to qualified native applicants as follows:

Faculty of Medicine	1 positions outside the quota in the MD program 1 position in Medical Laboratory Science
Faculty of Dentistry	1 position in Dentistry and 1 in Dental Hygiene
Faculty of Pharmacy	1 position
Faculty of Rehabilitation Medicine	2 positions in Physical and 2 in Occupational Therapy
Faculty of Nursing	4 positions in-pre-nursing

Five Year Projection: 1993-1997

(a) 14 graduates from the MD program

(b) A *minimum* of 11 students in the MD program. (Based on admitting a minimum of 2 students per year plus the student with deferred admission to 1993.)

Table 5: Lakehead University, Current Statistics

Intake	**Year**	**Entered NNEP**	**Admitted to BScN**	**Remaining in BScN**	**Graduated**
I	Jan-July '87	12	9	3	2
II	'87 to '88	12	8	1	
III	'88 to '89	12	7	1	
IV	'89 to '90	12	7	1	
V	'90 to '91	13	8	5	
VI	'91 to '92	14	7	7	
Totals		*75	46	18	**2
Percentage of Entrants			**100 per cent**	**46 per cent**	**24 per cent**

* The 11 students of the present (VII) intake have not been included in this summary. Since they are not yet eligible to enter the BScN program, the inclusion of this number would skew the percentages.

** It should be noted that, to date, only students from the first and second intake have been able to complete the entire five years of the program and therefore be eligible to graduate.

Integrating Science and Traditional Culture

*Rahael Jalan**

A high degree of professional control over health care is exercised by doctors, dentists and other health care professionals. In contemporary health care, the view is that only modern medicine, with its powerful array of medications and technological intervention processes, can remedy health problems most effectively. Experience and observation over the centuries, which constitute the traditional body of knowledge in health care and prevention of disease, have been largely ignored by the medical community. Traditional culture and ways of life are seen as backward and ritualistic, with no scientific basis. Modern society relies on observations made in the short period of time where immediate results can be demonstrated. Medicines are developed and approved on the basis of experiments conducted in a laboratory or controlled environment. The short-term results observed may be only part of the story. Often the longer-term ramifications are either overlooked or not fully monitored. In recent years, the long-term effects of some modern medical and technological processes have been under scrutiny. Understanding the potential of self-healing, community-oriented health care concepts such as education and prevention are taking root.

There is no doubt that scientific and technological advances have contributed significantly to the quality of life on the planet. However, in embracing the new, the old ways and traditions have been rejected as unscientific and at times have been outlawed. Some scientists are beginning to recognize and acknowledge the wisdom of the ancients.

---

* Indian Health Careers Program, Saskatchewan Indian Federated College.

Traditional healing practices were passed on by word of mouth through the generations. There is very little in the form of written documentation of the methods used. Ancient healers relied on natural remedies. The ancients also recognized the power of nature and spirituality. Today's environmental movements, which emphasize greater harmony with nature and its protection, have much in common with First Nations philosophy and practice. It seems that we have come full circle.

We are now poised at a point in history when the modern and the ancient could merge and forge a new path toward a more balanced lifestyle. To achieve a balance between the ancient and the modern, there needs to be an innovative approach to our system of education. Traditional learning from one's elders in the community and education in academic institutions should exist side by side. We need to move quickly in this direction. Otherwise, the vast repository of undocumented knowledge may be lost forever to the new generations.

Present Situation

In the present system of science education, there is the presumption that those with certain cultural backgrounds are not capable of learning science. There seems to be an underlying perception that First Nations students do not have a leaning toward maths and science because of their culture and background. A substantial number of students seem to suffer what could be termed 'maths and science anxiety'. This is not merely a problem with Aboriginal students; it is a general problem. Students are not taught a wide range of basic mathematical and scientific concepts at the elementary and secondary levels. Their analytical skills are not developed, and they find it difficult to work a problem through to its logical conclusion. Therefore, they do not have a firm grounding in the fundamental principles necessary to deal with the somewhat more complex concepts in maths and science when they enter university. The transition from school to university becomes very difficult for many students. This is more pronounced in the case of First Nations students because they are not encouraged to learn maths and science in the school system. The consequence of this can be seen in many areas where scientific learning is necessary, particularly in the area of health care.

Health care is a major concern for Aboriginal people, who are severely underrepresented in the health care professions. Consequently, they can rarely receive health care from individuals from their own communities who are sensitive to their culture and concerns. Isolated Aboriginal communities cannot attract doctors. This situation cannot be changed until there are sufficient numbers of Aboriginal doctors and other health care professionals.

There is a need to attract more First Nations students into the health care professions. Many Aboriginal students who come to university are reluctant to express their desire to become doctors because they have not been given the necessary foundation in maths and science and therefore feel that it is beyond their capabilities. They keep away from areas that involve maths and science. Moreover, students coming from a reserve find it difficult to adapt to the general system. To attract more First Nations students into these areas there has to be an overall effort to promote programs in maths and science in First Nations communities.

The SIFC Science Department

The science department at the Saskatchewan Indian Federated College, which is federated with the University of Regina, offers a program designed to meet this need. In 1985 the Medical Services Branch of Health and Welfare Canada, partly in response to the concerns expressed by the World Assembly of First Nations of 1982, funded an initiative by the Saskatchewan Indian Federated College (SIFC) for the purpose of developing and implementing "a health career program (HCP) that will prepare Indian students for a career in one of the health professions". During the ensuing years the program was established at the SIFC as the Indian Health Careers Program (IHCP).

One of the objectives of the program is to provide learning experiences that will enable students to enhance their understanding of First Nations culture, traditional First Nations medicine, current and future health care needs and the goals of First Nations people. To meet this objective, the program developed five Indian Health Science courses. These courses were designed specifically to meet two goals. First, they gave students information relevant to the health care system as it currently relates to Aboriginal people. Second, they were designed to enhance the students' understanding of the basis for traditional practices of health and healing: wellness, unwellness, and wholeness as practised by Aboriginal peoples of the Americas. Emphasis is also placed on examining and tracing the evolution of traditional religious philosophy and practices among Aboriginal peoples as a result of their interaction with non-Aboriginals. Students discover how these changes have affected the current practice of religion and healing.

However, the primary objective of the program is to provide first- and second-year pre-professional university level classes that will fulfil the admission requirements of post-secondary health science programs and give students transferable credits toward such programs. The IHCP had a choice of allowing its students to enrol in the university's maths and science courses or mounting its own offerings in these areas. Students had difficulty coping with the large classes in mathematics and science courses offered by the university. This led to the creation of the department of science at SIFC. The programs that the department offers are designed to give First Nations students a maximum of support and accessibility to training for the science careers of their choice.

The SIFC science department has worked continuously to improve the quality and effectiveness of the program by doing the following:

1. recruiting qualified and committed faculty members to teach the required pre-professional maths and science courses;
2. keeping introductory maths and science class sizes small to help beginning students meet the required academic standards;
3. providing academic support and enrichment to bridge the gap for those students weak in maths and science. Some classes meet five or six hours a week instead of the prescribed four hours per week. Professors are willing to devote considerable time to students outside class hours for purposes of review and tutoring. This also facilitates an informal setting for getting to know the individual student and helps students feel more comfortable in the classroom; and
4. designing the program with a commitment to presenting the curriculum with a strong First Nations perspective as well as articulating the relevance of such courses to contemporary First Nations concerns.

Our focus has been on teaching, remediation and research, especially into curriculum and program development. We would also like to place more emphasis on recruitment, retention, reformatting of courses and First Nations community involvement. For example, one of our immediate goals is to recruit a class of approximately 25 students for the pre-professional training required for most health professions. This, we envision, would provide the cohesiveness and camaraderie lacking at the present time.

During the past few years the department of science has faced severe pressure from budget restrictions and the shortage of faculty required to teach the necessary classes, while the demand for introductory maths and science courses in the pre-professional program, the secondary teacher education program, the health administration program and others has increased substantially. A high level of commitment by faculty and staff has ensured that existing program quality has been maintained.

Results

The effectiveness of this endeavour is reflected in the increase in enrolment in all the courses offered by the science department. We have seen an increase in the numbers of First Nations students who have indicated a desire and demonstrated the ability to learn maths and science. Many non-Aboriginal students have enroled in the Indian Health Studies classes. They wish to learn about the tradition, culture and healing practices of the First Nations.

From our experience in the evolution of the program, we have learned some important lessons. It is not that there are significant differences between

Aboriginal and non-Aboriginal students with respect to learning abilities. In teaching maths and science to First Nations students it has been our observation that, given the opportunity and encouragement, they are just as able as other students to deal with the complex concepts of mathematics and science. The problem is that First Nations students are not fully prepared and therefore not motivated to undergo professional training requiring maths and science.

To promote education in general there is a need to stimulate intellectual, moral, social and spiritual growth in children. It is necessary to encourage diversity and a healthy questioning attitude, rather than conformity and a mere acceptance of established norms. Cross cultural education and an understanding of the diversity of coexisting cultures will serve to enhance and promote tolerance and add to our wealth of knowledge.

Four Community Social Initiatives

Grand Lac Victoria Community

*Richard Kistabish**

Today, Grand Lac Victoria is still the only Indian band in eastern Canada that has not settled on a reserve. Its members live in Quebec in an area bounded on the north by the Abitibis, in the west by the Timiskamings, in the south by Maniwaki and in the east by the Atikamekw. In the 1980s, for the umpteenth time in its history, this community held a referendum on accepting reserve status (which the Department of Indian and Northern Affairs had offered on a silver platter). It was agreed, once again, that occupying the territory, nomadism and certain traditional activities were priorities. Nonetheless, the price of this 'freedom' is the daily petty annoyances imposed *ad nauseam* by both levels of government.

At the time of Confederation in 1867, the officer of the Hudson Bay Company stationed at Grand Lac Victoria wrote:

> Grand Lac is now the best paying single post on the frontier from Mingan to Rainy Lake.

Since then, wilderness logging, hydro-electric dams, the extraction of gold and copper from the earth, the collapse of the fur trade, hunting and fishing by the dominant culture – all these factors and many others have brought the economy of Grand Lac to its knees.

* Health Program Co-ordinator, Grand Lac Victoria Band Council.

At the same time, the group's socio-medical environment had also deteriorated gradually, to such an extent that in 1980, Chief Donat Papatisse decided to take drastic steps to solve all these problems. First, the few established services (community health representative, nursing), which had been managed by a neighbouring reserve, had to be repatriated to GrandLac. Then, the infectious phenomena that multiplied rapidly in the community had to be attacked head on: otitis, bronchitis, pneumonia, tuberculosis, intestinal parasites, and so on.

A multi-disciplinary team was therefore built gradually. They increased the ranks one by one: janitorial services, community organization, housekeeping, general practitioners, pediatrician, psychiatrist, co-ordination, NNADAP officer, escort-interpreter, social service and education liaison officers, and prevention worker. Over time, all the practitioners developed a systemic philosophical approach together: it is based on networking techniques and could henceforth gain widespread acceptance in the Aboriginal environment. Its premises are that everyone involved is equal (what the person who mops the floor says is as important as what the doctor says), all information circulates freely, no one acts alone, and each new member is carefully chosen by Grand Lac representatives.

In the meantime, with pathogenic germs relatively under control, the Grand Lac population tried to remedy the shortcomings in social services for Aboriginal people, that is, the isolation of a child in a sick environment and customary intervention *in extremis*. A formal complaint filed with the Youth Protection Commission on December 15, 1988, prompted an extensive two-year investigation. The report led to intensive departmental intervention and the appointment of a mediator to bring the two parties involved closer together. Social services eventually rallied behind the Grand Lac multi-disciplinary team and also adopted its work philosophy. Furthermore, a few psycho-educators and a child psychiatrist joined the network. Each child started receiving indispensable assistance. And what is more, groups of children and adolescents are taking a course in order to try to come to terms with suffering related to services provided in the past.

Between 1988 and 1992, the overall picture of the repercussions of violence and rape finally appeared clearly, with epidemic proportions. In view of the clear-cut image that emerged, a broad-based police campaign was undertaken in May 1992: the victims reported the horrors of their past together. At present, about ten assailants are in jail; a few others will be brought before the courts in the next few months. Here still, the team involved in this psycho-social operation has had to adjust to the Aboriginal analysis of the assailant-victim diad. This means that the victims usually want their assailants to receive a punitive sentence coupled with therapy. They know that there will inevitably be contact with them after their incarceration. Furthermore, one of the recently identified snags in this dynamic is the shortage of funding for therapy for sexual assault victims (and others); the amounts allocated provide only a few months of treatment – in most cases, a mere prelude to treatment. The patient is abandoned right in the middle of the intervention. The situation is particularly paradoxical in that it is often easier to obtain suitable treatment for an assailant in prison.

Some people will claim that this multi-disciplinary approach is expensive. But we will see that this is wrong if we look closely at the harvesting of the area's natural resources for more than a century: the federal government's granary has been filled for a long time by taxes on the sale of lumber from the upper Ottawa valley, legendary fortunes have germinated and ripened there, and yellow gold still flows into the coffers of the dominant culture. We are therefore talking about crumbs and petty cash to counter the after-effects of this extortion.

The free circulation of information is a key aspect of the teamwork with the Grand Lac population. In order to work, this dissemination must be done through osmosis. For example, when required, the victim and/or the wife of an imprisoned assailant should be informed of his progress in therapy. They come up against ridiculous obstacles posed by the Access to Information Act and supposed confidentiality. Serious social problems are the direct result of this obscurity and breakdown in communication. We cannot analyze this issue in detail in this brief summary. However, we cannot skirt it. That approach leads directly to a dead end. Basically, we are talking here about looking at individual rights as opposed to collective rights. The laws and rules of the game that currently govern these rights are dictated by the dominant culture. The balance between the individual and the group is quite different for Aboriginal peoples. The role of the Royal Commission is to initiate consideration of this difference and to suggest an appropriate adjustment to the individual/collective balance.

Three other recommendations for the Royal Commission would facilitate the work of multi-disciplinary teams similar to those in Grand Lac. Through its research, the Royal Commission could first shed light on the 1966-67 agreement (public health) between the federal and provincial governments concerning social services for Aboriginal people. This agreement simply must be reopened and updated.

Moreover, the Royal Commission could propose a mechanism guaranteeing real co-operation among social, health-care and legal services (probation, prisons, courts, parole and so on).

Finally, the Royal Commission could open the eyes of Aboriginal people to the disturbing incidence of fetal alcohol syndrome and secondary organic cerebral syndromes. And how many people are carriers of sub-clinical conditions that have never been diagnosed?

Métis Child and Family Services

*Carolyn Pettifer**

Our agency is one that has been out there struggling. We do have a political mandate from the Métis Nation of Alberta. We are a provincial agency. We are not an urban-based agency; we are an agency that meets the needs of the Métis children and families right across the province.

Although a lot of our services have been focused in the last nine years in the city of Edmonton, we have been working on getting those services out to all of the communities across the province. For us to do that, we have to be involved in a process whereby we can open the doors with the provincial government and with the federal government to allow us to participate and to enter into agreements to do our own work in the communities.

We have a framework agreement with the Province of Alberta and a subsequent Memorandum of Understanding with the Alberta Family and Social Services. That is to allow us to do joint planning, joint initiatives, talking about partnerships, talking about how we as the Métis community and the province can work together in better meeting the needs of Métis children and families across the province. It is a process, as well, where we can be involved very much more closely with the federal government.

---

* President of Métis Child and Family Services, Edmonton, Alberta, and founder of the agency at its inception nine years ago.

I think it is really important that an agency out there that is delivering services has a political mandate to deliver those services, especially when we are talking about entering into agreements with the province and/or the federal government.

The way the funding arrangements are designed right now, our agency basically works only on fee-for-service arrangements, and that is not good enough for us. We don't need to be involved with government when the programs and the directions are designed at the senior levels of provincial and federal governments and the Métis community doesn't have any involvement in the design and the development of those programs. The funding really limits us in terms of what we can do.

Our agency has about five different kinds of agreements: one with the City of Edmonton; two or three, I believe, with the province; and a couple with the federal government. We spend so much of our time and energy in seeking the sources of funds that we need to do our work.

Our approach is basically wanting to do a holistic, integrated approach to working with children and families. A lot of the work that we are doing is with families with the child welfare system, mostly in the area of support services. The funding arrangement there doesn't allow us to be involved in the way that we would like to be in doing the work with children and families.

In that sense, I think that being involved with changes to legislation, to regulations – to make change with any government requires politics. Politics is what makes change. So we feel very strongly that the work that we do with our politicians and the support they give back to us is really crucial for allowing us to take on the directions, to be involved in those changes.

We have had a lot of struggle with our agency, when we are talking about seeking the recognition by government to allow us to participate and involve ourselves in those changes.

The Métis community has a lot of human resources. There is an abundance of people that we have to work with. Our people have been brought up and exposed to all of the social ills faced by other Aboriginal people around the country. A lot of us have survived and overcome and are successful, but we have been exposed and we know the conditions, we know the problems and we know the issues. We know the kinds of things the families are feeling – the pain and all the social problems they go through. I think a lot of us, because of exposure, can relate to those and, as a result of that, we can share some of our pain, some of our healing processes with those individuals.

Feelings of self-worth, self-identity are all very important. The basis for a healthy, supportive environment is a strong family, our children being brought up with strong feelings of who they are and self-esteem. Those kinds of things are what need to be instilled in our children and in our families if we are going to be healthy mentally, physically, emotionally.

Those are just some of the areas we are working in with our families – the holistic approach. But, as I said, we can't operate in an integrated, holistic way without the funding arrangements that go with that.

If I can give one solution to the whole issue, it would be to say to all of those federal government departments that piecemeal funding is not the way to go. Let's take all of those pieces of funding from all of those governments, federally and provincially, and put them in a pot. Sign a federal-provincial agreement with the Métis community, and you can rest assured that we will come up with our own solutions and our own unique approaches to working with children and families. And we will be successful.

If you are looking for a solution, let's involve the Métis community in the process and in a manner that we agree to how we should be participating, not in a manner that the federal or the provincial government chooses or decides how to involve us. Allow us the opportunity to talk and dialogue about a process for participation and our involvement and partnership.

Community Development, Sobriety and After-Care at Alkali Lake Band

*Joyce Johnson and Fred Johnson**

In the spring of 1992, the Alkali Lake Band received funding from Health and Welfare Canada through NADAP's Community Based Research Component to conduct research on alcohol recovery. The primary objective of this research was to determine what were the most effective factors in achieving and maintaining sobriety among the residents of Alkali Lake. The quantitative research component is entitled "A Study of Sobriety and After-Care at Alkali Lake Reserve – 1993". The project also included a separate historical study of the social policy initiatives used in the sobriety movement from 1972 to the present. When completed, this research will be published and made available to other communities that have not yet achieved sobriety or started their healing interventions.

The problem that must be addressed is the disease of alcoholism. It is a disease that is medically recognized as having no cure; it can only be controlled through abstinence. To deal effectively with this problem and its effects, a detailed knowledge of the disease is required. One of the reasons it is so difficult to deal with is simply that very few people are truly knowledgeable about alcoholism and how to deal with it, and they know little or nothing about after-care and the effective healing interventions that are essential to maintaining sobriety.

This lack of knowledge about alcoholism is reflected in the shocking statistics on Aboriginal social problems. The suicide rate for Aboriginal youth (age 15 to

* Counsellors, Drug and Alchol Programs, Alkali Lake Band Council, British Columbia.

19) is six times higher than the national average. The number of Aboriginal children in care and the number of Aboriginal adults in jail are also six times the national average. While many Aboriginal communities have made substantial progress and reached high levels of social, economic and cultural development, many others are still caught in a trap of poverty, hopelessness, and alcohol. It is for those communities that this research was conducted.

In 1985 a film was produced entitled *The Honour of All – The Alkali Lake Story*, which was seen throughout North America. As a result we receive phone calls and letters on a regular basis, usually from people who have seen the film and for whom a spark of hope has been ignited. Then they want to know how Alkali Lake accomplished this and whether more information is available.

The study was conducted in two parts. Part I is an historical summary that documents the actual interventions used by Andy and Phyllis Chelsea to turn the community around and parallels the events portrayed in the film. Part II focuses on the subject of alcoholism itself: what the Alkali people found to be helpful in sobering up and maintaining their sobriety through an after-care program. In this study the subject of sobriety (and the maintenance of sobriety through after-care), is distinguished from the action of ceasing to consume alcohol. Quitting drinking and maintaining sobriety are presented as two separate and distinct subjects.

In the Alkali Lake experience, the first step took place on a community level – through the authority of the band chief and the band social worker. The second step was undertaken on a personal level – tendering the healing process that is required to maintain sobriety. The Alkali Lake experience has shown that both these stages are necessary – the community-level interventions and the personal after-care components are both essential to the community healing process.

Based on the historical study of the interventions used at Alkali Lake between 1972 and the present and the data gathered in the 1992 research, several conclusions emerge:

1. ***The confrontation intervention*** was used to get people to stop drinking. The key elements of this method are the provision of choices, expression of concern and follow-through on the ultimatum. Using the steps correctly results in the ultimatum not appearing as force, and people feel they have made the choice themselves.

2. ***After-care.*** The treatment alone is not sufficient to maintain sobriety. Many aspects of after-care must be developed to facilitate a healing process. Without after-care the risk of relapse is high, or the person remains a 'dry drunk', perpetuating the same behaviours while sober as they did while drinking. From the historical study, the personal growth training undertaken in 1981 was significant in moving people past the plateau stage, out of the dry drunk syndrome, and into individual programs of personal healing and

personal growth. It was after the personal growth workshops, attended between 1981 and 1985, that the community reached 95 per cent sobriety. The healing must be an ongoing and intensive process, and it must occur in the community.

3. ***Alcohol and Case Work.*** Based on the effectiveness of the confrontation intervention and the success of after-care initiatives at Alkali Lake, it is felt that people in the helping professions should have more training in alcoholism and how to work effectively with alcoholic clients. The research submits that the alcoholic client and the alcoholic community do not constitute a hopeless situation but can respond to a combination of sober leadership, structured interventions, and resources for healing and after-care.

4. ***Family Support.*** The statistics showed that family was the biggest factor is people's decision to quit drinking. Based on this finding it is recommended that social workers acquire more training in (family) systems theory and a greater understanding of holistic (and medicine wheel) models.

5. ***Spiritual Support.*** The historical research shows there was virtually no practice of Aboriginal spiritual ceremonies prior to the late 1970s. Yet it is estimated that today close to half the adult population (about 100 people) participates in traditional practices such as the sweat lodge and the pipe ceremony. The practice of the traditional spiritual ceremonies was purposely revived and relearned from outside resources during the past 15 years at Alkali Lake. From this it can be concluded that this type of specific planned intervention to revive and relearn Aboriginal spiritual ceremonies played a significant and substantial role in the recovery of the Alkali Lake community.

Summary of Research Findings

Question 1

Which interventions did you use to become sober?

- Family support (25% of all responses) and personal growth workshops (20 per cent), were the two main interventions used to quit drinking. Treatment centres, at 12 per cent, and AA meetings (11 per cent) were also used.

Question 2

Which interventions were most effective?

- The most effective factors identified in the interventions used to quit drinking were self, at 24 per cent, followed by family, at 17 per cent.

Question 3

Please explain why.

- The reasons for effectiveness were stated as spiritual support, at 28 per cent, and family support, at 23 per cent.

Question 4

What significant event or thing caused you to want to be sober?

- The reasons for wanting to become sober were identified as family, at 48 per cent of all responses, and spiritual, at 31 per cent.

Question 5

What has helped you to stay sober?

- The factors used to maintain sobriety were spiritual support (including AA meetings and sweat lodges), at 25 per cent, and support groups (other than AA), at 18 per cent.

Question 6

What have been the most effective factors in your after-care program?

- The most effective factors in an after-care program were spiritual support (including AA and sweats), at 34 per cent, and support groups (other than AA), at 19 per cent.

A Model for Delivery of Health and Social Services to the Atikamekw People: Theory, Practice and Necessity

*Louis Hanrahan**

This presentation takes a quick look at a community services delivery model developed with the intention of facilitating an integrated approach to community health and social services practice in the three Atikamekw communities of central Quebec.

In 1983-84, shortly after having come together under a new umbrella organization known as Atikamekw Sipi, the three Atikamekw bands – Manawan, Wemotaci and Opiticiwan – announced their intention to take over the provision of social services to the Atikamekw people.

The bands passed by-laws giving them authority to dispense all social services to the residents of the three communities. This authority was then transferred to Atikamekw Sipi. The Atikamekw operated under what they considered to be their legitimate authority. Accordingly, no agreements were signed with provincial authorities at any level, even as concerns statutory services pertaining to youth protection and young offenders.

The Atikamekw were able to secure the financial means to provide social services through an agreement worked out with the local DIAND authorities. This agreement stipulated that all funding for social services provided to Atikamekw clients would be transferred to Atikamekw Sipi. Before the takeover of social services, funding arrangements had been make between the individual bands and Health and Welfare Canada for the administration of prevention services such as

* Former director, health and social services, Conseil de la Nation Atikamekw.

NADAAP and the Community Health Representative program. These programs were later transferred to Atikamekw Sipi.

The initial funding allowed for the hiring of a twelve-person team, which included seven community workers and professional supervisory staff. Branch offices were set up in each of the three communities as well as in two neighbouring towns. Initial services were geared around voluntary services applied to the solution of social problems. They also, inevitably, included the reception of youth protection related complaints, follow-up in such cases and referral to outside services when needed. When the health prevention and promotion workers came on board, an integrated multi-disciplinary team approach was developed.

An Integrated Approach

Parallel to the undertakings to secure financing and assert jurisdiction, some effort was devoted to developing a service delivery model that would be more appropriate to the culture, situation and needs of the Atikamekw population. This model was founded on the principles that helping was not only a professional responsibility, that the problems were a collective responsibility, that all those people charged with particular responsibilities concerning the development of the communities must work together and with the community and, finally, that the communities had within them the resources to address most problems and issues facing them. Tied to these principles were the underlying assumptions that the Atikamekw had the right to do things their own way, the right to make their own mistakes and, especially, the right to decide on their own priorities. It was also understood that Atikamekw Health and Social Services were to be free from political interference.

Decision Making

To ensure community participation in the decision-making process, health and social services committees were set up in each community. These were to be tied to and named by the band council and were to advise it on health and social services matters. They would also advise the health and social services agency on needs and provide feedback on service delivery. Early plans to involve these committees systematically in case planning and decision making were never implemented.

Accountability

Atikamekw Health and Social Services would be accountable to the Board of Directors of Atikamekw Sipi who were essentially the elected chiefs; they were also accountable to the individual band councils through their local health and social services committees. It was hoped initially that accountability to the board of directors of Atikamekw Sipi would be assumed through a national health and social services council that could become more familiar with the health and social services field and follow activities within it more closely. This was never done.

Financing

In principle, funds would have been managed globally in keeping with the practice model. This was not possible, however, because of the large number of funding agencies and programs (both federal and provincial) and the varied, if not contradictory, conditions imposed by them.

Service Delivery

The core of the service delivery approach was the integrated effort of a multi-disciplinary team.

Integrated Approach

The integrated approach was aimed at ensuring a concerted effort toward the prevention and solution of problems and operated on several levels at once. It necessitated multi-disciplinary planning, case discussions, and intervention. It allowed for the design of specific responses to specific situations.

One of the more interesting aspects of this approach was that it allowed for an exchange of responsibilities between workers if required. In other words a CHR could follow a youth protection case if the client preferred or if there was the possibility of conflict of interest. This interchangeability of roles also facilitated the set-up of a 'round-the-clock social emergency service.

Professional Profile

The model of the highly specialized professional 'helper' or person who 'made' you better was not considered appropriate for the Atikamekw context. It was therefore decided to work with community workers who would all have community development as a common field of expertise. In addition they would have only partially specialized knowledge of another particular field of activity. It was hoped this would avoid professional jealousies and segregation.

Training

This is not to say that community workers were not to be trained. To the contrary, an innovative university-level program was set up specifically to support this integrated professions approach. It was a three-year bachelor degree work/study program which, although accredited by l'Université du Québec à Chicoutimi, was run by l'Institut éducatif et culturel Atikamekw-Montagnais which set curriculum and hired instructors. The program was designed around a common core program in community development in an Aboriginal setting.

This occupied all of the first year and decreasing parts of the second and third years. Specialized courses in social work, community health and alcohol and drug abuse prevention completed second- and third-year instruction.

Clientele

Fundamentally, though intervention may often have to be centred around specific individuals, the health and social services team was to see their clients in as broad a context as possible. Their preferred focuses of attention were consequently to be the community, the extended family and the nuclear family.

Practical Obstacles

It is obvious that the full implementation of a model such as that just described would have necessitated a fair bit of control over all aspects – legal, financial, and professional – of the management of health and social services. It would in fact have been possible only under a complete takeover of jurisdiction which, of course, was never possible. Other factors also impede the implementation of the model.

Conforming With Provincial Legal Requirements

Before 1988 Atikamekw workers called on the legal system only when absolutely necessary, and legal requirements were met on a case-by-case basis with all the flexibility the law allowed. All other cases were handled voluntarily.

In 1988, DIAND used its financial powers to impose the signing of agreements with the provincial social services agencies, with the effect of making the Atikamekw agency a ward of the two provincial agencies that it had, until then, dealt with on an equal footing. This situation resulted in the erosion of the autonomous practice of Atikamekw workers. The problem has now been exacerbated by the recent adoption in Quebec of strict bureaucratic guidelines monitored through the production of paperwork in order to reduce waiting lists. This has had the perverse effect of slowing down actual case management productivity by Atikamekw workers, although the latter never had a waiting list problem.

Unfortunately the 1900 agreements facilitated the use by Atikamekw workers of the long arm of the law. The number of cases brought to court and of youth placed in outside institutions and foster homes increased significantly.

Low Adaptability of Youth Protection Legislation

Despite the obligation for Aboriginal groups to conform to this law and the very evident cultural differences involved, no efforts were made to adapt this law to Aboriginal reality.

Severity and Prevalence of Problems

One constant obstacle was the severity and prevalence of problems. The volume of cases was always very heavy, and some problems were too severe to treat through only partially specialized personnel.

Limits of Model

These include a rather limited range of professional competencies and ultimately a limited choice of professionals on the part of clients. Also, without the involvement of the judicial element, the level of authority vested informally in a few individual workers over the destinies of some families would ultimately be unacceptable. It is important, then, that such a model be linked to the development of a local judicial authority.

Lack of Clear Health Objectives

This process would have been greatly facilitated had goals with respect to the attainment of individual and community health been set and shared with and by the population.

Limits of Personnel

Several workers had histories of personal problems, which at times affected both their work and the public's perception of them. This of course limited their professional effectiveness.

Financial Limits

The agency was on the one hand underfunded, considering the volume of services, and on the other required to adhere to inflexible conditions. There were also effects on the delivery of services. These included very heavy caseloads for individual workers and the resultant professional fatigue. Most important, however, financial limits restricted our capacity to set up adequate professional supervision and support of workers at the local level.

Limited Training Opportunities

Though the training program described above was quite successful, it was not possible to make it a permanent program because of university regulations, and it was cancelled.

Low Priority of Health and Social Services Programs

Once a partial (administrative) takeover of health and social services had been achieved, Atikamekw authorities at both the national and the local level tended to view health and social services as a relatively low priority item.

Favourable Elements

Despite all the difficulties just outlined, some measure of success was very definitely achieved, to a great extent because of the following elements.

Dedication of Personnel

Team spirit was high, and support for members who suffered momentary downturns was always strong. Another very important factor that played in favour of success was the involvement of health and social services personnel at all levels of the community, both as volunteers and as elected officials.

Relative Flexibility of Provincial Agency Representatives

The provincial officials with whom formal and informal arrangements were made were willing, for the most part, to accept the most liberal interpretations possible of legislation and procedure.

Conclusions

Despite this list of difficulties, implementation of the practice model was fairly successful. It was possible to achieve good progress in the development of healthier communities, though on both the individual and the community level there are many ups and downs and a lot remains to be done. It is nonetheless possible to identify specific factors that would greatly improve the workings and results of what we have called the integrated approach:

- Programming should be centred on clearly stated health goals that have been set through needs analysis and community consultation.
- The model is best applicable in the context of complete autonomy, which includes at least the pertinent judicial powers.
- It would be preferable to combine health and social services funds into one global budget.
- The core integrated team should be backed up by easily accessible specialized professionals.
- Efforts should be make to encourage youth to pursue studies in related fields in order to ensure continuity without relying completely on special training programs.

Four Community Health Initiatives

The Inuulitsivik Health Centre and its Maternity Project

*Aani Tuluguk**

The Inuulitsivik Health Centre (IHC) was incorporated in 1982 under terms of reference that were set in Chapter 15 of the James Bay and Northern Quebec Agreement. IHC initially took over the management of former federal nursing stations in the seven communities of the Hudson Bay region of Nunavik (Northern Quebec). Mandates as a hospital centre, a social services centre and later a community health centre were added. We are thus a truly multi-service organization, and much emphasis is put on multi-disciplinary team approach to medical as well as social interventions.

The Inuulitsivik board of directors is composed mainly of elected representatives, one for each of the seven villages and four from among the staff. Elections are held normally every three years, and board members' terms are renewable. As any other public health and social services establishment in Quebec, the health centre is provided with a global budget base onto which specific program funds – distributed through the regional council – are then grafted. The latter portion has been increasing in relative size over the past few years as this is the approach now favoured by the provincial ministry of health and social services. Home care and mental health are examples of programs funded in this fashion.

* Inuulitsivik Hospital and Social Services Centre, Povungnituk, Quebec.

The maternity project was developed at the time the 25-bed hospital was being built in 1985-86. With support from the Native Women's Association, a tour of the communities was organized to gather the points of view of the population concerning maternity services. A strong desire was expressed at the time

- to bring deliveries back to the communities; and
- to involve Aboriginal personnel in the provision of perinatal services without compromising safety and quality of care.

The choice we made was to develop a project whereby a maternity centre would be established in Povungnituk using resources allocated to the new hospital but under a working model that would be exportable to other communities at a later stage. Inuit midwives would within it be trained locally and progressively become the primary care givers in team with our physicians and nurses.

The midwives are active members of the Council of Physicians, Dentists, Pharmacists and Midwives (CPDPM), an advisory body to the board of directors that concerns itself with issues of quality of care within the establishment. The Perinatal Committee, which is chaired by a midwife, meets weekly to review prenatal files and issue recommendations with regard to risk grading, place of delivery and perinatal care plan. It also develops practice guidelines and protocols on behalf of the CPDPM in the area of perinatality. More than 775 deliveries have been done in Povungnituk since the opening of the maternity program in October 1986, and since July 1991 one Inuit midwife has been granted full privileges for this practice, so we can truly say that nearly one-third of deliveries are now done entirely in Inuktitut with only local staff in attendance. Three more Inuit women are involved in our training program at this point.

The health centre is finally awaiting news from the ministry for the construction of a new nursing station in Inukjuak that would include space for a maternity service there. Plans have also been made for a similar project in Salluit, a community of approximately 900 people.

As a health centre we have many of the necessary tools to involve Aboriginal people in the provision of services in their own communities. What we need now is more openness and flexibility from professional corporations, regulation makers and the school system to allow more or most of the training to take place in the North, using available professional resources there. It would also be helpful if interprovincial barriers to professional mobility (a problem more acute in Quebec) could be dropped to allow us the possibility of recruiting people with specific skills and interest in this process. It is our belief that just as we have been able to train clinical midwives (as well as audiology technicians – another one of our projects), so could we just as effectively train X-ray, laboratory, and dental and medical records technicians, as well as nursing staff, using apprenticeship models.

Anishnawbe Health

*Priscilla George and Barbra Nahwegahbow**

Anishnawbe Health is a culture-based multi-service health centre located in downtown Toronto. It is incorporated as a non-profit corporation and began providing health services in 1989. It is governed by a nine-member board of directors elected from and by the Aboriginal community. A staff of thirty includes administrative staff, street workers, counsellors, AIDS education worker, registered nurses, physicians and other clerical and program staff.

Core funding is provided by the Ontario Ministry of Health, and additional project funding comes from the City of Toronto and other provincial government ministries. The federal government provides no funding whatsoever to help us meet the healing needs of our community.

The community served by Anishnawbe Health is large, diverse and scattered over a huge geographical area. Estimates of the Toronto Aboriginal population put it at somewhere between 50,000 and 70,000. Many different Aboriginal nations from across Canada are represented: Okanagan, Micmac, Cree, Ojibwa, Mohawk, Métis and Inuit to name a few. Some are long-time residents of Toronto, some were born there, many are newly arrived, and still others are simply passing through. Our client base also includes those who travel on a regular basis from First Nations communities outside Toronto to participate in our traditional programs. Our clients come from a wide range of economic and social circumstances, from the homeless street people to those who have the means to live fairly comfortably.

* Respectively, president and executive director, Anishnawbe Health, Toronto, Ontario.

But the people served by Anishnawbe Health have something in common – they're looking for a sense of Aboriginal identity and a sense of belonging to the Aboriginal community. They're suffering from the effects of the oppression that Aboriginal people have lived under for too long and they manifest it in many different ways – mentally, emotionally, spiritually and physically.

In order to facilitate healing/empowerment, Anishnawbe Health does two things:

- we help people gain an understanding of our history as Aboriginal people – our political, social and economic situation; and
- we help people learn our traditional ways by providing access to ceremonies, elders, traditional healers, teachings, etc.

For Anishnawbe Health, being a culture-based health centre means that traditional healing approaches and traditional healers are at the core of the organization and provide the primary methods of healing our people. It means that western medical practitioners play a secondary role and act as support or 'helpers' to the traditional healers.

Traditional healers, elders and traditional teachers are brought into Anishnawbe Health on a regular basis. The demand from the community for access to these people has been overwhelming. Traditional healing is certainly cost-effective because it does not entail hospital stays, surgery, costly prescription drugs, costly and invasive tests, or referrals to high-priced specialists. Traditional healing is a very empowering process for the individual and his/her family since they become active participants in their own healing, e.g., gathering and preparing medicines.

There are some serious challenges that we face in terms of meeting our community's demand for traditional healing:

- The scarcity of traditional healers, teachers and elders who are credible and who are willing to travel to a large urban centre such as Toronto to work with our people.
- The token recognition given to the value of traditional healing by government departments such as the Ontario Ministry of Health and federal Medical Services Branch as evidenced by the financial resources that are made available – our annual budget for physicians is almost $300,000, while the budget for our traditional healing program is $45,000. Medical Services Branch continues to reject all of our applications for funding assistance to bring healers into our health centre.
- Our own people have been so damaged by the colonization process that they either fear or place little value on our own traditional healers and our healing approaches.

Because we are an urban health centre, the major issue that requires immediate attention is acknowledgement of federal responsibility for status First Nations people living off-reserve. Our own political leadership needs to ensure that this gets put on the agenda. Historically, those of us who make our homes in urban areas are forgotten in political negotiations. We sometimes feel our rights get sold out to gain concessions for our brothers and sisters on-reserve. But, like them, we also need to assert our Aboriginal rights so that we can regain our political, social and economic health.

The Kahnawake Mowhawk Experience: Responsibility for Controlling Our Own Health Care Services

*Keith Leclaire**

The Kateri Memorial Hospital Centre is a community medical initiative presented by the Mohawks of Kahnawake. The history of the Hospital, which began in 1905 in Kahnawake, was presented with special focus on the 1955 community struggle to keep Kateri Memorial Hospital Centre open when closure appeared imminent. Also highlighted were the 1980 events leading to the construction of the new facility.

The development of a nation-to-nation agreement, the continued development of an unincorporated institution under community control, and the need to ensure accountability directly to the community over a regional health structure were presented.

Discussion of the need to ensure First Nations health be a federal responsibility was highlighted. Emphasis upon the Hospital's position that the federal government transfers federal health funding to the province via the *Established Programs Financing Act* and the *Canada Assistance Plan* were discussed.

Health and Welfare Canada's current Indian Health Transfer initiative was touched upon. Kateri Hospital and the Mohawks of Kahnawake view this process as simply allowing First Nations to take over programs with preset policies and regulations. In short, Health and Welfare Canada's Health Transfer initiative allows administrative authority to transfer program dollars from one program to another. Actual health services control is not transferred.

---

* Director of Administration, Kateri Memorial Hospital Centre, Kahnawake, Quebec.

Factors contributing to Kateri's smooth operation were highlighted. Participatory management practices, the development of a mission statement, philosophy, goals and objectives at the various departmental levels, good communication between 130 staff and 12 departments and a focus upon employee skills enhancement summarized these factors.

Suggestions to allow other communities to learn from Kateri's experience noted the following major points.

- When there is no political action taking place at the community level, make it happen.
- Develop and nurture a core of Indian health advocates to deal with the provincial and federal bureaucracy.
- Strengthen the skills of community people, especially in assertiveness with the bureaucracy and in planning for training, competency and evaluation.
- Make sure outside planners know that you are obligated and prepared to do whatever is necessary to achieve your goals. In other words, "walk your talk."

To accomplish these things, community planners must ask:

- What is achievable and what is not? Unrealistic expectations lead to failure, which makes a poor foundation for future success.
- Are human resources consistent with organizational needs? If needs change, do we have the resources to adapt?
- Do we have the proper space to be productive? Kateri's 1986 move to the new building precipitated a 36 per cent increase in out-patient use of the facility.
- Have we considered the feasibility of a fund-raising arm? The Kateri Hospital Foundation was created two years ago in response to the Hospital's need for additional funding from outside the community.

The presentation concluded with a clear understanding that Kateri Hospital's process has been long, slow and sometimes very frustrating. As there must be both a time to laugh and a time to cry, there must be a balance to compensate for the hard times and the good times.

The Nuu-Chah-Nulth Experience: A Descriptive Review of West Coast People's Struggle to Rebuild Healthy Communities

*Richard Watt and Simon Read**

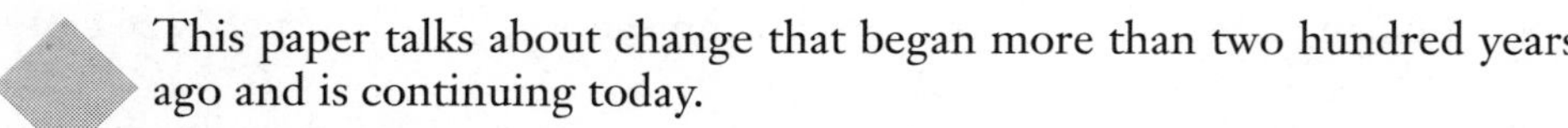

This paper talks about change that began more than two hundred years ago and is continuing today.

Over the past three hundred years, history has taken the Nuu-chah-nulth nations from healthy self-sufficient populations of tens of thousands to a colonialized state of a few thousand, through to the beginnings of recovery of self-government.

At no time did the Hawi'i (Hereditary Chiefs) enter into treaties that define the basis for coexistence of Nuu-chah-nulth-aht with the occupying populations.

The Nuu-chah-nulth Tribal Council is in its third decade of working toward the restoration of self-government, using a two-pronged strategy. One side is the constitutional and political process, which will result in the first government-to-government treaties for the Nuu-chah-nulth nations. The other, which is clearly an interim step, is to acquire the maximum degree of control over all existing government services.

In taking control of programs, three major issues stand out that have received concentrated attention from the Nuu-chah-nulth Health Board.

* Nuu-chah-nulth Health Board, Port Alberni, British Columbia.

One is the need to overcome the consequences of five generations of colonial government, which are reflected at all levels, from the number of suicide attempts to the shortage of culturally trained and professionally trained health professionals.

The second is the need to reconstruct the Nuu-chah-nulth system of wellness out of the fragments that have survived through the generations, against the weight of dependence that has built up on the medical model of treatment.

The third is the amount of effort expended in trying to path together a holistic approach out of the assortment of program and funding sources with their inconsistent objectives and requirements.

The original holistic view of wellness, embodied in the words *thlim?uxtih* and *esahk*, is described and related to the impact of colonization and institutionalization.

The Nuu-chah-nulth health transfer is placed in the context of the expanded involvement in health services, which has continued since the early 1970s, and the changes that are continuing today.

Efforts to address the issues of developing health providers, restoring mental wellness, and managing financial and jurisdictional issues are described.

In the short term, issues to be resolved include control over non-insured health benefits, better services to urban members, provision of personal home care, follow-up on residential school issues, increased funding from the provincial health care system, and further development of health and social services based on a traditional model of family responsibilities.

In the longer term, we look forward to the day when there is a Nuu-chah-nulth government operating with a secure resource base. We expect this to emerge through negotiations under the British Columbia Treaty Commission process. We suggest that interim measures should take into account the reconstruction that is needed to repair the damage of a hundred years of attempted deculturation.

The antagonistic approach of the present criminal justice system is an obstacle to dealing with the many family violence issues in our communities. We believe that traditional systems of maintaining balance in the community need to be reconstructed, including laws developed from their traditional base.

The Nuu-chah-nulth Tribal Council has initiated a process of dramatic change in which health and social services play a major role. Rapid changes will continue, and the health and social services roles will change as well. We foresee the emergence of a generation of healthy self-sustaining communities to follow the present generation of change.

KEYNOTE SPEAKERS

Global Nutrition and the Holistic Environment of Indigenous Peoples

*Harriet V. Kuhnlein**

This presentation began with a series of slides that set the stage for the audience to remember the richness and beauty of the traditional food systems of Indigenous peoples. During the presentation, the foods shown and the area the foods are from were explained. The presentation emphasized four major functions that Aboriginal foods and total diets contribute to Aboriginal peoples:

- Food is an anchor to culture and personal well-being.
- Food is the direct link between the environment and human health. It is the avenue by which a healthy environment can provide complete nutrition and a sense of integration and wellness.
- Food is an important indicator of cultural expression, and
- Food is an essential agent to promote holistic health and culture.

Declining Use of Traditional Food Systems

It is becoming more and more clear that traditional food systems derived from the local, natural environments of Indigenous peoples are on the decline throughout the planet. For a variety of reasons and external pressures, foods made available through industrialization and market economies are replacing traditional foods in the diets of Aboriginal peoples.

* Ph.D., R.D., Centre for Nutrition and the Environment of Indigenous Peoples, McGill University.

One small but significant example of this phenomenon is the use of cow-parsnip (*Heracleum lanatum*) by the Aboriginal people of the B.C. west coast. This is a traditional green vegetable harvested in the spring, with care taken to remove the caustic outer peel. It provided a welcome change from winter diets. Its taste and nutrients are similar to celery, and it is remembered by Nuxalk elders (who call it *xwiq* in their language) as a pleasant taste treat.[1] However, during this century, the use of cow-parsnip has been slowly declining, to the point that it is rarely used today by Nuxalk women. The elders still remember it, but younger women often do not even recognize the plant or know how to prepare it. The vegetable was never used preserved, but was used fresh in season (see Figure l).

Another example of the declining use of traditional foods in favour of foods from markets is taken from the work I contributed to with the community of Broughton Island, a community representative in many ways of the Inuit communities of Baffin Island in the Eastern Arctic. The Baffin Inuit have a rich and

Figure 1

Nuxalk Use of Cow-parsnip (*Heracleum Lanatum*)

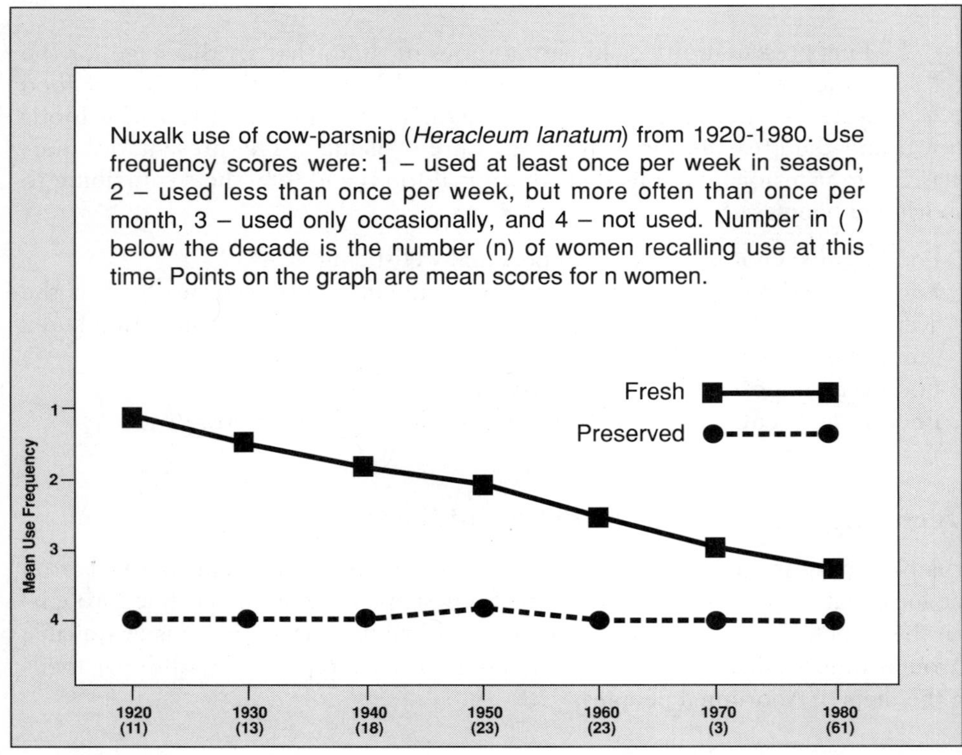

Source: Kuhnlein, H.V., Turner, N.J. Cow-parsnip (*Heracleum lanatum Michx.)*: An Indigenous Vegetable of Native People of Northwestern North America. J. Ethnobiol. 6:309-324, 1986.

varied traditional food system, but today the use of foods provided through commercial outlets provides the majority of daily calories to people of all ages. Figure 2 shows that for women in the 20 to 40 years of age group, approximately 70 per cent of their annual average dietary energy is derived from market foods. Even in this remote area of the Canadian Arctic, people are buying the majority of their foods, rather than taking them from the traditional natural resources. There is variability across the seasons, with the season providing the most market food calories being October and November, and the season providing the least being June-July, when substantial traditional food harvesting is taking place.[2]

In the Western Arctic, another community where we have looked at the extent of use of traditional foods is Colville Lake, Northwest Territories. This small community of about 60 people is considered even more remote than Broughton Island because there is less access to supplies of market foods. Here the Sahtú

Figure 2

Use of Market and Traditional Foods by Adult Women, Broughton Island 1987-1988 (as a % of Total Energy Intake)

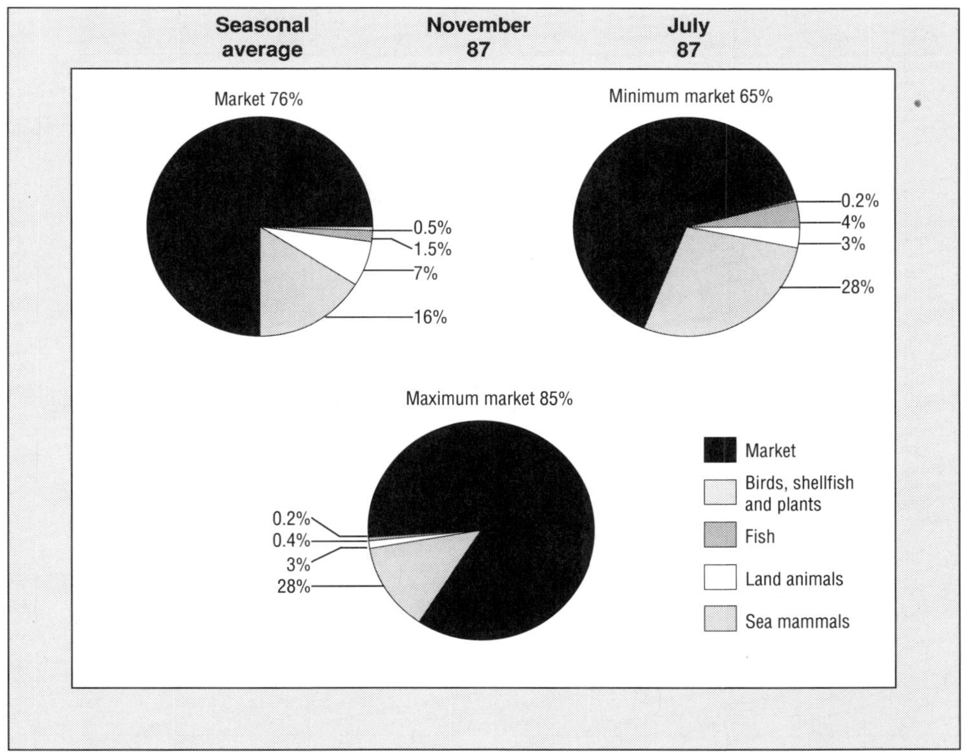

Source: Kuhnlein, H.V.(1989). Nutritional and Toxicological Components of Inuit Diets in Broughton Island, Northwest Territories. Contract report to the Department of Health, Northwest Territories, Yellowknife, Canada.

Dene/Métis maximize their use of market foods in the spring season, May and June, when their harvest of traditional foods is most limited.[3] As Figure 3 shows, in winter and summer when they are having more traditional foods, 30 per cent of calories are still coming from market foods.

It needs to be emphasized that even though a large percentage of calories comes from the use of market foods, the people in these communities are still deriving a major portion of their essential dietary nutrients (protein, essential fatty acids, iron, zinc, and other essential nutrients) from the use of the traditional food resources. It is not too difficult to understand why this is the case when we look at a list of the most frequently used market foods, as shown in Table 1.[4] The list of the foods used most often is remarkably similar in all of the Aboriginal communities where I have worked in the last 10 to 15 years. What we see are low-cost, quick-energy, and low-nutrient quality foods. It is not surprising, then,

Figure 3

Use of Market and Traditional Foods by Adult Women, Colville Lake 1988-1990 (as a % of Total Energy Intake)

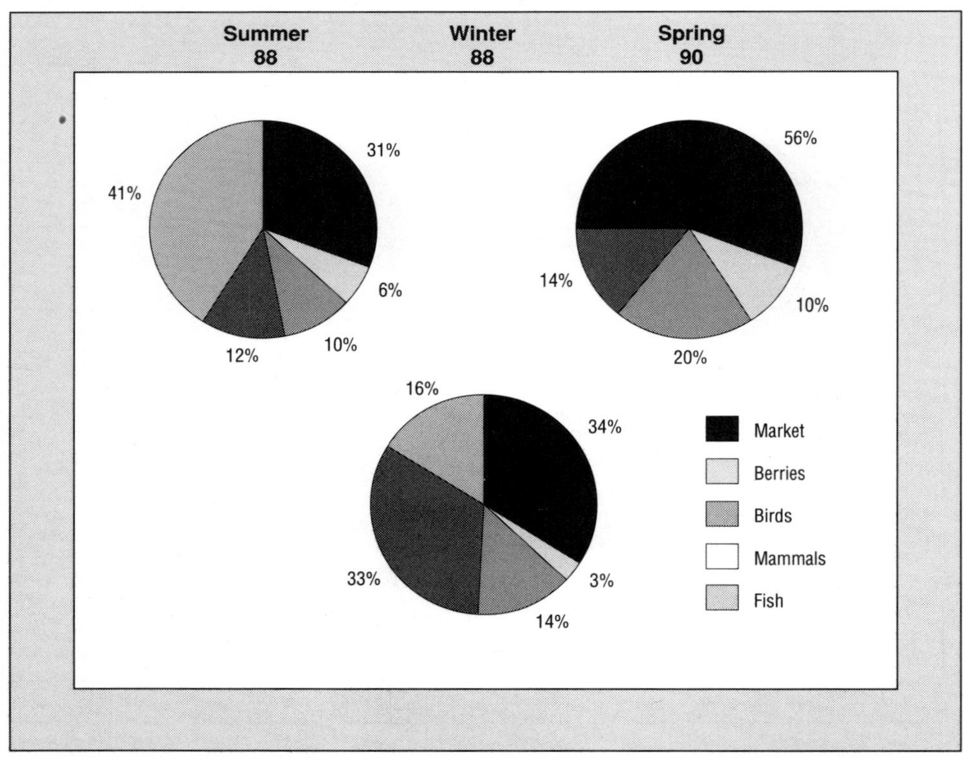

Source: Kuhnlein, H.V.(1989). Dietary Evaluation of Food, Nutrients, and Contaminants in Fort Good Hope and Colville Lake, Northwest Territories. Contract Report to the Department of Health, Northwest Territories, Yellownknife, Canada.

that the nutritional status of Indigenous peoples declines when they stop using their traditional animal and plant foods taken from the natural environment and replace them with foods such as these. This is especially evident when there is a circumstance of poverty and low expendable income to drive the supply/demand market equation to provide higher-cost, more nutritious foods to remote communities such as fresh meats, vegetables and fruits.

Table 1

Most frequently consumed market foods: all Broughton Island surveys

Reports[a]	Food item
217	Tea
194	Sugar
142	Bannock, biscuits
129	All fruit 'ades', Kool-Aid™ (dry mixes)
108	Crackers, pilot biscuits
82	Evaporated milk
61	White bread
46	Ready-to-eat breakfast cereals
42	Coffee
40	Butter
39	Cola-type carbonated beverages
31	Non-caffeinated carbonated beverages, popsicles
30	All types of chips
29	Non-dairy coffee whiteners
28	Luncheon meats, sausage, salami
27	Chicken (stewed, broiled, baked, fried)
26	Eggs, fried or boiled
26	Vegetable Fat, Crisco™, hardened shortenings
26	All noodle soups: canned, dried, or instant
23	Mashed potatoes, instant or homemade
22	All jellies, james, jelly candies, gum drops
21	Beef, ground or steak (assumed 20% fat)

a Foods were coded only once for each 24-hour recall record. 'Reports' is the average number of records for all surveys, where the mean total of foods recorded was 319.

Source: Kinloch, D., Kuhnlein, H., Muir, D.C.G. Inuit foods and diet: a preliminary assessment of benefits and risk. The Science of the Total Environment 122:247-278, 1992.

Considering the reasons in the broadest, global view for this unfortunate nutritional health circumstance where people are replacing their highly nutritious traditional foods with low-nutrient-density market foods, there is a complex but recurring rationale. Most importantly, this involves food industrialization, market economies, and colonization in one form or another. There are population pressures on the land and sea resources; education in its broadest sense and exposure to others; media and private enterprise advertising; and lack of access to traditional food resources because of limited time, energy or equipment for hunting, fishing or harvesting. Other reasons are migration from rural to urban areas; changing food preferences and health beliefs, in part because there is an imperfect transfer of the wisdom of the elders to younger generations; and health personnel on reserves and in communities and hamlets who have little knowledge and interest in the traditional culture, which includes the environment/wellness dyad. These are all part of the problem, with each community and individual experiencing differential effects from these varied components of the rationale.

My friend and colleague, Laurie Montour, from Kahnawake and Walpole Island, described the knowledge of traditional foods in Aboriginal communities today when she wrote, "Sadly, though, there is the realization that the foods themselves, and the skills and practices in using them, are slowly dying. There is a triple threat: the loss of knowledgeable elders, leaving no one to teach; the loss of culture, leaving little incentive to learn; and the loss of healthy ecosystems, leaving no foods available to take even if one wanted to."[5]

Following on this, the more recent knowledge and publicity about environmental contamination have caused another serious, if not critical, wound to the use of traditional food systems. At a time when our knowledge of the human health effects of specific contaminants is far from complete, people in communities are being frightened away from the use of their traditionally known culturally-relevant food resources. Concerns about mercury, PCBs, cadmium, toxaphene and other organochlorine contaminants are under intensive review in this country, because of the impact these contaminants may have on the health of Aboriginal peoples who still take some of their food resources from the natural environment.

To illustrate, again using the hamlet of Broughton Island as an example of Baffin communities, review of the extent of traditional food use across seasons demonstrated the variety of foods used and their complex patterns of use. Analyses of the various foods for PCBs permitted a calculation of the seasonal and average annual intake by age and sex (see Figures 4 and 5). The project demonstrated that while the use of traditional foods is substantial, and critically important for nutrition, the intake of PCBs is worrisome, but still within accepted guidelines for tolerable daily risk on a population basis.[2]

Figure 4

Total Inuit Food Consumed Per Day
Total Population (adjusted), Broughton Island, July 87-May 88

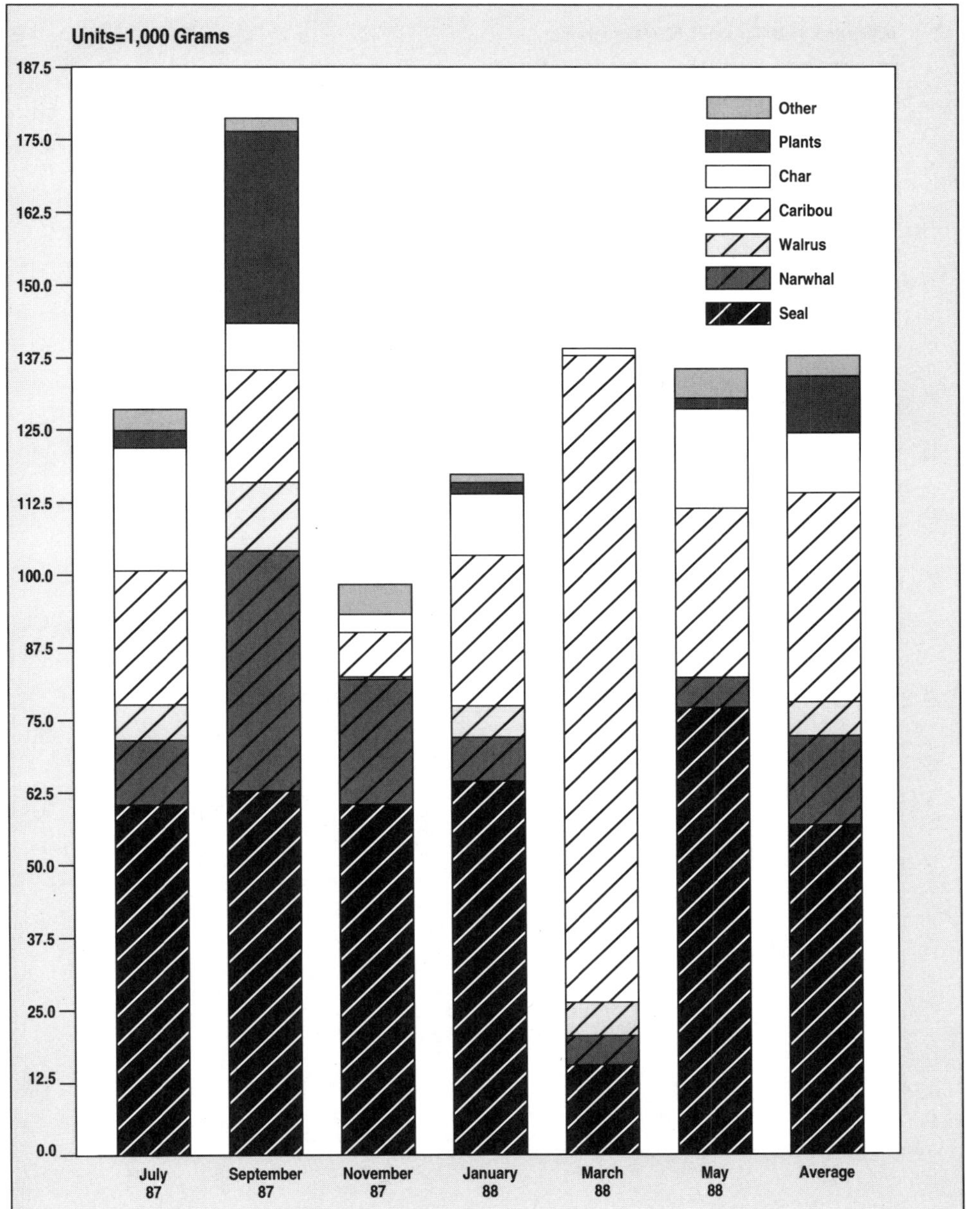

Source: Kuhnlein, H. Nutritional and Toxicological Components of Inuit Diets in Broughton Island, Northwest Territories. McGill University, 1989.

Figure 5

Total PCB's Consumed Per Day
Total Population (adjusted), Broughton Island, July 87-May 88

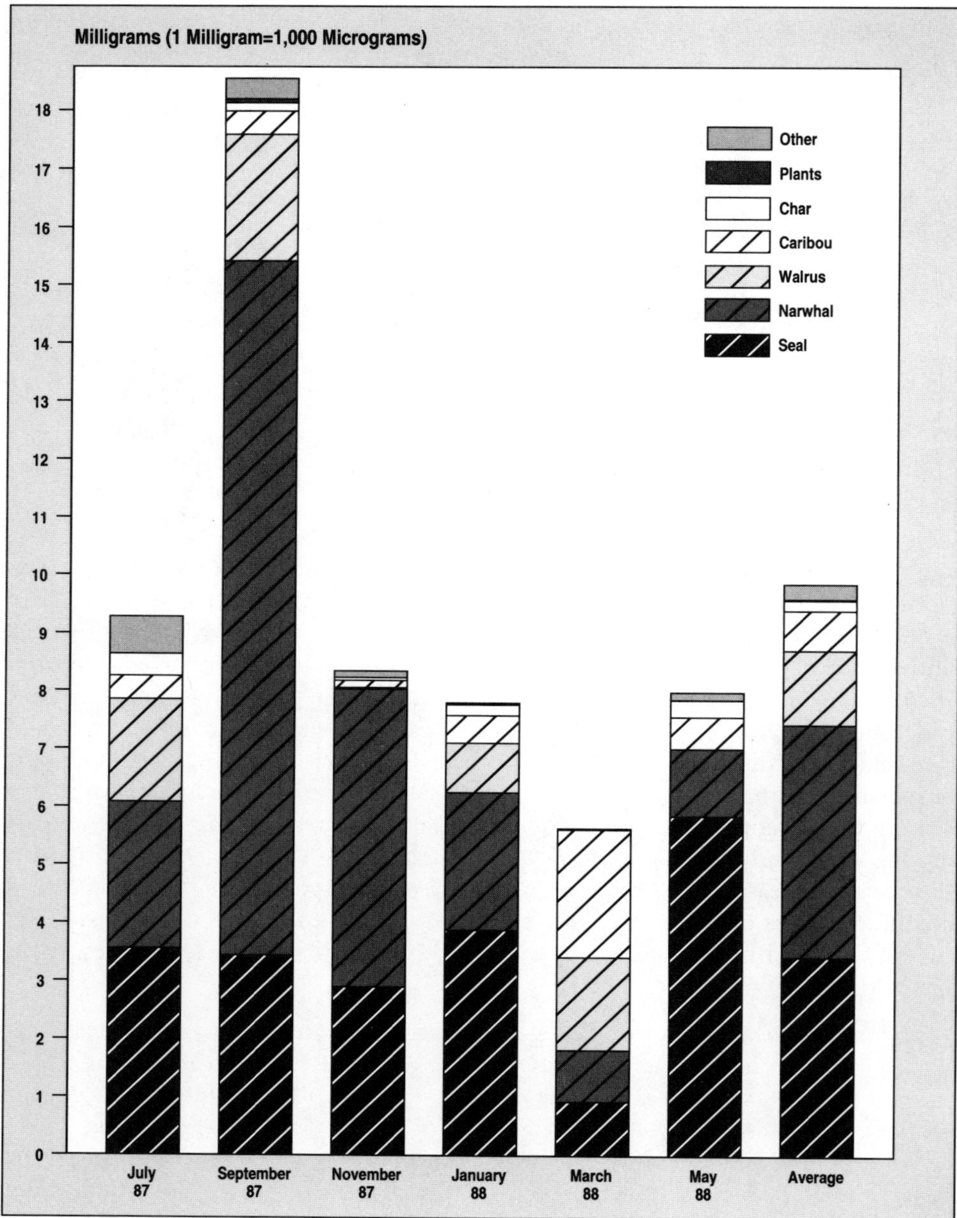

Source: Kuhnlein, H. Nutritional and Toxicological Components of Inuit Diets in Broughton Island, Northwest Territories. McGill University, 1989.

Clearly, research of this kind is needed, not only to identify severe ecosystem illness and to prevent human health effects, but also to devise guidelines for intake that consider the benefits of the foods to individuals as well as the risks of contaminant intake. Another important effect of this research is the stimulation of national and international action to stop polluting the planet. It is unfortunate, but a reality, that the food systems of Aboriginal peoples are the best sentinels for this kind of inquiry and will be a most effective motive for political action.

What I want to emphasize here is that traditional food resources of Aboriginal peoples, and the use of these foods, are important for so many reasons. The declining use of these foods is not just a symptom of a larger system that is failing, but it is a major organ in the system of environmental and cultural well-being that needs immediate and vital attention. This is so for Indigenous people globally, wherever the forces of deculturalization and environmental destruction are powerful. Finding solutions to return traditional food systems to the control and benefit of local Indigenous peoples would contribute greatly to the prognosis of planetary health, which affects all of humanity now and in the future.

Changing Nutritional Environments of Indigenous Peoples

The loss in use of traditional food systems, the simultaneous increase in use of high-energy, low-nutrient-density industrialized foods available through market networks, and the coincident changes in lifestyle have resulted in well documented changes in disease patterns of Indigenous peoples. This is true for rural and remote communities, but also for people close to and in urban environments. The rich, the lucky, and the well educated may be able to find a healthy diet among the foods of well stocked urban markets, but that is not to say that it happens. The diseases of the so-called western diet and lifestyle are striking rural and urban, rich and poor alike. Chronic diseases that were unknown among tribal peoples and those of non-western cultures are now on the increase among them and building into an impressive list. Obesity and diabetes, the cardiovascular diseases, cancer, infant morbidity and mortality in higher frequencies, alcoholism, loss of teeth and clear eyesight, and rampant infections are all part of this diet and health picture that has emerged for Indigenous peoples in the last 100 years.

In the non-industrialized world, in countries such as India, China and Guatemala, where Indigenous peoples are still fighting the battle of getting enough food energy and protein, these chronic diseases are not of the same magnitude, of course. However, the wealthier segments of those societies are finding themselves afflicted with the western-lifestyle diseases and are realizing that these are certain to follow upon development or migration to find the so-called better way of life.[6]

Is there something that can be accomplished for better health of Aboriginal peoples by paying greater attention to the benefits of traditional food systems? Surely, it is not reasonable to expect a return to the past, to the way people were living and eating 100 years ago. In my view, to answer this question, the best approach is to take a cold, hard look at what's going on and to try to reverse the trends, or at least to try to steer the ship.

It is time for action and leadership to stop the global loss of traditional food system knowledge and the loss of tangible and meaningful links to the environment and to human health and social well-being that are unique to Aboriginal peoples living on their traditional lands. It is time for Aboriginal peoples to take back the traditional food systems and to use them to their best advantage as decided in every community. At this time traditional foods are slip-sliding away with every passing generation, and with the loss of every elder who has lived close to the land. It is also time to take back traditional knowledge of the environment and how it gives health to people in their food. This is teachable information for the schools and should be insisted upon in the information offered in health centres and in the training curricula of health professionals serving Aboriginal peoples. When it comes to issues of health, traditional food systems and food contaminants, it is time to strike a balance between loss, demoralization and scare tactics on the one hand and, on the other, assuming the collective and personal knowledge and control needed to make a difference for confidence in the total food system – both traditional and market foods – for community health promotion.

Demedicalizing the Approach to Food and Nutrition

One of the suggested topics for this keynote address was the demedicalization of health. In my view, there is no better place for demedicalization than in the area of nutrition. The medical networks of academics, policy makers and practitioners, as we know them internationally, focus on disease: how to find what's wrong, and how to fix it; how to make the human body well again after it gets sick. A tiny fraction of the financial and personnel resources for medical teaching, research and practice goes to finding what is right in an individual or a community and keeping it that way. This concept goes beyond current practices of health promotion that emphasize eating a healthy diet and getting more exercise using southern Canadian health education techniques; it means looking at the existing community with its local culture and environmental realities and building on the positive elements already there. Indigenous cultures have always held a holistic view on the intertwining of environment, culture and health through the traditional food system and all it offers – nutrition, outdoor activities, community spirit, sharing, etc. – the emphasis being on what is right and healthy and how to get people to take better advantage of it.

Two examples of this concept of the need for the demedicalization of nutrition are offered for your consideration. The first goes back to my days as a nutrition graduate student and my dissertation research with the Hopi. At that time there was very little scientific documentation on the nutritional values of the traditional Hopi foods. In fact, that was partly why I was there. At the same time, (mid-1970s), there was an increasing and alarming rate of diabetes on the reservation. Because the traditional Hopi foods are often made of corn, especially blue corn, and because there was no documentation on carbohydrate, protein, fat, and calorie contents of foods such as piki and nokviki, the physicians in the local Indian Health Service clinics were admonishing the Hopi to avoid all traditional Hopi foods completely ("they're just starch"), to take their insulin, and to eat only a carefully prescribed diet of imported foods. What was happening was that people who fell into diabetes because of lifestyle changes were driven even further away from the diet and lifestyle that could make them well again. Fortunately, with increased knowledge on the nutrient profiles on the Hopi foods, and improved methods of dietary counselling, this is no longer the blanket recommendation on the Hopi reservation.[7]

The second example concerns childhood blindness in developing countries, particularly in tribal communities, which is caused by vitamin A deficiency. Every year a half million new cases of childhood blindness are caused in large part by insufficient quantities of vegetables, fruits, and animal foods in children's diets because of lack of access to land to grow foods, environmental destruction, and poverty so severe there is not enough food to eat. The solution to this problem that is now promoted by physicians in the World Health Organization is to give capsules of vitamin A at the time of immunizations. There is only passing mention that vitamin A capsules are not a sustainable solution to this severe nutritional problem affecting the whole community, that the real answer lies within the traditional food system in each local environment, knowledge how to use it, and access to it. The medical band-aid will not solve the real problem. In fact, it is probably impeding the real solution to the problem of an unhealthy ecosystem by instilling a complacency that something is being done.

In both of these examples, the medical solution is not what is going to make the difference for a sustainable nutrition and environment. The difference will be made in finding what is right in the traditional knowledge of the environment and the foods it provides, putting that knowledge forward, and implementing it for the health of the people.

A Strategy to Promote Traditional Food Systems

The Aboriginal leadership in Canada is highly regarded internationally for its success in promoting and protecting the cultural traditions, rights and responsibilities of Canadian Aboriginal peoples. For the situation of declining use of traditional foods to be turned around, it will take strong leadership at both the national and the local community level. It will take commitment on the part of entire families within communities.

This kind of grassroots movement for community recognition and documentation of their traditional knowledge has already been taking place in several areas in Canada. Port Simpson, Nuxalk Nation, Shuswap Nation and the Mohawks of Kahnawake, among others, have begun to implement traditional knowledge of food, environment, culture and lifestyle into the elementary school curriculum. The knowledge and wisdom of the elders regarding the environment and its integration with food, culture and self-identity is an important concept. It needs to be documented carefully for future generations and put to use with the best communication techniques available within communities and for sharing among communities. An essential aspect in the training of young people is the knowledge and respect for an environmentally sustainable food system, from both traditional and market foods. This kind of training comes best from the home and the community, as well as the school system. The subject matter is suitable for curricula in the elementary through the secondary schools.

At the professional level, health career programs for Aboriginal people should be fostered, and these should clearly include the professions in nutrition and dietetics. Training within these programs needs to include substantial information on the integration of environmental integrity with culture and nutritional health, and how Aboriginal foods promote health in the local environment. At this moment there are fewer than a half dozen practising Aboriginal dietitians/nutritionists in Canada. Improving this statistic will greatly assist the solution to the problem of nutrition education in a sustainable environment for Aboriginal peoples.

Finally, in my view, it is critically important that health professionals who seek employment in health services for Aboriginal clients be well informed about the contributions and values that the local environment and culture, and the traditional food system, offers to the community and to the individual. This holistic approach includes the best of Aboriginal values on health and social issues, and it is a real service to communities for health professionals working there to build on these concepts and practices.

The integration of knowledge on environmental quality and cultural identity to promote the understanding and reasonable use of traditional food systems will greatly enhance quality of life and self-care for Indigenous peoples.

Notes

1. Kuhnlein, H.V. and N.J. Turner (1987) Cow-parsnip (*Heracleum lanatum*): an indigenous vegetable of Native People of Northwestern North America. J. Ethnobiol. 6(2):309-324; Kuhnlein, H.V. (1992) Change in the use of traditional foods by the Nuxalk of British Columbia. In: Pelto, G.H. and L.A. Vargas, eds. *Perspectives on Dietary Change. Studies in Nutrition and Society*. Special issue. Ecol. of Food and Nutr. 27(3-4):259-282.
2. Kuhnlein, H.V. (1989) Nutritional and Toxicological Components of Inuit Diets in Broughton Island, Northwest Territories. Contract report to the Department of Health, Yellowknife.
3. Kuhnlein, H.V. (1991) Dietary Evaluation of Food, Nutrients, and Contaminants in Fort Good Hope and Colville Lake, Northwest Territories. Final report to NHRDP.
4. Kinloch, D., H.V. Kuhnlein, and D.C.G. Muir (1992) Inuit Foods and Diet. A preliminary assessment of benefits and risks. The Science of the Total Environment. 122:247-278.
5. Kuhnlein, H.V. and N.J. Turner (1991) *Traditional Plant Foods of Canadian Indigenous Peoples: Nutrition, Botany and Use*. Gordon and Breach Science Publishers. Foreword, viii-ix.
6. International Conference on Nutrition. Proceedings. WHO and FAO, Rome, December, 1992.
7. Kuhnlein, H.V., D.H. Calloway, and B.H. Harland. (1979) Composition of traditional Hopi foods. J. Am. Dietet. Assoc. 75:37-41.

References

Schaeffer, O. (1977) Changing dietary patterns in the Canadian North: health, social, and economic consequences. J. Can. Diet. Assoc. 38: 17-35.

Eaton, S.B. and M. Konner. (1985) Palaeolithic nutrition: and current implications. New Eng. J. Med. 312:283-289.

Brand, J.C. et al. (1990) Plasma glucose in insulin responses to traditional Pima Indian Meals. Am. J. Clin. Nutr. 51:415-420.

O'Dea, K.(1984) Marked improvement in the carbohydrate and lipid metabolism in diabetic Australian Aborigines after temporary reversion to traditional lifestyle. Diabetes 33:596-603.

Nuxalk food and nutrition Handbook and *Kanusyam a snknic* "Real Good Food." Nuxalk Food and Nutrition Program. Nuxalk Nation Council, Bella Coola, B.C., 1985

Diamond, J.M. (1992) Diabetes running wild. Nature 357 (June 4):362-363.

Illness Care, Health, and the Economic Base

*Robert Evans**

One of the ways in which academics try to learn about things is to undertake to talk about them and then, hopefully, when they are through, they may have learned something from their audiences.

I think that is an important point as backdrop to this talk. I am not a specialist on Aboriginal issues. I cannot tell you the kinds of things that you really do need to know.

What I propose to do is to provide a sense of what I think the overall background is nationally and internationally that has a powerful impact on both the constraints and opportunities on what it is you are trying to do here – that I do have some awareness of and have spent some time thinking about. Then I think it clearly is up to you to translate that into doing things or not doing things and achieving results.

It would be both arrogant and naive for me to pretend that I could tell you your business. Although, as a professional economist, I have my share of both of those qualities, I am not prepared to get into this in quite that way.

When I was a member of the B.C. Royal Commission on Health Care and Costs, studying the B.C. health care system. Again, we were all acutely aware that the problems in this particular area were of extraordinary complexity and largely beyond our reach and required another commission to deal with them –

* Professor, Department of Economics, University of British Columbia.

and here you are. You have another commission. I guess that's a way of passing the intellectual buck.

The two parts to the title that I gave this talk reflect what, to me, seemed to be – I suppose one hesitates to use the phrase 'two solitudes' – two separate administrative intellectual trends that are going on in health care, really quite separate from each other and with not a great deal of overlap. There are some very interesting and very important things going on in what I have called the illness care system, and there is a separate discussion and a separate evolution of ideas and, to some extent, policies going on in response to the WHO definition of health and the notion that the promotion of health requires a much more holistic concept of the individual in society. The phrase 'new paradigms' floats around a lot – although one of the things that makes it so popular is that nobody knows what it means – the notion that there is something more to health and something more to the promotion of the well-lived life than simply supporting the illness care system.

That notion, I think, is developing and evolving really with not a great deal of contact with what is going on in the illness care system.

What I want to do is I want to start by describing, obviously far too briefly, what I think is happening in the illness care system, and I think that has powerful implications for what may and may not be optimal strategies for trying to pursue broader definitions or broader concepts of health. So I will start with the illness care system – that I can actually get some numbers on – and then try to switch over and say, "Okay, so what."

The first point that I would make is that I do not use the illness care system label in any critical sense. It is my experience with people in the holistic approach to health that they tend to use that as a epithet, as a slur. They say, "It's not a health care system at all; it's an illness care system," as if that is something you should be ashamed of.

I do not myself think there is anything to be ashamed of in providing care to people who are ill. That seems like a perfectly decent and proper thing to do. It would be a good idea if, in addition, you did things that actually helped them to get well, but that often happens. Critics from outside tend to concentrate a great deal on the shortcomings of the illness care system, but I think we need to recognize its very real strengths and effectiveness as well.

That is not a criticism, but it is a statement, I think, that the illness care system is good in taking care of illness. It's a good thing to do. You shouldn't expect it to do everything that is involved in the promotion of health. There are some real risks there that I will get to a little later on.

The illness care system, as we know it – the conventional, the mainstream, what is referred to as the health care system in Canada – is, of course, as you all know, in crisis at the moment. This is not a surprise. It has been in crisis for as long as I can remember – and I have been in the field for about 25 years. I expect it always will be.

Being in crisis is part of the negotiation process whereby the people who provide health care in a society and, to some extent, the people who use it, negotiate their claims with the rest of society. In a publicly funded system – which means virtually all of them in the modern world – there is a continuous dialogue with the rhetoric of crisis that could be described – as it has been by one of my colleagues, Jonathon Lomas at McMaster – as "orchestrated outrage." It is the continuous outrage of the people in the system at the inadequacy of the resources they have got.

In the last 30 years we have expanded that system in real terms per capita four times, so it is now 400 per cent larger in real terms than it was 30 years ago. That has had no impact on the crisis rhetoric. The rhetoric is just part of the normal operations of the system, I suggest to you. If you think back, you will certainly see that it has been around for a long time. And it turns up in almost every other system as well, perhaps every other system in the developed world.

However, that being so, I think we are at a time when something has changed in Canada and in the rest of the world. All across Canada we have had within the last five years major commission reports, inquiries, premiers' councils, a wide variety of investigative agencies that have recommended major reforms – and this hasn't happened in 20 years. This is a new event, at least new in recent years.

It is interesting that exactly the same thing is happening all over Europe and in the South Pacific. The Americans, of course, are trying to reform their system, but then well they should. In those systems that actually run reasonably well, there is the same process in the same time period happening everywhere, so there is nothing unique to Canada. All of a sudden, within about the same five-year period, every country that has had a reasonably effective, universal, comprehensive, relatively cost-controlled system is suddenly getting very interested in reform. So we are dealing with a phenomenon that is obviously something broader than simply the present Canadian experience.

We are very much part of this general trend, but I think we need to reflect upon the fact that we are part of something that is happening everywhere, very recently, and quite suddenly. Something has changed, and it isn't something within health care systems themselves. It is something outside them. And the something is not very far to seek.

If you want to see what is really causing the crisis in health care, you look at the data on the general economy. You can look at that in Canada, or you can look it all across the western European world, and you find that somewhere around 10 years ago there were some quite significant changes in the level of economic growth in most of those economies. The British are an exception, but then their growth was so low in the earlier years that you couldn't see much of a drop. But in western Europe, as well as in Canada, something changed.

I want to show you some images of that. They are very simple, and they are remarkably stark. They surprised me when I started fooling around with these charts. As is appropriate for an economist in the forecasting business, I am very shortsighted, so I have to check my transparencies. I can't see them as well as you can.

What that shows – this is just straight Statistics Canada data, straight out of the publications – is real output, domestic product, total output for Canada – 'real' meaning adjusted for inflation, 'per capita' meaning divided by population. That is your basic measure of the economic resources available per capita in Canada and how they have been evolving over time.

I have plotted a trend for them from 1960 to 1980, the simplest possible plot, a log linear trend – and anything who knows anything about this game will realize the low intellectual level at which I am working. If you follow the trend from 1960 to 1980 and project it through to 1991, you get the nice smooth curve there. The remarkable thing is that the reality lies bang on the curve for 20 years. That is a long time to be that tight on the curve. Then the next fun part is what happens in the early 1980s. We come off the curve and we don't get back on. We manage to get back in parallel with it for a while, and then we hit another recession. By the end of that period, the actual is about 25 per cent below the trend value. That is the external economic reality, the external environment we are working in.

You can do a lot of qualifications to that. All statistics are, to some extent, false. But that is the broad outline.

The next transparency tells you exactly the same story but in an even more dramatic form. This is the actual value of output per head relative to its trend value. You can see that over the 20-year period it bounced around within 5 per cent either way of its trend value, then it collapses in the early 1980s and then it collapses again at the end of the 1980s.

That has something to do with funding difficulties for new programs, because that is your overall economic base in the country. It doesn't say that new programs of various sorts shouldn't be priorities; it just says that the competition is getting tough.

If we now relate that to health care – this is all just straight Department of Finance stuff – a very common statistic that is used by the people who say that health care costs are out of control is that we are spending more and more of our income on health care over time. Well, there is some truth in that but, as usual, it is far too simple.

What did happen to health spending relative to income, and what would have happened if we hadn't gone into the collapse of the early and late 1980s? In the next slide, the upper line is the reality; the lower is what would have happened if we had continued on our previous growth path.

You can see that the reality was a steady growth here, flat in the 1970s and then, with the recession, an explosion of share, levelling out, another big bounce with the new recession. If there hadn't been those two recessions, if we had stayed on the previous trend, we would have had a pretty well-contained, a not doing anything terribly special kind of health care system. Don't quote me on that. It was doing lots of special things, but it wasn't doing anything special in terms of its economic impact.

That is total health care. Now let's focus on hospitals and doctors alone, not because they are all that matters but because they are what is funded through the universal public health insurance systems.

This goes back to the post-war, and it does that because the data go back. If there had been data available, I would have plotted the other one back, too.

Now you see the really dramatic, steady increase from the late 1940s all the way up to 1970, flatten out, drift off, and it would have kept on drifting slightly downward except for recession, recession.

The reality happened. There is no getting around that. But the point about it is that what we seem to have here is an external environment that deteriorated markedly and an illness care system that did not respond to that change, that continued to behave as if it were still in the high-growth environment. There seems to have been enough inertia built up in that system over the previous 20 years – and, if we had time, I could go through some of the details of what that inertia is, what forms it takes – that the health care system has not adapted to the new environment.

That means a lot of conflict. That means that the control processes, the attempts to limit that growth, have to be imposed tighter and tighter as the overall economic environment deteriorates. Even trying to do that, you can see the realities; you have these pressures. This is the dilemma of the Minister of Finance of a health care system in which expectations are very powerfully driven by past performance and past experience that says we have to keep on growing, and the economy is supposed to be there to help us keep growing. If the economy is inadequate to help us keep growing, we just have to expand our share of what is there.

That is, as you see, what happened during the 1980s, and I think that is what powers the recent pressure for reform throughout the health care systems of Canada and, indeed, of most of the OECD world. I am not going to take you through one of these sets of transparencies for every one of the 18 countries in the OECD, but they would look roughly similar. I think the Canadian ones are particularly dramatic.

I will give you a flavour of the international environment. Here are the two outlines – the United States, the country of the cost explosion, the United Kingdom, the country of the Chief of Nasty, and, in the middle, the average of all OECD countries – western Europe, Australia, Japan, New Zealand, Canada and the United States, all averaged: parallel to the United States up to the late 1970s, flattens out, parallel to the U.K. from then on.

The Europeans figured out how to limit their costs; they decided to do it, and they did it. The United States didn't; they haven't yet. They are trying to trace every disaster to us. The British were always Chief of Nasty – my background is British. Canada following the U.S. right down the line, just a little colony of the U.S., goes into universal health care; everything changes; we flatten out; we hit the OECD average; and then we come unglued with the recessions.

What is the relevance of all this? The relevance of all this is that I think the mainstream system is going to be tied up for some time to come, wrestling with its own problems of restructuring. You don't have to go much farther than this morning's news programs on the closing of Shaughnessy [a Vancouver hospital].

What that says is this: In this kind of environment, how do you do new things? How do you go out as a Royal Commission, for example, as we did, and get told by all kinds of people about priorities for different, new and important things to do in an environment where it is very unlikely that the overall globe is going to be able to go?

The answer is this: You are going to have to manage better the resources that you now put into the illness care system and you are going to have to transfer them, if you really want to, out of that system and over to other sorts of community-based programs. That was essentially the message of our Royal Commission and, in one way or another, I think that has been the message of all the royal commissions. You translate that to where the rubber meets the road – the Commissioners have all gone home by then – and it says that you close Shaughnessy. Suddenly, there are a whole lot of people who work at Shaughnessy. They have jobs.

Every dollar of spending in health care is, by definition, a dollar of somebody's income – an accounting definition. That is not an estimate. That is not an economist's viewpoint; that's an accountant's viewpoint. That is reality – that's a stretch right there, isn't it? It really is the case; trust me on this one.

If you want to change priorities, which is a nice phrase, or redeploy resources, which is another nice phrase, what it means is that you have to take employment away from somebody and give it to somebody else, or you have to tell somebody, "The job you have been doing for some years and feel reasonably confident at and know what you are doing and, by the way, happens to be where you like to live, doesn't exist any more. There's another job opening up somewhere else that will be quite different. You're going to be nervous as all get-out figuring out how to do it, but that's what we really want done and, if you want to work in this system, that is where you are going to have to go."

Those kinds of statements don't resonate with a lot of the people in the system already. They would be much happier to say, as they have said for 40 years, "There are new needs, of course, but there are also old needs. So keep on funding the old needs and also add on more resources to do the new important things." We have done that for most of the history of our system, and we are probably not going to be able to do it any more. That's the message here.

That was why in the B.C. Commission we said, "Business as usual is not sustainable." We don't know that; that's a statement about the future. But it does look like the world has changed in a way in which that is going to be very tough.

So how does that flip over into the second part of my talk, holistic health care and all that? There is a very important distinction, I think, that needs to be made here between broadening the definition of health and broadening your concepts of the determinants of health. I will try to run through that carefully.

The WHO back in the late 1940s defined health as a state of complete physical, mental and social well-being and not merely the absence of disease or infirmity – in other words, virtually all good things. This is the well-lived life.

In some sense, you could call a healthy life a well-lived life. I am not going to argue with the philosophy behind that, but I am saying that is really pretty difficult to operationalize, and it is not at all clear that the illness care system, either in its present form or in some extended form through funding preventive interventions by clinical people or something of that sort, is an appropriate mechanism for achieving that. It's likely to be very expensive and it's likely to be ineffective.

Take a very clear-cut, unambiguous, well-known example. It is now pretty well agreed – and there is a recent report out from LCDC in Ottawa to confirm – that there has been virtually no pay-off to the research done and the treatment done on most kinds of cancer, particularly lung cancer. Huge resources go into this area; not much comes out in terms of benefits.

We know why most people get lung cancer; they get it because they smoke. What we don't know is a whole lot about why they smoke, although we know there are some very interesting correlations with social status, sense of control, empowerment or non-empowerment – nice and controversial stuff, but really some pretty powerful stories coming through. We also know it has something to do with whether there are people in the business of trying to addict children to smoking, which is when most people take it up. Yet, what we do is we spend our money on supporting biomedical researchers in our universities. What's the point?

When that came out a week ago, the coverage in the newspapers was: Hey, we gotta do more about prevention but, of course, we certainly shouldn't cut back on biomedical research because that is good; that is a good thing to do. It doesn't happen to do any good in terms of outcome, but, gee, we should keep it going anyway because there are folks with white coats and neat looking labs and we've got to do those things. It's important. God demands it.

That is what I meant about the difficulty in addressing the obvious, saying, "Look, if this is not working and that looks like it might work, maybe we should close some of this down and move the resources over there." It is very hard to get that thinking going.

What I think has happened in the holistic area – in the new dimensions of health care – sorry, that was a very important Freudian slip; I did not mean to say that – the new dimensions of the determinants of health, the things that matter to your health are very narrowly defined, not only in the WHO definition but things like mortality and morbidity are conventionally defined. What we are now learning is that they depend far more on your social environment, also on your physical environment obviously, on your social status, on your sense of where you fit into your community.

The hard evidence is now coming in – not in terms of fuzzy things like people feel good and report it on a questionnaire – but whether they are dead or alive. Mortality rates actually depend on things like social status and social networks, and you can show that pretty clearly and you can replicate it in animal experiments. You can go into the lab and show the same darn thing, and it is really quite remarkable.

So what do you do about that? I think the real danger is that you take this new perception that a much wider range of determinants affect health, narrowly defined – don't get drawn too far into very broad definitions of health that are too difficult to get agreement on. Stick to very narrow ones, where nobody can deny we are talking about health. We are talking about very narrow mortality and morbidity measures that are dependent upon very much broader conditions than simply the health care system.

The trouble, I think, is that the people who are worried about holistic health have tried to define conditions and problems as diseases. Alzheimer's was invented as a disease about 10 years ago. It used to be just senility, and then it became a disease. Once it was a disease, it was eligible for biomedical funding; it was eligible for public support in a whole variety of ways. Alcoholism – is it a disease or not? People insist it's a disease. Why does it matter? It's a hell of a problem. It matters because, if it's a disease, then it comes under the health care system, under the illness care system. It becomes eligible for different kinds of funding; it becomes eligible for different public attitudes.

Defining a problem as a disease looks like a very good way of raising its status and raising the resources that go to it, but there is a price to be paid for that. The price to be paid is, first, that it falls into the standard illness care framework of who gets to define the problem, who gets to identify its dimensions, and who gets to be paid for providing the solutions. You maybe didn't want that. The example of lung cancer, it seems to me, is a good one. It is clearly a disease, but we are not addressing it in a very effective way.

The thing I am adding to that with those transparencies is that it may not be such a hot idea in the future, as it has been in the past, to try to get your very real problem classified as an illness. The sharks are getting pretty hungry in the illness care system; things are much tougher there than they were ten years ago, and that is going to continue. There is no real reason to believe that we are going to get back on that growth trend.

I think what it says is this: Be awfully careful about defining problems as diseases in the hope that will elevate their status and get you better results. It may well not. It may well backfire on you.

Secondly, be pretty careful about defining health itself too broadly. I think you can get a lot of mileage out of defining health pretty narrowly, but really focusing hard on the very broad determinants of that health. The evidence really is good on that, so that you can now start to say: Look, the things that matter for people's health, in the narrowest sense – not the airy-fairy sociologist sense, but in the narrow sense of who lives and who dies and in what condition they do that. The things that matter are far, far broader than the illness care system, and the problem is to try to hold that system under some kind of control so that you can free up resources to do other things.

DAILY SUMMARIES

Opening the Round Table

Elder Glen Douglas thanked local chiefs and elders for allowing the Round Table participants to be guests on their territory. He opened the gathering with a prayer, ending by underlining the importance of the health and social aspects of the lives of Aboriginal peoples. Royal Commission Co-Chair Georges Erasmus thanked Elder Douglas for setting the tone for the next three days.

Mr. Erasmus said that since the Royal Commission was created in August, 1991, it has taken a holistic approach to its work, trying to integrate all the issues under its large mandate. He said that exploring social issues, health and healing were the core of the Commission's work.

When Christopher Columbus 'discovered' the continent 500 years ago, Aboriginal peoples were healthy and had a holistic approach to living. They believed life was a journey to learn the full meaning of being human, and their values and norms reflected this approach to life. After contact with the Europeans, the lives of Aboriginal peoples were characterized by a loss of control over their destiny; only within the last few decades have Aboriginal peoples begun to regain control over their lives.

Mr. Erasmus said the subject of health and social issues is important because it means coming to terms with the pain that many Aboriginal people experience daily. In their travels across the country, commissioners have heard countless people stress that what is needed now is a process to become healthy. Mr. Erasmus is inspired that the solutions to these health and social problems are coming from Aboriginal peoples themselves; in particular, he noted the strong leadership of Aboriginal women. The healing process will involve Aboriginal peoples reasserting control over their lives, he said.

Royal Commission Co-Chair René Dussault began by noting that the round tables were important forums that bridge information coming from two sources: public participation and research. The round tables help the commissioners focus on policy orientation.

Mr. Dussault briefly reviewed what the Commission has heard during its last two rounds of hearings. Aboriginal peoples, he said, believe that health means something more than the absence of disease, more than ensuring adequate health services. Health, from an Aboriginal perspective, refers to the core of a person, the vitality that animates people, their families and communities. "Where it exists, it reverberates" through all aspects of Aboriginal society, touching education, employment, justice and family values. The key is that health is a holistic concept in which all aspects of society are inter-related. The solutions to social problems, therefore, start with a critical analysis of the medical and social services available to Aboriginal peoples.

"Aboriginal people have the right to receive the same quality of health care" available to everyone else in Canada, stressed Mr. Dussault. He listed five elements of a solution to health and social problems in Aboriginal communities:

- comparable standards of medical and social services for Aboriginal and non-Aboriginal peoples;
- a focus on raising the self-esteem of Aboriginal peoples;
- a recognition of traditional culture and traditional approaches to healing;
- a holistic approach to critical problems in Aboriginal communities; and
- Aboriginal and community control of programs.

Mr. Dussault added that the non-Aboriginal world will also benefit by the solutions offered by Aboriginal peoples.

Frank Rivers welcomed the delegates and representatives from First Nations on behalf of the Squamish Nation Council. He added his hope that the submissions made to the Royal Commission would offer solutions to the health and social problems facing Aboriginal peoples.

Round Table Chairman Dr. Louis T. Montour reminded the participants of the significant task that lay ahead during the following days. Much work has already been accomplished in the area, including numerous presentations to the Commission in its previous rounds of hearings, and many studies on Aboriginal communities over the past years. Dr. Montour wondered why there has been so many studies and so little change – in one community, 26 private consultants were conducting studies at one time. The recent events in Davis Inlet that received widespread attention are an example of the conditions faced in many Aboriginal communities across the country, he added.

Dr. Montour quoted from a presentation made previously to the Commission about the problem of family violence in Aboriginal communities: "Provide children with examples of the right thing to do. Give them a reason to live, not to die."

Solutions to health and social problems must be culturally appropriate, he continued, and the major focus must be on healing. Health problems and social problems are not end points but symptoms of a larger illness – and for the symptoms to go away, the cause of the illness itself must be identified and treated. For that reason, "Indian medicine is politics," he said – communities will become healthy only if governments are serious about dealing with the underlying issues.

Dr. Montour concluded that the illness in Aboriginal communities is characterized by loss – loss of control, loss of culture. "Language is culture," he reminded the gathering, and healing must include "using, learning and saving your language." Aboriginal people must negotiate a new social contract, and the Round Table is one opportunity to contribute to that process.

Panel Presentation of Discussion Papers

Aboriginal Health Policy for the Next Century

Moderator Dr. Jay Wortman introduced the first two panelists of the morning; each presented a discussion paper commissioned for the Round Table. John D. O'Neil, Associate Professor of Medical Anthropology at the University of Manitoba, reviewed the themes of his discussion paper. He said there are differing models and perspectives, in Aboriginal health, about what constitutes health and healing, and Aboriginal theorists have shown that prevailing scientific models are grounded in eurocentric philosophic traditions.

Mr. O'Neil recalled his experience at a debate in Australia, where he was "struck most dramatically" by the level of discussion about theories and perspectives of Aboriginal health. There is international collaboration among Aboriginal societies to confront common health concerns, a cross-fertilization and sharing of ideas.

Most scholars agree that European-introduced disease was a major factor in the catastrophic decline of the North American Aboriginal population, yet contemporary epidemiological data is often presented in a way to suggest that these contact epidemics were an intrinsic characteristic of Aboriginal culture. For example, the high infant mortality rates in Aboriginal communities are usually presented within a context that distorts historical reality, distorts evidence that prior to contact, morbidity and mortality in Aboriginal societies was probably quite low.

Many Aboriginal communities have "Fourth World health conditions", characterized by a dramatic increase in chronic diseases such as diabetes, heart disease and cancer. The development of a society is usually characterised by a decline in infectious diseases and an increase in chronic conditions, but Aboriginal communities across the world suffer the worse of the chronic conditions on a scale unknown in non-Aboriginal communities.

The French philosopher Michel Foucault developed theories about how colonial surveillance systems have been used as mechanisms to control different segments of society; Mr. O'Neil suggested that the way in which data are collected on Aboriginal people reflects a colonial perspective. He added that statistics on Aboriginal communities are well-developed but information is lacking on the situation of urban Aboriginal peoples.

He recalled how students in medical school are introduced to the situation in Aboriginal communities by being shown slide after slide listing statistics about the poor health of Aboriginal people. A graduate student made the important point that the way in which the information was presented served to reinforce the stereotype that Aboriginal communities were sick and powerless. "We must see Aboriginal communities as healthy places" with positive lifestyles and values, he stressed.

Health care workers need to reflect on the fact that their science is embedded in the enlightenment period of western culture. In North America, there is a monopolistic approach to medicine – for example, Canada is only beginning to look at licensing midwives – whereas Britain and other countries take a more pluralistic approach. "We need to embrace traditional medicine," said Mr. O'Neil, and the lessons of traditional medicine will enrich all society, not just Aboriginal communities. He added that traditional medicine is the foundation of Aboriginal culture, and the statement "medicine is politics" is even more true in Aboriginal communities.

Mr. O'Neil noted that the history of development of health care services in Aboriginal communities has been very brief; there has been tremendous growth within the last decade, and "we need to be positive and optimistic about this development." The history of damage has been hundreds of years long, and the situation will not improve overnight.

Mr. O'Neil concluded by underlining the importance of three themes: resolving the jurisdictional conflict between the federal, provincial and municipal governments for health services to Aboriginal peoples; the link between health issues and sustainable economic development; and the focus on community healing. The movement to heal communities is very powerful, and everyone should support the process.

Challenging the Way We Think About Health

Karen Ginsberg, Information Management Unit, Royal Commission on Aboriginal Peoples, presented the next discussion paper on behalf of author Rosemary Proctor, Deputy Minister of the Ontario Ministry of Community and Social Services. Ms. Proctor had noted a recent *New York Times* article which announced that the prestigious U.S. National Institutes of Health was establishing a new Office of Alternative Medicine. To her, this article illustrated the importance of the bridge between traditional understandings and approaches to health, and those embodied in the dominant culture.

For some years, there has been a change in the way people think about health, illness, curing and caring. Ms. Proctor believes what is happening is a change in the model which defines health and disease – how health is thought of, and how illness is treated. The paradigm shift is a revolution, and since it is essentially a process of redefining how one sees the world, it is often resisted by people who prefer the old definitions.

In the white western world, medicine has been rooted in the 'germ' theory of disease – illnesses are caused by specific germs, or other causal agents. Within this framework, disease is defined as a dysfunction or inability to function, and the cause originates outside the individual. Health is then defined as the absence of disease. For nearly two centuries, this model has influenced the way people through much of the world think about health and disease. "It fundamentally influences what we call health care," Ms. Proctor noted.

The causation model was never situated in a social or economic context. It is generally seen as timeless and without boundaries, rooted in "proven scientific evidence." It does not acknowledge that modern medicine has engulfed, and in many ways discredited and eliminated, traditional forms of thinking about health and health care in different parts of the world.

However, a new framework is gradually emerging to challenge the causation model of disease and health. Ms. Proctor calls this new model the "environmental paradigm, because it explains illness and disease in terms of all aspects of our world environment and of our bodies themselves." The environmental framework sees human beings as adapting to their environment in effective and ineffective ways, and simultaneously altering their environment in beneficial or harmful ways. Within this model, health becomes a goal statement: the presence of physical, social and mental well-being. Disease is therefore seen as emerging from the interaction of the individual and the social environment.

This paradigm shift engages the public individually and collectively. "It engages us in our communities, in our particular historical and social consciousness." Health promotion and prevention become key concepts in the new model. There is scope for individual responsibility for health, and collectively, "we have a responsibility to prevent disease or improve the chances of achieving health."

The new framework is being expanded by efforts to recover or rediscover aspects of traditional healing. Healing circles, for example, link people's spiritual and social well-being with the physical and emotional problems they experience. The work going on now in Aboriginal communities, finding ways of integrating traditional healing with modern medicine, will help further the development of new ways of understanding human health.

After the presentations, there were questions from the floor. Elder Glen Douglas wondered if Bill C-91, recently approved by Parliament to protect patent medicines, would prevent the use of traditional Aboriginal medicine. "This would be very ominous to us," he stressed. Marie Fortier, Acting Assistant Deputy Minister, Health and Welfare Canada, responded that the intent of the bill was to extend the period that new drugs are protected by patent, and the scope of legislation has not been expanded – there is no new jurisdiction over traditional medicine.

David Newhouse, Native Studies professor at Trent University, said that "if we are to make headway, we need to accept the new definition of health," as the presence of physical and social well-being, and he questioned if policy makers would truly embrace the new definition. Karen Ginsberg responded that the "new definition" has been in place for many years but ignored. Now, however, policy makers "can no longer neglect" the broad definition of health, and many are discovering that linking health to other social issues can help allocate resources more efficiently.

An Inuk woman from northern Quebec explained that her people are governed by the James Bay Agreement, signed by the federal and provincial governments, Hydro-Quebec, the Cree and the Inuit. "We have the highest rates of youth suicide and STDs, and family violence is rampant," she said. Under the Agreement, her community was given a hospital and a large budget for health services, but no budget for community services. She believed that many of her community's problems are related to the lack of recreational and other community services. The moderator noted that her comments underlined the importance of linking illness with issues of health prevention and promotion.

Panel of Elders

The moderator, Marlene Brant Castellano, began the session by introducing the four elders and the topic of traditional understandings of Indian, Métis and Inuit health and healing. She stated that "within our tradition is the key to health, and particularly, the key to healing the spirit."

Ms. Brant Castellano shared two stories: the first was told to her by a woman who had been in a residential school and who had suffered much despair in her life as a result of that experience. In a dream, the woman heard the elders call out and tell her, "Go back to your mother, you need to go home." Initially, the woman said she could not understand this as an instruction regarding her own health, but later she realized it meant going back to her traditions, culture and to Mother Earth.

The first panelist, elder Jean Aquash, an Anishnawbekwee from Walpole Island in Ontario, began by thanking the Creator, and the spirit of the people of this land, for inviting her to the Royal Commission on Aboriginal Peoples. Ms. Aquash is originally from Ontario but has been living in Alberta since 1985. She takes paternal lineage from her father's clan, the Thunderbird clan. She did not understand clanship until she began to look down the traditional path.

Health is an important issue to discuss, she said, expressing her concern about child sexual abuse, family violence and suicide within her community. In her own study and work, she reaches out for healing. As a child, she was made to go to residential school, and later, when she began to look for answers to her life, she had to do much of it by herself, alone.

Ms. Aquash shifted to a different way of thinking in 1975 through her experience in the sweat lodge. "Since this experience, I have made many spiritual commitments. My commitment is to a power greater than myself."

"The spirit is in everything. We have just evolved within each other," she said. Ms. Aquash has come to understand this through her learning, and has recognized that the old people have helped her understand the meaning of living.

Ms. Aquash said "we are a walking medicine wheel" essentially made up of four parts: mental, spiritual, emotional and physical. "In order to have holistic healing, we must first look at our pasts and dramatic experiences." Ms. Aquash said her first step was to think about her mind; receiving help from Alcoholics Anonymous helped her do this. "Because I treated my body badly I did a lot of fasting, and I've learned to give my body youthful agility through cleansing."

Now she is acting upon her emotions – the last part of her healing journey. She discovered that dealing with emotions had a lot to do with the beginning of her life. "I felt that I was less than, not good enough, and that no one could be close to me, and that I couldn't be close to anyone else." She explained that these emotions were related to feelings of abandonment and rejection that resulted from being placed in a residential school. "A lot of things that I didn't have in the beginning of life marked a path for me."

Since her spiritual awakening, Ms. Aquash has been open to other forms of healing. Through her work with Bear Woman and Associates, she has recognized the importance of emotional healing. "All mankind must find original purpose and walk in integrity of their truth."

Ms. Aquash concluded by speaking to the importance of emotions and spiritual growth. "We must first learn what is unconditional love and exercise this love around us." She believes in the commitment to spiritual practices. "All of us are bigger than what we see. The only thing that holds us back is our past experience. If we walk through this we will come to the light of unconditional love."

The second speaker, Norman Chartrand, the provincial elder for the Manitoba Metis Federation, said that after reading the material for the session, he was fearful because the papers were very academic. For most of his life, his learning has come from listening, observing and doing. "Written material was not part of my learning process," he said.

Health, Well-Being and Economic Conditions

"Health and well-being of Aboriginal peoples is closely related to poor economic and environmental conditions and social dislocation," and "if we are to overcome these difficulties, we must learn to communicate," Mr. Chartrand said. During his childhood, his community survived through caring and sharing, and medicine provided by the Métis community – knowledge passed on from generation to generation.

Mr. Chartrand recalled that in the past, most Métis families had their own gardens which allowed them to have food year 'round. "Much of this way of life is lost," he said. Referring to current conditions in some Métis communities, he noted that housing is no longer the same and many Métis do not have the money to live the 'new' way.

Looking to the future, he said that "the Métis must have the strength to hold on to the old ways that were good. We must not make any big changes just to please other people." He stressed the importance of the Métis remaining with the old traditions in order to keep the Métis traditions alive.

"Many solutions can be found in not just doing things, but in stopping certain things," he said. For example, "they must stop taking our children and they must stop taking our lands and our fish – our means of making a living. We must also hold on to our famous traditions of humour, laughter and dancing because these traditions have also helped us to survive."

In his opening remarks, elder Glen Douglas, a member of the Lower Similkameen Indian Band, said that "I'm here to tell you in 15 minutes what took me a life time to learn."

Mr. Douglas emphasized the need for balance and harmony to achieve health and well-being. Balance and harmony can be found within the medicine wheel, a very important teaching tool. In addition to the four states of the human condition – physical, emotional, mental and spiritual – the medicine wheel also contains the four seasons and the four stages of human development. Mr. Douglas offered an example of the child who becomes unbalanced through witnessing the abuse of his mother. When the child goes to school, he is incapable of paying attention to what he needs to learn. Again, he emphasized the importance of balance and harmony.

He further stressed the importance of balancing and integrating the four components of the human condition. The role of the elder is very important in this process. For example, elders teach about the mind and the body. Mr. Douglas said it is important to strengthen the heart for the "great journey between the heart and the mind." Another important teaching role of the elders, he said, is passing on the oral tradition. "When we listen, we hear what the elders are saying; when we watch, we learn from their example," and "we are all role models," he said. "When we hit our wives, our children will follow."

Mr. Douglas highlighted the interconnectedness of comprehension, retention and recall. From the mind, he said, we learn the universal laws of honour, respect, caring, and language. From these universal laws comes sharing: what the earth has shared with us and what our parents and elders have also shared with us.

He said that it is very important to know who we are, what territories we are from, and what resources we have, because it is from our people and our land that we get our medicines for healing. For example, the sweat lodge is important for cleansing and performing prayers.

Dreams and vision quests tell us about our responsibilities. One responsibility is not harming ourselves or others. "I believe the Creator is our government," and government is based on consensus and longevity. In contrast, western government is based on money, power and greed, he said. Gifts from the Creator should not be used in bad and evil ways. Unfortunately, "there are some people who are selling our ceremonies and traditions in Europe." These people, he said, "talk the talk but they don't walk the walk."

Mr. Douglas said he broke the word of his elders when he used alcohol. He drank because of his experiences in residential school and the war. Drinking helped take the pain away, "but eventually, I had to recover from that too." Mr. Douglas read a poem he had written during this time in his life which captured his thoughts throughout his recovery process.

In his parting words, Mr. Douglas highlighted some of the difficult things he has had lived through. The *Indian Act*, he said, is "one of the most genocidal pieces of legislation that has disallowed our traditional ways to healing." Expressing his hope in hearing the voices of Aboriginal people, he said he found it "peculiar that part of the Commission (instead of all) is Native", and asked: "Is it just tokenism?"

Daisy Watts was the final elder on the panel. Ms. Watts is an Inuk from Kuujjuaq in northern Quebec and spoke to the audience in her own language. She spoke first about the traditional medicine that her people have used for centuries. For many generations of the Inuit, plants have been of primary importance. She said that although older people have been using plants for medicine for many years, younger people are just beginning to use them. She recalled an elder telling her a story about a young woman who had suffered from severe bleeding during childbirth. It was the use of a special plant that enabled the woman to recover fully.

In speaking about her community, Ms. Watts said the elders are especially concerned about the younger people. "We hear things about what the young people are doing that is not good. Every time we hear of an untimely death, accident or suicide, we are deeply saddened."

In her closing remarks, Ms. Watts related her personal experience of heart surgery that had saved her life. "I would have died if it were not for modern medicine and the help of God."

The moderator opened the floor to questions and comments. The first speaker, Dr. David Young, said it was paternalistic for society to continue saying that Aboriginal medicine must be brought up to the western standards, when in fact, there are many areas where Aboriginal medicine does a better job. He remarked that it would probably be more useful for our society to create ways to empower Aboriginal healers.

Glen Williams, from a healing circle in Vancouver, believed churches should be called to account for their involvement with residential schools. "The church must be held accountable" for the healing process needed by Aboriginal peoples recovering from their experiences in residential schools, and the Aboriginal leadership should initiate this healing process. Mr. Williams also raised the issue of the misuse of Indian medicine by pharmaceutical companies. He recommended the implementation of training programs for Aboriginal youth interested in learning and maintaining traditional ways. In conclusion, he said, he would like to see more work done, on a national and international level, to develop policy on environmental issues.

Global Nutrition and the Holistic Environment of Indigenous Peoples

Dr. Harriet V. Kuhnlein, Professor of Human Nutrition at McGill University, is also the Director of the Centre for Nutrition and the Environment of Indigenous Peoples in Canada, United States and Guatemala. She began her keynote address by presenting a series of 25 slides from Aboriginal communities in Canada, the United States and Guatemala. She asked the participants to consider four major functions that Aboriginal foods and total diets contribute to Aboriginal peoples:

1. Food is an *anchor* to culture and personal well-being.

2. Food is the direct link between the environment and human health. It is the *avenue* by which a healthy environment can provide complete nutrition and a sense of integration and wellness.
3. Food is an important *indicator* of total cultural expression.
4. Food is an essential *agent* to promote holistic health and culture.

Declining Use of Traditional Food Systems

"It is becoming more and more clear that traditional food systems derived from local, natural environments of Indigenous peoples are on the decline throughout the planet," said Dr. Kuhnlein. For a variety of reasons and external pressures, "foods made available through industrialization and market economies are replacing traditional foods in the diets of Aboriginal peoples."

Dr. Kuhnlein cited the example of the cow-parsnip, used by the Aboriginal people of the B.C. west coast. Although this green vegetable was remembered by Nuxalk elders as a "pleasant taste treat," in this century the use of cow-parsnip has declined to such an extent that many young people of this community do not even recognize the plant or know how to prepare it.

Communities such as Broughton Island in the Canadian Arctic also show a declining use of traditional foods in favour of foods from markets: despite a "rich and varied traditional food system...the use of foods provided through commercial outlets provides the majority of daily calories to people of all ages." Even in the Western Arctic, in communities as remote as Colville Lake, the residents will have a 30 per cent calorie intake of market foods during the winter and summer seasons, when traditional foods are more plentiful.

Despite a reliance on market foods, said Dr. Kuhnlein, the people of these communities "are still deriving a major portion of their nutrition (protein, essential fatty acids, iron, zinc and other essential nutrients) from the use of traditional food resources." This is readily understood by considering the "low-cost, quick-energy and low-nutrient quality food" that is transported to these communities – tea, sugar, evaporated milk, soft drinks and white bread. When traditional foods are replaced by foods such as these, the nutritional status of Indigenous peoples rapidly declines.

The reasons for this "unfortunate nutritional health circumstance" include:

- industrialization
- market economies
- colonization
- population pressures on the land and sea resources
- media and private enterprise advertising
- lack of access to traditional food resources
- changing food preferences and health beliefs

- lack of interest and knowledge in traditional culture on the part of reserve health personnel

Dr. Kuhnlein quoted her friend and colleague, Laurie Montour, from Kahnawake and Walpole Island:

> Sadly, though, there is the realization that the foods themselves [traditional], and the skills and practices in using them, are slowly dying. There is a triple threat: the loss of knowledgeable elders, leaving no one to teach; the loss of culture, leaving no one to learn; and the loss of healthy ecosystems, leaving no foods available to take them even if they wanted to.

Added to these concerns is the issue of environmental contamination, which, according to Dr. Kuhnlein, has placed a "another serious if not critical, wound to the use of traditional food systems." Although "knowledge of human health effects of specific contaminants is eons away from being complete," said Dr. Kuhnlein, "people in communities are being frightened away from the use of their traditionally known culturally-relevant food resources."

Research is needed, stressed Dr. Kuhnlein, "not only to identify severe ecosystem illness and to prevent human health effects, but also to stimulate national and international action to stop polluting the planet." Unfortunate though it may be, the food systems of Aboriginal peoples can act as sentinels for this kind of inquiry and "will be the most effective stimulant for political action."

"The declining use of traditional food resources is not just a symptom of a larger system that is failing," said Dr. Kuhnlein, "it is a major organ in the system of environmental and cultural well-being that needs immediate and vital attention." This holds true for all Indigenous peoples, around the globe.

Changing Nutritional Environments of Indigenous Peoples

Dr. Kuhnlein addressed the "well-documented changes in disease patterns of Indigenous peoples," listing obesity, diabetes, cardiovascular diseases, cancer, infant morbidity and mortality in higher frequencies, alcoholism, loss of teeth and clear eyesight, all of which have "emerged" in the health picture of Indigenous peoples in the last 100 years.

Action and leadership are needed, she said, and Aboriginal peoples must "take back" the traditional food systems and use them to their best advantage. This means taking back traditional knowledge of the environment, too, she added.

Demedicalizing the Approach to Food and Nutrition of Aboriginal Peoples

"In my view," said Dr. Kuhnlein, "there is no better place for demedicalization than in the area of nutrition." This means focusing on what is right in an individual or a community, rather than focusing on what's wrong. Medical "band-aids" do not solve nutritional problems: "the difference will be made in finding what is right in traditional knowledge of the environment and the food it provides, putting that knowledge forward, and implementing it for the health of the people."

A Strategy to Promote Traditional Food Systems

In conclusion, Dr. Kuhnlein alluded to the high international regard given to Canada's Aboriginal leadership, for "their success in promoting and protecting the cultural traditions, rights and responsibilities of Canadian Aboriginal peoples." She felt that following factors needed to be addressed:

- strong leadership at both the national and the local community levels
- commitment on the part of entire families within communities
- communicating to younger generations the knowledge and wisdom of the elders regarding the environment and its integration with food, culture and self-identity
- training within the home and school environments
- encouraging careers in health for Aboriginal people

Should these factors be achieved, said Dr. Kuhnlein, self-care and quality of life for Indigenous peoples will be greatly improved.

Panel Presentation of Discussion Papers

Suicide in Aboriginal Peoples: Causes and Prevention

Peter Ernerk, Executive Director of the Inuit Cultural Institute, welcomed the participants in English and Inuktitut. He introduced Dr. Clare Brant, who discussed his paper on the causes and preventions of suicide in Aboriginal peoples.

Dr. Brant called suicide a "gruesome topic." Although his many years in the field of psychiatry has lead some people to assume that he is no longer affected by the prevalence of suicide, this is not true, he said; he is very alarmed by the distressing trend of suicide in Aboriginal communities.

Dr. Brant, quoting the nineteenth-century pathologist Ramon Cajal, said that "every disease has two causes – the first is pathophysiological and the second is political." He listed the following statistics:

- the Aboriginal suicide rate is three-and-a-half times higher than the Canadian rate
- the suicide rate for Aboriginal people is highest in the age group 15-24 years old

Dr. Brant offered more statistics from a 10-year study in North West Alaska. Following is a list of characteristics of people who committed suicide and attempted suicide during the years 1970-1980:

Characteristics	Male	Female
Age	23.2	22.0
Education	10.5	9.5
Unemployed	78%	82%
Never Married	92%	77%
No Occupation	61%	79%
Household Income Less Than $10,000/year	77%	88%
Alcoholic or Alcohol Abusers	77%	65%

Death by "misadventure" (for example, a car accident), was not included in the statistics but it could be, if consistently dangerous behaviour was considered a prelude to suicide. Also, said Dr. Brant, any study done now would include questions on sexual abuse, because the link between sexual abuse and suicide is strong.

Referring to the "never married" category, Dr. Brant suggested that, in the case of a young woman becoming pregnant, having the child and not marrying the father because she did not want to lose her "mother's allowance," the man involved would feel "redundant," and "disposable." Consider his humiliation, Dr. Brant continued, when he realizes he cannot provide for his family. Consider, too, how the woman feels, when she makes a very personal decision based on stark economic realities.

"There has always been a widely recognized and accepted statistical correlation between socio-economic class and suicide in North American culture," continued Dr. Brant. As well, television is seen to have a deleterious effect on self-esteem. He listed eight psycho-social stresses affecting mental health:

- inadequate housing
- employment/welfare
- no recreational facilities or programmes
- poor access to education and health resources
- disorganized band administration
- absent or inadequate transportation
- disorganized and inadequate social services, including family and child services
- absence of counselling services

Prevention Strategies

Prevention strategies can be divided into three categories: primary, secondary and tertiary. The term tertiary refers to "dealing with the suicide attempts which will involve usually temporary hospitalization to deal with physical injury, crisis intervention counselling on an emergency basis, evacuation to a locked psychiatric facility, treatment of depression and other mental illnesses, alcohol detoxification and rehabilitation, pharmacotherapy and psychotherapy."

Secondary prevention consists of "early identification of those people at risk." Primary prevention, "which would remove the causes of poverty, powerlessness and anomie, are infrequently discussed and rarely implemented."

In conclusion, Dr. Brant stated his firm belief that "the Native people of Canada have the emotional and intellectual resources to deal with the triad of poverty, powerlessness and anomie" that results in "depression, substance abuse and suicidal ideation and plan."

Racism/Sexism and its Effects on Aboriginal Women

In place of Professor Emma LaRocque, who was unable to attend the conference, Jo-Ann Daniels, a co-founder of Women of the Métis Nation, presented the major points of Ms. LaRocque's paper.

"Eight out of 10 Aboriginal women in Canada are sexually abused," began Ms. Daniels, and at a recent gathering of Métis women, only seven out of the 150 present were able to say that they had not experienced violence at some point in their lives. Ms. LaRocque's believes that when the European patriarchy was imposed upon Aboriginal peoples, violence against women increased dramatically. In particular, sexual violence against women increased as women became objectified by men.

Ms. LaRocque's paper explored at length the long-term effects of racism, sexism and colonization, and the way Aboriginal men have internalized the values of the dominant white culture. While sexual assault is prevalent in all cultures, said Ms. Daniels, the apathy shown to it on reserves must change. And to effect change, myths need to be disproved. An example of a harmful myth is that sexual violence was tolerated in Aboriginal communities in earlier times.

Offenders need to be responsible for their actions, continued Ms. Daniels, and there needs to be more compassion for and understanding of the problems of the victims. Sentencing and the parole system are far too lenient, she said. "When will the victims receive the help they deserve?"

Ms. Daniels discussed the possible causes of sexual violence; the idea of the rapist as victim was considered – and rejected. If all the people who were victims in turn became victimizers, then the millions of women in this position would be causing harm to others.

Sexual violence is a very complex issue and, despite the lack of agreement on the cause, there must be a total rejection of sexual violence by society.

Ms. Daniels suggested three courses of action for violence prevention:

- Aboriginal youth need to experience a socio-economic revitalization in their communities, to give meaning to their lives. This should include vocational choice as well.
- Schools must present Aboriginal history in the present, not the past. Young people need reassurance and knowledge of their history.
- Recreational development: massive efforts are needed in all Aboriginal communities.

All teenagers must respect themselves and respect women, said Ms. Daniels. "Rape devastates," she said, and the most terrible result can be suicide. When violence occurs, spiritual needs must be attended to. When children are young, it is essential to support their hopes and dreams; without positive thoughts, children literally cannot see a future.

"Aboriginal women cannot be partners in self-government until they are accepted as equals," stated Ms. Daniels. This means that all Aboriginal people must look violence squarely in the face and deal with it honestly. It also means learning to differentiate the levels of violence and handing out appropriate judgements. It could mean changing the *Young Offenders Act* and it should mean establishing long-term rehabilitation programs.

After the presentations, there were questions from the floor. One participant asked Dr. Brant if there is a causal link between children who have been raised in foster care and subsequent suicide attempts. Dr. Brant replied that disturbing childhood experiences such as loss of or separation from a primary caregiver often produces a damaged child and a skewed adult. We are still seeing the fallout from the children's aid system, he concluded.

Another question, also directed to Dr. Brant, focused on the link between suicide and a residential school experience. Dr. Brant did not have statistics available on this subject but said that the age of the child when he or she began to attend a residential school seemed to be quite important: the younger the child, the more devastating the separation from her or his parents. In general, said Dr. Brant, an early residential school entrance meant a "ruined" child, and this same child, when he or she reached adulthood, did not know how to parent a child.

Dr. Michael Monture referred to the high incidence of unwed pregnancies in Aboriginal communities in northwestern Ontario. Young women see pregnancy as a way out of difficult or violent situations, said Dr. Monture. "Is there anything we can do to change their perception?" he asked. Dr. Brant agreed that young Aboriginal women often do try to "escape" unhappy home lives by becoming unwed mothers. Unfortunately, they are often disappointed by the outcome, which can be as difficult as the original situation, he added.

Round Table 1: Holistic Community Health Strategies

Dr. Jay Wortman, a consultant with the Medical Services Branch of Health and Welfare Canada, said he sensed in the room a pent-up desire to speak, and felt the round table was structured to allow for that. He asked participants to introduce themselves.

Alwyn Morris, a Mohawk from the Kahnawake Reserve and an Olympic gold and bronze medallist, has worked with young people for eight years.

Katie Rich has been Chief of the Mushuau Innu Band Council at Davis Inlet for a year.

Dr. Yvon Allard is a member of the Manitoba Metis Federation and a cardiovascular researcher at St. Boniface Hospital.

Jean Goodwill is a registered nurse, former consultant with MSB, and current board member of the Indian Hospital and Health Committee member of Standing Buffalo Reserve, Fort Qu'Appelle, Saskatchewan.

Dr. Irwin Antone is an Oneida, a practising physician, and assistant professor at the University of Western Ontario.

Dr. Edward Connors is of Mohawk and Irish descent. He consults for the Sacred Circle of Ojibway Tribal Family Services, a youth suicide prevention program.

Maggie Hodgson is Executive Director of the Nechi Institute on Alcohol and Drug Education in Edmonton.

Madeline Dion-Stout is Cree, a registered nurse, and Director of the Centre for Aboriginal Education, Research and Culture, Carleton University.

Martha Montour is a registered nurse and a lawyer, attending on behalf of the Native Women's Association of Canada.

Roda Grey is Inuk. She is National Health Coordinator for the Pauktuutit and a member of the Inuit Women's Association.

Aani Tulugak is an Inuk woman from northern Quebec. She is General Director of the Innuulitsivik Hospital and Social Services Centre at Povungnituk.

Dr. Wortman opened the discussion by restating the fundamental questions:

> What is preventing the application of holistic community health strategies to deal with critical situations such as youth suicide, family violence, addiction and other serious ills? How can we support holistic community health strategies to deal with critical situations? Why has this not been done? Who should take these steps?

He suggested holistic strategies don't work because they are preventive, but the Aboriginal community is dealing with crises like suicide and family violence requiring treatment; this dichotomy makes it difficult for decision makers to assign priorities to various aspects of health care.

Ms. Montour expressed pleasure in seeing women at the table because traditional healing practices were cultivated by women, and women must be involved in the decision making that surrounds their implementation. She said the government must stop sending to reserves mainstream medical professionals with no knowledge of traditional culture or practices, and begin funding other models of health care.

Dr. Connors felt the problem was less intrinsic to the holistic approach than to a lack of holistic thinking. Today's young people were raised by non-Aboriginal caretakers, he said, and are unaccustomed to thinking holistically. Consequently, when the elders give them holistic solutions to problems like suicide and violence, they do not understand and are unable to implement them. They are unable to "see the vision the elders have tried to share."

Community health strategies assume a pre-existing sense of community, said Dr. Allard. But this requires a group of individuals with a strong sense of self, common history, and roles in the community. All too often, there is a collection of people living in the same area but not necessarily working together.

However, even "the use of the word community is a step in the right direction," said Ms. Dion-Stout. She discussed the need to understand "all our poverties, not just the socio-economic ones." These are "all of our basic, unmet, human needs." For example, Aboriginal people are made poor by discrimination, and this poverty leads to pathology. Information is vital to understanding these poverties. "Our health is determined by the information in our society that describes our situation," she said.

Ms. Dion-Stout defined herself as something of a "heretic" in her belief that many biomedical strategies haven't worked. But she pointed out that not all traditional practices have been effective, either. For example, she said, "we enshrine the phenomenon of extended families, and I too believe in them, but studies have shown that extended families also hide sexual abuse." She stressed the need to make room for a variety of belief systems, to recognize the good and bad in traditional as well as biomedical practices.

Taking Control

Mr. Morris stressed the need for First Nations people to "take control of our own destiny." Ultimately, he said, government funding is allocated by our own leaders. Who says that just because high school in the non-Aboriginal community takes place over a five-year span that it must do the same in the Aboriginal community? It's a hard world out there, he said, so why not better prepare the young people by stretching high school out over an extra year-and-a-half and keeping them in their communities a little longer?

We are at the centre of an "expanding cultural revival", Mr. Morris continued, "so why aren't we taking control of it?" When Aboriginal leaders are faced with decisions like "who gets a house this year and who doesn't," it's "no wonder they are paralysed." Aboriginal people "must become visionary," he said, by setting their own priorities instead of leaving it up to outsiders to do so.

Ms. Goodwill identified two factors interfering with the effective application of holistic community health strategies. The first, she said, is that communities have always had to grapple with two government departments, one for social services and the other for health. But, "they don't talk to each other," she said. "They must be forced to bang their heads together."

Her second point addressed the need to take health care outside the buildings in which they are housed. When the problem of Aboriginal drug abuse was identified, treatment centres began popping up all over the country. People were admitted and got terrific treatment, but then went home to communities with no support systems. Two weeks later, they were back where they started.

Although he expressed full support of a holistic approach to medicine, Dr. Antone expressed his concern that many communities don't know anything about traditional ways of healing. "Many of them are gone and may be lost forever," he said. He identified a "lack of sincerity" among health care providers and community members who "talk and talk and talk and never go beyond talking." Talk used to lead to community action, he said, but this may be one of the traditions that has been lost.

"I hear many people talk about the need for funding of traditional practices," he said, but if we look back to traditional times we see that "there was no funding." Dr. Antone stressed the need to be sincere and innovative, and to make people accountable. He pointed out that what works in one place may not work in another. And he said there is no reason why "western and traditional medicine cannot be interwoven and practised hand in hand."

"We're burning out our people"

In preparation for her role at the Royal Commission, Ms. Tulugak solicited ideas from professionals and community members. Doctors, midwives and social workers identified lack of funding, personnel, training and treatment facilities in the North as major obstacles to implementation of community health strategies. Community members said: "There are too few people working in health care who understand what we're doing, too few who have completed the circle of healing. Because of this there is too much pain in our community. We're burning out our people."

Ms. Tulugak told of visiting a family who had experienced a suicide in the past year. They told her they didn't want to talk about it, they just wanted to forget. "But we cannot heal without talking," she said.

Community members also identified a lack of resources in the North. When people require treatment, she said, they must go to Montreal. Due to language and cultural barriers there, people come back discouraged. But there are no provisions for treatment facilities under the James Bay Agreement which "governs all our money," she said, just as there are no provisions for daycare centres or recreation facilities. For community health strategies to be successful in the North, there must be funding for resources, as sense of personal responsibility for health, and a willingness among people to deal with their own childhood pain.

Ms. Grey agreed that communities must own their problems, but questioned how this would be possible without funding and resources. It is frustrating, she said, and she found herself wondering if these meetings would be worth it. "They cost a lot of money," she said, "and we need money."

"February 14 is a day when we give gifts to loved ones," began Ms. Rich, "but this February was a sad time for us." Overcome with emotion over the recent near-suicides of six Davis Inlet teenagers, the room was silent for several minutes before Ms. Rich decided not to continue.

"One way we get strength is through our own mythology," said Ms. Hodgson, "but it also stands in our way. We must be aware of our culture, but we must also be aware of the culture we're creating." When the churches came, she said, one of the things they brought was gambling. Ms. Hodgson said when she learned of a 62 per cent rate of long-term sobriety in her community, she wondered what percentage of those people spend hundreds of dollars each month on gambling instead of on their families.

"We go to bingo to socialize and be with others like ourselves," she said, "but we are recreating our culture, and not always to our own advantage." It's been shown, she said, that teenagers develop their addictive behaviours early. Yet they are the ones being left to care for younger children while their parents go to bingo. The parents are saying they work hard, they deserve a break, why shouldn't they spend some money on themselves. But these are the same excuses they used for their alcohol use.

Abandonment is a theme running through Aboriginal culture, Ms. Hodgson said, first through the residential schools, then through alcoholism, and now through bingo. "We're missing the mark," she said, "when we create sobriety but do not address the issue of addiction."

In closing this segment, said Dr. Wortman, "each panelist has spoken. Although Katie Rich said little, her silence probably spoke loudest of her pain and the pain of her community." Dr. Montour then opened the floor to questions and comments.

Responding to Dr. Antone's comments about the interweaving of traditional and modern healing practices, Ms. Jorgensen pointed out that this has already happened although it hasn't been acknowledged. She gave examples of aspirin and cancer drugs which originally came from bark, and said it is time for western practitioners to acknowledge their debt to Aboriginal healers. Dr. Wortman pointed out that Aboriginal contributions to healing comprise more than "boiling the heck out of bark", but include understanding the connections between mental and physical health.

Dr. Connors said that in the past, elders gave healing to their communities in return for support. Today, he said, the elders continue to provide the healing they always have, but the rest of the community doesn't support them as in the past. Unfortunately, he said, today's elders "can't buy gas with tobacco."

Mr. Keith LeClaire, a Kahnawake Mohawk, identified three levels of discussion. On a personal level, he said, there is a need for communication and to rebuild support mechanisms to deal with the pain and anger. On a community level, we must "look at our own communities and ask what we have and how we can use it before asking for more money." On a federal level, Aboriginal people need to be in charge of the allocation of their health care dollars. It's hard to develop programs, he said, when you start talking to one agency, and they bounce you to a second and a third "like a ping-pong ball."

In response, Dr. Allard described how the Métis implemented their own community health strategy 150 years ago by creating St. Boniface hospital, which has been funded entirely by the Métis and Francophone communities. But last year, in keeping with provincial health care reforms, the government took away the pediatric, gynaecological and geriatric wards. "The Métis get no funding," he said. "This facility was created by the community and is now being dismantled by the government. We feel powerless to prevent these 'reforms'."

As a Métis who works for the federal government, Dr. Wortman said he sees people in Aboriginal communities everywhere being confused about where government funding originates, how it's allocated, and so on. He said it's difficult to motivate people when they can't figure out the mazes they must navigate, and acknowledged that this is an issue that needs to be examined.

"The realities haunt us all the time," said Mr. Morris. People leave the reserve to make life better for their people, become immersed in non-Aboriginal society, and then try to go home. But once they get there, he said, they are ostracized for joining the mainstream system. "Once we leave our homes to become leaders in a non-Native political system," he said, "we can never lead in our own communities."

Dr. Isaac Sobol, a non-Aboriginal physician serving the Nisga Valley, commented on the loss of the traditional knowledge base. As an "outsider", Dr. Sobol wondered if there was information to which he was not privy, but said he sensed there has been a loss of knowledge, and asked if there is a will to rediscover and reintroduce traditional practices. "People watch TV," he said, "and see commercials about Robitussin DM. Then, when they come to me, they want Robitussin DM."

Dr. Sobol recalled discussions he'd heard about increasing the numbers of Aboriginal students in medical schools, but questioned whether there was talk of teaching traditional practices at university. He pointed out that the medical system is tied to the pharmaceutical industry, and that doctors are pharmaceutical sales people. This is a problem with the whole society, not just Aboriginal communities, he said, but it impedes the effective implementation of holistic community health strategies. "I've heard talk of calendars which would picture Aboriginal athletes, doctors and actors as role models. But where are the calendars showing healing elders as role models? This, too, is an impediment to holistic health care," he said.

Ms. Goodwill felt that traditional knowledge exists in most communities but is very well hidden. Ms. Aguash of the Enoch First Nation concurred, saying she knows some people who have the knowledge but don't share it due to scientific patenting. They'd rather use it for themselves.

Dr. Wortman noted that although the question had not been answered, it had generated a good discussion. A recurring theme seemed to be the appearance of a vicious circle. He asked: "How can we form healthy communities when individuals within the community are suffering so much? But how can individuals heal themselves without the support of a healthy community?"

Plenary Session

Dr. Louis T. Montour, a Kahnawake Mohawk, physician, and Director of Professional Services at Kateri Memorial Hospital, opened the plenary session with a personal comment. As a physician, he has been asked many times by non-Aboriginals for his view of Aboriginal medicine. When he turned the question back to them, they generally came up with stereotypes about shaking beads and smoking grass.

Dr. Montour, however, described Aboriginal medicine as part of a lifestyle. If one is immersed in the culture, the healing works well, but if one is detached from the culture, it's ineffective, he said. Medical intervention is needed to help people survive long enough to commence their healing journey, he said, identifying respect, caring and sharing as the essence of traditional medicine.

Mr. Tuma Young of the Mi'kmaq Nation said that although traditional teaching is geared to prevention, people have always had crises and traditional practices were intended to deal with them, too. He felt that one thing hindering their use in crisis situations is people refusing to take responsibility for their actions. For example, he said, he hears a lot about violence against women as a women's issue when it should be a men's issue because men are the ones committing the violent acts. This kind of self-responsibility, he said, grows out of self-respect, a respect that says, for example, if you're going to tell teenagers to stop smoking, you have to be willing to take that step yourself.

Dr. Brant, a practising psychiatrist on his home reserve and Assistant Professor at the University of Western Ontario, recalled a story of a patient from a reserve outside London. The youngest of several children who had become quite successful, this man was caring for his elderly mother. She was cranky and mean and constantly reminded him what a failure he was. For two years, despite transportation difficulties, the patient visited Dr. Brant twice a week without progress.

One day, the patient disappeared. When the Dr. Brant saw him six months later at a social event, he looked wonderful, had lost weight, had found a girlfriend. His former patient told Dr. Brant that he had consulted an Aboriginal healer who had told him someone must have cursed him out of jealousy because he was so good-looking and intelligent and came from such a good family. To lift the curse, the elder told him he must throw a feast for all 90 members of his clan.

But this would cost a few thousand dollars, which the man didn't have. So he had to return to his reserve, go off welfare and get a job. He lost weight, met his girlfriend and six months later, though he hadn't saved enough money to throw the feast he was still saving for it, and enjoying life in the process. This, said Dr. Brant, was a fine example of the way traditional healing practices work.

Okanagan elder Glen Douglas identified denial as a major obstacle in solving Aboriginal health problems. He said: "I see myself as three people. I am who I think I am. I am as you see me. And I am who I really am in the darkness of my sweat lodge where I don't role play for anyone. It's there that I can't deny who I am."

A second problem identified by Mr. Douglas was that many people with the knowledge of traditional practices won't use it for fear of being charged with practising medicine without a licence. He told a story about a man who, in 1938, went to hospital with appendicitis. The doctor said he would need surgery in the morning, but the man said no and sent for a traditional healer. When the healer arrived, he put a red bandanna over his eyes, did his work, and the man got up and walked out.

When the surgeon arrived at 6 a.m., he was angry and went looking for the man. Finding him and the healer in a pool hall downtown, he had the healer arrested. In court, the healer was asked what he had done to the man. The healer asked for a pitcher of water. When it arrived he put the red bandanna over his eyes,

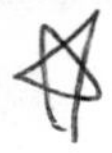

cupped his hands around his mouth and inhaled. The level of the water went down. Then he exhaled, and the level of the water went up. He told the court: "That's what I did. I inhaled the poison out of that man's body."

He then challenged the doctor to try and do the same thing. The doctor said nothing. The healer challenged him again. The doctor declined. The case was dismissed.

Mr. Douglas's last point involved suicide prevention. He said he had lost two nephews and a daughter, and even though he worked in crisis intervention he was unable to help them. "Suicide is very hard to stop," he said. "Sometimes I think about it myself." But he said he has learned to think about priorities, to decide what's most important at any time, and this is a valuable lesson for anyone.

Dr. Connors said he felt that although traditional knowledge has suffered and has gone underground, it is now surfacing again. But it will only flourish when people in western society begin to show their respect for it. At Lake of the Woods Hospital, there is an Aboriginal healing program, but it did not come about at the suggestion of Aboriginal healers — it was created because the hospital wanted them and invited them. Dr. Connors pointed out that, as long as society thinks that healers can do their thing on the side for free while doctors and psychiatrists get paid for their work, Aboriginal knowledge will stay underground. But when that situation shifts and the worth of Aboriginal healers is acknowledged, our society will begin to heal itself.

David Newhouse, an Onandaga and Chair of the Joint National Committee on Aboriginal AIDS Education an Prevention, felt that an important point had been overlooked in the afternoon's discussion. He said that western society has a hierarchy of different kinds of knowledge, and the knowledge and practices of traditional cultures tend to fall at the bottom.

To illustrate this, he talked of a recent experience while sitting on a board created by the Ontario NDP to consider regulation and training standards in the health care field. The Traditional Chinese Healers' Association asked to be regulated, but were rejected because "their practices were not based on a body of knowledge which meets western standards." The Chinese healers pointed out that their practice is 5,000 years old, while western medicine has only been around for 200 years. This shows, said Mr. Newhouse, that "we must begin to consider the question of validity of different kinds of knowledge if traditional health practices are to be taken seriously."

Regarding family violence and suicide, Peter Ernerk, Executive Director of the Inuit Cultural Institute, said that it is "time to take control of our lives and make changes in our own communities." The Northwest Territories now has four suicide prevention specialists, as well as volunteer-staffed crisis lines. He said men must be encouraged to get involved in reducing family violence.

Dr. Montour summarized the plenary by pointing out that we are suffering from a clash of two cultures, one based on traditional values, the other on colonialism and profit. "To get healing," he said, "we must have acknowledgment of the damage that has been done and reconciliation between the two cultures."

Mr. Douglas led a closing prayer in which he gave thanks for the opportunity to meet and share knowledge, and asked for help in guiding each other on a healing path.

Day 2

Panel Presentation of Four Community Social Initiatives

Métis Child and Family Services, Alberta

After Elder Glen Douglas conducted the opening prayer, Round Table Chairman Dr. Louis T. Montour requested a minute of silence to observe the recent death of Derek Decook. In his opening remarks, Dr. Montour emphasized the need for moving ahead and finding solutions. He challenged the panelists to assist in this process and introduced the panel moderator, Alwyn Morris. Mr. Morris is a Mohawk from the Kahnawake Reserve and an Olympic champion.

Carolyn Pettifer, a Métis and president of the Métis Child and Family Services, has worked with the Alberta Métis community for 10 years. She was involved with the initiation of a non-profit housing project in Ontario, but her biggest challenge, she said, is working within the Métis community. "I would rather work in the community and outside the system," she commented.

Ms. Pettifer expressed a need to establish a process to encourage Métis participation and involvement in the direction of future work with provincial and federal governments. A good friend once told her to "get out there and push for process. We must be directly involved in policies and programs that affect our community."

She stressed the need for service organizations to be mandated by Métis political organizations, especially now, when "arrangements with governments really limit us in terms of what we can do." "[The Métis] feel very strongly that our political work is crucial and that it allows us to be involved in political changes that affect us," she said, adding that "there should be more Métis participation at this Royal Commission, and I look forward to a Métis Round Table so that our health and social issues can be adequately discussed."

"The Métis community has a lot of human resources and many of us have survived, overcome difficulties and have been successful," she said. "If we are going to be healthy, self-esteem must be instilled in our children, and our families must provide a supportive environment to make us strong."

"I would like to tell all governments that piecemeal funding is not the way to go," said Ms. Pettifer. "If all these bits of money were collected up, put into a pot, and given directly to the Métis community, we could find our own solutions." Returning to the issue of participation, she stated, "it is we who must decide how we will participate, rather than having the provincial and federal governments deciding how they want us to participate."

Grand Lac Victoria Community

Richard Kistabish, the second panelist, began his presentation by thanking the Royal Commission for the invitation to speak. Mr. Kistabish has been Assistant Adviser in charge of co-ordination for the Grand Lac Victoria Band Council and has co-ordinated professional social services.

Mr. Kistabish explained that his community has no reserve and no legal status. "We are still nomadic peoples who preserve our traditional lifestyles – we are not sedentary," he said, pointing out that "many governments object to how we obtain our supplies and services."

In 1980, when Mr. Kistabish was President of the Algonquin Council, the chief visited him to discuss the "deplorable conditions of the community". Together they determined that a bicultural or holistic approach would be useful in their community. In defining 'bicultural', Mr. Kistabish explained, "we seek all the resources we can get, and we seek them from both cultures."

A multi-disciplinary team of 27 people was established to work with the community. Team members included social workers, a liaison, counsellors, a drug addiction specialist, a nurse, two physicians, a community health physician, a paediatrician, a psychiatrist and two psycho-educators. Special services included family violence prevention programs which served male offenders as well as female victims. The band also received housing, a dispensary and premises for the their council.

"Although the cost of this approach may seem expensive," he said, "when you look at our history and what was taken from us ... it really is not expensive at all.

When we speak about change, it is critical that we take our past into account – this is what we are trying to do in our multi-disciplinary approach to working with the community."

Mr. Kistabish emphasized the importance of denouncing abuse as a step toward community healing. "In the early stages of our process we obtained co-operation from the Quebec Provincial Police – despite the Oka crisis – to send a clear message to the community that the abuse must stop." This was done with the support of the community, he affirmed.

The multi-disciplinary team's work was guided by several objectives:

- *Health and Social Affairs:* The team wanted to rid the community of any illnesses that could be cured by a couple of days in hospital. For example, it was discovered that school officials had mistakenly identified many children as learning disabled, when a great number of them had suffered hearing impairment or loss due to chronic ear infections. The school boards were embarrassed when the scope and nature of the problem were accurately identified.
- *Tradition:* Expressing his personal opinion, Mr. Kistabish said that "religion is for personal and community development – not for curing and healing".
- *Economic Development:* Restoring the economy of the community is critical.
- *Environment:* "It is vital that once you've healed yourself and your community," said Mr. Kistabish, " ... you must also heal the earth."

Mr. Kistabish criticized the administrative practices of the federal government's provision of therapy for child sexual abuse. "Their insistence on paying for individual therapy, and putting a cap on it, I find truly unbelievable", he said. He likened this practice to a surgeon, who in the middle of heart surgery, turns the electricity off and leaves the patient on the operating table.

"You can't leave people open after they have begun a healing process because of monetary reasons," he said in closing.

Alkali Lake, British Columbia

Joyce Johnson, a council member of the Alkali Lake Indian Band, began her presentation with a brief history of the band's study on sobriety and after-care at Alkali Lake reserve.

In the spring of 1992, the Alkali Lake Band received funding from Health and Welfare Canada to conduct research on Alkali Lake's recovery from alcoholism. She said the primary objective of the research was to determine what were the most effective factors in achieving and maintaining sobriety in the community.

"The problem of alcohol must be addressed," she said. "Alcoholism is a disease that has no cure, but can only be controlled." A major difficulty in solving the problem of alcoholism is that "few people are truly knowledgable about [it] and how to attain and achieve sobriety."

"This lack of knowledge about alcoholism in Aboriginal communities is reflected in the shocking statistics on Aboriginal social problems", she stated. For example, the numbers of Aboriginal children in care, and the numbers of Aboriginal adults in jail are six times higher than the national average. Ms. Johnson reported further that "the unemployment rates are double ... and accompanied by living conditions that are described as being at the level of 'third world' standards."

Ms. Johnson made a distinction between 'quitting drinking' and 'maintaining sobriety'. Because they are separate and distinct stages, "they both require a specialized knowledge of alcoholism and an understanding of how to deal with the persons and families affected by the disease". In the Alkali Lake experience, the issue of stopping drinking was first raised at the community level; the second phase of the healing process occurred on a personal level, and comprised the 'after-care' phase of alcohol recovery," she said. Ms. Johnson pointed out that the after-care phase is critical to community healing and development.

The use of confrontation and spirituality intervention, used during the sobering-up and after-care phases was discussed. Ms. Johnson explained that "after-care must be developed to facilitate a healing process" and that "without attending to after-care, the risk of relapse is high, or the person remains a 'dry drunk', perpetuating the same behaviours while sober as they did while drinking." Personal growth, family support and spiritual support were deemed essential in the process of achieving sobriety.

Fred Johnson, a counsellor with the Alkali Lake Band, gave an emotional account of his personal experience of attaining sobriety. As a leader, he said, fear is one of the largest problems he had to face. He explained that "it was not until I looked at my own sexual abuse issues that I began to understand why so many of our people are on the streets abusing and killing themselves." He said he "still cries when hears about the residential school experience."

"It is very important for our leaders to be sober and healing so we can go the distance in helping our people," Mr. Johnson said, and for the government to be respectful in their dealing with Aboriginal people. "We have been through hell and we want you to respect our people".

Mr. Johnson raised the issue of land claims, noting that "this is another hurt my people must deal with." He said that "my traditional territory is a large piece of land, but the reserve we live on is very small ... it is my hope that the Commissioners and the people in Ottawa can do something to change this situation."

Atikamekw Health and Social Services Project

Louis Hanrahan, former director of Health and Social Services for the Conseil de la nation Atikamekw, observed that "my presentation will be more reserved, in comparison to others who have been more emotional, and more realistic. I believe this demonstrates the limits of non-Native intervention and participation."

He added that his presentation reflected the situation of the organization until 1990 and did not reflect events that have taken place since that time.

Mr. Hanrahan gave a brief historical and geographical overview of the Atikamekw communities. There are approximately 3,500 Atikamekw people living in central Quebec, in relatively isolated communities. In 1984-85, they grouped together in an effort to create co-ordinated community services. The band attempted to adopt solutions that would establish their right to control the provision of social services.

An integrated approach, using a 12-member team, was used to implement this initiative. Their work focused on the needs of the community, family and individuals. Mr. Hanrahan said "the team looked for ways to organize services that were culturally appropriate and holistic in nature." The helping of others, he said, was viewed as a sharing rather than a professional activity. Ten members of the community, who earned bachelor degrees in community work at the University of Quebec at Chicoutimi, participated in the initiative. "We didn't believe that professionals were appropriate to carry out this work," he said. "Instead, people with experience in community development were deemed more appropriate. We also recognized that the community had the necessary resources to participate fully and develop their own priorities, and that this was their right."

Mr. Hanrahan cited several factors that influenced this work. He explained that service users were more comfortable with people who were not social workers. The team's ability to work in the community without formal agreements with other services was another important factor. "Agreements were only made on an individual basis", he said. If the team was unable to solve a problem, a community agency was called in to assist. People's involvement at all stages of the work "enabled important social service issues to be dealt with," he stated.

Mr. Hanrahan said that "the biggest problem was the unforeseen severity and prevalence of the problems. We also didn't have clear objectives, but instead aimed at solving very specific problems." Some of these difficulties contributed to the team's inability to maintain control of the work, he said.

In conclusion, Mr. Hanrahan acknowledged that what they were trying to do was complex. He contended that the financial conditions, loss of control, and heavy reporting requirements to several different agencies were all factors creating insurmountable difficulties. Although they wanted to avoid legal control and intervention, Mr. Hanrahan said that "instead, we gave too much power to individuals" who were involved specifically in protection and offender services.

Question Period

A speaker reaffirmed the importance of "Indian people helping Indian people" and stated, "that governments should be making resources available to Indians throughout the land." Elder Douglas addressed the issue of youth participation. "It is like our women, who are half of the population ... we have denied them their voices. We have learned paternalism through the *Indian Act*. We have mistreated our women and children and now is the time to do more than give them mere lip service."

A speaker asked the Alkali Lake presenters if there was an organized teaching program to allow them to share their success with other communities. Ms. Johnson said some statistical studies were available but a lack of analytical documentation of the Alkali Lake experience made it difficult to share their success. Another member of the band expressed her concern "that the process not become to complicated ... It was a simple process, one of sharing and caring."

Panel Presentation: Four Community Health Initiatives

Kateri Hospital, Kahnawake, Quebec

Moderator Peter Ernerk introduced Keith LeClaire, a Kahnawake Mohawk, to present his discussion paper on taking control of health care services at Kateri Hospital, Kahnawake, where he is Director of Administration. Opened in 1905, Kateri Hospital is located on Mohawk land nine miles outside of downtown Montreal. It is a 43-bed facility with a 90 per cent occupancy rate last year, serving 18,000 outpatients per year. It is staffed by, and serves, a mixture of Mohawk and non-Mohawk people.

Kateri is governed by the great law of peace, said Mr. LeClaire, which consists of four themes: peace with oneself and one's surroundings; respect for oneself and others; being of good mind by being positive and creative in thought and action; and responsibility and accountability to oneself and others.

In 1955, the administration of Kateri went bankrupt and the government threatened closure. The community around the hospital – especially the women of the community, and particularly June Deslisle – refused to accept this, choosing instead to take responsibility. "No matter how long it takes," said Mr. LeClaire, the experience of Kateri Hospital is proof that "you can make things happen."

In the absence of government funding, Kateri was maintained by volunteers who brought in food, cleaned the facility, laundered the linens, and so on. With the leadership of the women of the community the hospital slowly built its credibility.

In the 1980s, the hospital needed a new building. Although the climate toward non-Francophone residents, and Aboriginal people in particular, was repressive, the board of 11 directors implemented a four-step plan of action. First, they determined, there was a need to create community awareness of the importance of the new building; second, they worked to have hospital board members elected to the tribal council; third, they lobbied for the council to enter into negotiations with the province; and finally, they established a nation-to-nation agreement with the provincial government, respecting the positions of all concerned.

Although many people were uncomfortable with this process, and in expressing their discomfort ignored the great law of peace, Kateri endured. Mr. LeClaire expressed the hospital's debt of thanks to Myrtle Bush, Franklin Williams and Donald Horn, who were primarily responsible for negotiations.

Because Kateri is not integrated into the provincial health system, but is directly accountable to the Mohawk community, there are fewer bureaucratic stumbling blocks to its administration. As there was no surrender of land to the province, there is not even a provincial flag flown over the hospital.

At the federal level, Kateri is perceived as a provincial responsibility because 90 per cent of its funding comes from the province. It is clear, said Mr. LeClaire, that the federal government has no wish to be responsible for Aboriginal health, but "I believe they should be," he said.

At the provincial level, Kateri is perceived as fulfilling its responsibility to its community members. At the local level, it is seen as a Mohawk institution, fully accountable to the community from which it sprang.

Mr. LeClaire stressed the advantages of avoiding the obligation to adhere to the pre-set policies and regulations of a funding body like the Medical Services Branch. "From a holistic perspective, the transfer initiative is not to our benefit," he said, because it implies that Aboriginal people will bound by a "pigeonhole" approach to funding, eliminating any ability to "pick the programs we prefer."

Several factors contribute to Kateri's smooth operation. Participatory management means that department heads play a major role in establishing priorities. Development of a mission statement, philosophy, goals and objectives at the departmental level, to be integrated into the overall plan, provide a sense of grassroots participation. Recently implemented changes have led to the preparation of an application for hospital accreditation. Good communication among and between the 130 staff, 12 departments, board of directors and the community is facilitated by monthly meetings at departmental and committee levels. LeClaire highlighted the importance of Kateri's employee skills enhancement program. "Better skills make better people, and better people make a better hospital," he said.

Expressing his wish that others learn from Kateri, Mr. LeClaire advised:

- When there is no political action taking place at the community level, make it happen.
- Develop and nurture a core of Indian health advocates to deal with the provincial and federal bureaucracy.
- Strengthen the skills of community people, especially in assertiveness with

the bureaucracy and in planning for training, competency and evaluation.

- Make sure outside planners know that you are obligated and prepared to do whatever is necessary to achieve your goals. "In other words," he said, "walk your talk."

To accomplish these things, planners must ask:

- What is achievable and what is not? Unrealistic expectations lead to failure, which makes a poor foundation for future success.
- Are human resources consistent with organizational needs? If needs change, do we have the resources to adapt?
- Do we have the proper space to be productive? Kateri's 1986 move to the new building precipitated a 36 per cent increase in out-patient use of the facility.
- Have we considered the feasibility of a fund-raising arm? The Kateri Hospital Foundation was created two years ago in response to the hospital's need for additional funding from outside the community.

Mr. LeClaire concluded that Kateri's process had been long and slow, requiring all members of the community to work together within the law of peace. "I began my journey in Kateri Hospital with the help of a physician and a nurse from our community," he said, "and I look forward to Kateri helping me to commence my next journey."

Innuulitsivik Hospital and Social Services Centre, Midwifery, Povungnituk, Quebec

Aani Tulugak narrated a slide presentation on midwifery services at Innuulitsivik Hospital in the community of Povungnituk on the Hudson Bay coast. Innuulitsivik is a 25-bed regional facility serving a population of 4,000 in seven communities.

When the women of the area learned that funding for a hospital was being provided under the James Bay Agreement, said Ms. Tulugak, they "were determined that it not further deteriorate our culture, values and traditions, but that it serve as a tool and stepping stone to our full participation in the provision of health and social services." They wanted a place to learn about their bodies, nutrition, reproductive choices, pregnancy, childbirth and childcare, as well as "a welcoming place for abused women."

When the hospital was provided with an obstetrics budget, the community chose not to hire an obstetrician, but to bring in two white, professional midwives to train three Inuit women in their skills. The midwifery training is intensive and ongoing, and includes weekly sessions with the pregnant women of the community. These sessions provide a time for women to socialize, learn the skills needed to achieve and maintain their own health, identify additional areas of interest, and even learn communications and public relations skills that better enable them to deal with the outside world.

In addition, said Ms. Tulugak, pregnancy provides an opportunity to involve the men. The hope is that by involving and educating the men, their violent outbursts against women will decline. Men are invited to participate as much as possible in prenatal learning, delivery and family planning. Any man choosing to participate in the birth process at the hospital can have his airfare to the community reduced by half.

Elder, traditional midwives are also involved in the training of both the white and the Inuit midwives, so that the community is better able to retain its traditional healing values.

Quality of care at Innuulitsivik is overseen by the Council of doctors, dentists, pharmacists and midwives. The midwives are full partners in the Council who do not act in subordination to it, but with its authority. A midwife sits on the Council's Executive Committee, which is responsible for

1. review of perinatal files around the 32nd week of gestation, as well as at any other time requested;
2. elaboration and review of rules and regulations;
3. review and evaluation of training programs; and
4. establishment and review of the goals and objectives of the perinatal program.

When white staff are hired they must come expecting to teach their skills, said Ms. Tulugak, but staff and community members must also take responsibility for their own learning. (On the other hand, she said in response to a question later, they must also come "knowing that this is the way our hospital works, and if they want to work here, they must work this way, too.")

Just as the midwives are providing support to the community in ways that extend beyond the hours of delivery and birth, the community must support the midwives, said Ms. Tulugak. Their families must understand their need to get up in the middle of the night and go to work, sometimes for many hours.

Although the government continues to call the Innuulitsivik's midwifery services a "pilot program", said Ms. Tulugak, those who work there know that it is in the community to stay. "People are happy with the program, and better health is being achieved for our women and children. We are giving people the best service possible," she said, and that is success.

Anishnawbe Health, Toronto

In introducing herself, Priscilla George said that there were only three things she considered important for people to know about her: that she is an Ojibwa of the Saugeen First Nation, Turtle Clan. Her Ojibwa name means Rainbow Woman and, "when you think about it, a rainbow has no light of its own. It simply reflects, refracts and disperse the light that shines on it. As President of the Board of Directors, I am not responsible for the light of Anishnawbe. I simply reflect, refract and disperse the light of the others there."

Although Anishnawbe Health has existed since 1989, it has undergone massive change recently, she said. A management crisis two years ago shook the confidence of funders and precipitated a "taking-stock process". This culminated in a vision statement which affirmed that the Centre would no longer be 'culturally-sensitive', but 'culturally-based'; that is, it would operate on holistic principles of Aboriginal healing which derive from a philosophical understanding that everything needed to live, and the teachings needed to understand life, are provided by nature.

Anishnawbe's core funding is provided by the Ontario Ministry of Health, with additional funding coming from the Ministry of Citizenship and the City of Toronto. The city hosts a "large, diverse and scattered Aboriginal community of 50,000 to 70,000 people," she said. These people represent nations from across the country, live in all parts of the city, and come from a wide range of socio-economic circumstances.

"They all have one thing in common," she said. "They are looking for a sense of Aboriginal identity and belonging, and they are suffering from the oppression of colonial society which is manifested in many ways. They come to Anishnawbe for two things," she said, "an understanding of their history, and to learn traditional ways."

The original focus of Anishnawbe Health was on western medical practices, said Ms. George. There was a great deal of discussion about culturally sensitive services, and much time spent on cross-cultural training. Within the culturally-based model, however, western doctors play a secondary role to Aboriginal healers, who provide the primary means of treatment.

This model, said Ms. George, cannot be clearly defined or described because it is new, and as such it is constantly emerging, evolving and exciting. It involves an ongoing process of innovation and creativity, creating new programs and recreating old ones.

One tremendously successful program has involved bringing in an Ojibwa medicine man for two five-day sessions of diagnosis and treatment. On each visit, he treated 100 people, some of whom travelled hundreds of miles for the benefit of his healing. The irony of rural residents travelling to an urban centre to experience the healing power a medicine man whose way of life is rooted in traditional practices was not lost on the staff at Anishnawbe.

On each occasion many of the people he saw had been undiagnosed, misdiagnosed or over-medicated by western doctors. It cost the Centre only $30 per person he treated. This does not begin to account for health care dollars saved in cancelled surgeries and tests, missed appointments with specialists, and unfilled prescriptions, Ms. George said.

Anishnawbe staff played a vital role in the success of his visits, explained Ms. George, practising the correct protocol for inviting and welcoming him, cutting through red tape that allowed him to visit people in Toronto hospitals and care facilities, accompanying those who were apprehensive about receiving their first traditional treatment.

It is clear by the response to his presence and services that there is still a widespread belief in the value of traditional healing, said Ms. George. Yet there are few traditional healers around, and even fewer who are willing to leave their communities and travel to urban centres.

Other programs include an elder counselling service, traditional talking circles, Aboriginal language programs, writing workshops, issue-focused weekend workshops, AIDS awareness and HIV testing programs, and an extensive street work program run by six street workers and 200 volunteers and reaching 200 people per week by providing food, blankets, condoms and a needle exchange.

Anishnawbe also employs two physicians who hold clinics at many locations around the city and are on call 24 hours a day, 365 days a year, as well as nurses who provide family support services, after school programs and the like. In total, some 2,500 people per week use the services of Anishnawbe Health.

Ms. George stressed that it is not possible to provide traditional services without providing opportunities for staff to increase their knowledge of Aboriginal traditions, and incorporate them into their daily lives. An ongoing program focusing on personal empowerment and cultural integrity has precipitated "intensive personal growth" among staff and board members, who are looking forward to two healing retreats in the near future. Board and staff commitments to personal healing have been essential to the change and growth at Anishnawbe.

Two years ago, Anishnawbe faced the challenge of uprooting the western healing practices which had taken hold, leaving traditional healing in a low priority position, said Ms. George. She felt this had happened because:

- people fear the unknown;
- funding is more easily granted for medical doctors than traditional healers;
- society places a higher value on those with academic training than those with knowledge rooted in tradition;
- traditional resources and healers are scarce; and
- there is a lack of familiarity with the protocol for dealing with traditional healers.

Obtaining funding is an ongoing challenge, said Ms. George. The government will no longer provide funds for people to travel to their own reserves to seek healers from their own nations. Although responsibility for Aboriginal health belongs to the federal government, status Indians living off-reserve are historically forgotten in political negotiations. Ms. George stressed the need for urban Aboriginal people to assert their rights to regain their political, social and economic health through places like Anishnawbe Health.

Nuu-chah-nulth, British Columbia

Speaking on behalf of Richard Watts, Chairman of the Nuu-chah-nulth Health Board in Port Alberni, Simon Read began by acknowledging the Salish Chiefs for allowing the Royal Commission to take place in their territory, thanking the Commissioners for the opportunity to talk about Nuu-chah-nulth, and extending Mr. Watts's apologies for not speaking in person.

"Nuu-chah-nulth Chiefs have never signed a treaty recognizing a basis of co-existence," said Mr. Read. This, and building community self-government have been the focus of the Chiefs for many years. Self-government encompasses many things, he said, one of them being health and medical services. The health transfer initiative fits into a tribal council strategy formulated in 1981 because it allows for internal rather than external control.

Mr. Read identified three issues of concern to the Nuu-chah-nulth Health Board:

- The need to undo the effects of five generations of colonial government. "In the past 12 weeks," he said, "we have experienced 42 suicide attempts in a population of 3,000, one of them completed."
- The reconstruction of wellness in communities. "Traditional systems are skeletal," he said. "We must use them as a framework on which to rebuild our communities."
- The patchwork of federal and provincial funding sources. "It takes much time and energy to make the process work," he said.

Traditional healing is a way of life, said Mr. Read. "We need to encourage people to seek out their own life path" by drawing on the elders within their families and communities. Along this process, people confront their own issues. The Health Board has a role in helping them through this time, and encouraging them to return to a traditional view of health.

There are no qualified physicians from First Nations in British Columbia yet, and few First Nations nurses, Mr. Read observed. It is important for young people to enter these fields. To that end, career material encouraging elementary and high school kids to think in those directions has been distributed. But, he added, education in these fields "must be grounded in our own systems."

Mr. Read identified the short-term issues as control over non-insured health benefits; availability of home care options; follow-up work on residential school issues; assumption and integration of government programs; and development of better urban services for the 50 per cent of the Nuu-chah-nulth population living off-reserve.

In the long term, Mr. Read identified two key issues: problems with the justice system in dealing with abuse issues that should be dealt with in the community; and treaty negotiations aimed at providing a resource base to support Nuu-chah-nulth health services.

In closing, Mr. Read recalled the words of an elder who said, "when attempting to cross a strong-flowing river, you must test each step along the way. Some of the stones that look the strongest are the ones most likely to give way."

Health Economics

"I am not a specialist in the area of health economics with regard to the First Nations community," said Professor Robert Evans in his opening remarks. "What I can provide is a sense of national and international economic trends, which have an impact on what is being discussed at this conference." Mr. Evans stressed that he does not assume knowledge of First Nations' political and personal agendas.

Mr. Evans spoke at length about the illness care system (ICS), which he emphasized was not a critical term. Actually, he said, ICS, the dominant tack of western medicine, is "good at taking care of illness," but quite removed from a holistic approach to health. When the World Health Organization defines health, they could consider a broader system, he suggested, something more than just the continued support of ICS.

"The conventional, mainstream health care system in Canada is in crisis," said Mr. Evans. There is an "orchestrated outrage" on the part of health care workers and users, who despite a continuous dialogue, cannot manipulate an unwieldy system. In the past 30 years, he continued, the expenditure on health care per capita has grown by 400 per cent.

Canada is not the only country experiencing difficulty with its health care, stated Mr. Evans. The United States, countries in Europe and many other nations are recommending reforms to their systems. The time frame is also similar: in the past five years, countries around the world have exhibited a desire for health care reforms.

"What is causing this crisis?" queried Mr. Evans. Approximately 10 years ago, changes in the level of economic growth in western Europe and Canada occurred. Mr. Evans showed a graph of the growth of Canada's real GDP (Gross Domestic Product) from 1960-1991, illustrating that it did not keep pace with other economic factors. As the economic environment deteriorated, conflict resulted in the health care system. The effects of this conflict are still being felt, said Mr. Evans, especially when available monies for reform do not match the high levels of expectation.

There is mainstream support for health care reform, said Mr. Evans, which will continue its lobbying despite setbacks (e.g., the closure of Shaughnessy hospital). The management of the system of health care must improve.

While the interest in reform is keen, said Mr. Evans, when priorities change, someone or something must go without. The accommodation of new and old needs is problematic: creative solutions must be sought.

Research which focuses on the presence of disease has not proven as illuminating as was expected, said Mr. Evans. For example, there has been "virtually no pay-off" on the studies of people on reserves who have lung cancer. While the major cause of lung cancer – smoking cigarettes – has already been proven, the reasons why people begin to smoke have only just begun to be studied. In this case, research has had no effect on the outcome of an individual's health. The prevention of cigarette addiction would yield greater health to more people than any type of cancer treatment. As well, the issue of tobacco advertisers, and their targeting of young people as future smokers, must be addressed.

Panel Presentation: Discussion Papers

Funding Policy for Indigenous Human Services

Moderator Dr. Jay Wortman introduced the panelists. Kim Scott, a Senior Policy Analyst for the Royal Commission on Aboriginal Peoples, and the former Director of Health and Social Services at the Kitigan Zibi reserve, began her presentation by thanking the Musqueam and Salish nations for hosting the conference on their traditional territory. "I am comforted and pleased to see so many familiar faces here," said Ms. Scott.

"I am going to talk about the distribution of health wealth in Canada," began Ms. Scott. She described the CAP (Canada Assistance Plan), which, in its delivery of social services, takes a narrow focus and doesn't provide the same range as provincial agencies. The IHAs' services (Indigenous Health Authorities) are also restricted. The hope for CAP, said Ms. Scott, is that it can reconcile federal and provincial government responses. If the provinces do not agree with the federal government on the extension of services to reserves, then First Nations peoples will not receive the same broad services as other Canadians.

Ms. Scott discussed the transfer initiatives from the federal government: "In response to the growing pressure from Indigenous groups to move away from the paternalistic delivery of human services, the departments of Health and Welfare, Indian and Northern Affairs, and, to varying degrees, provincial governments have developed mechanisms to allow the transfer of administrative control for human services to local IHAs." Aboriginal communities are taking more control in this process. Ms. Scott also referred to the Health Programme Transfer (HPT), which "allows communities to access funding for the transfer process which includes pre-transfer planning, a health needs assessment, negotiations and transfer implementation."

While the short-term community evaluation of HPT recognizes its contribution of "greater financial and programmatic flexibility", the funding policy has also been criticized because it "does not allow for program evolution or enrichment." Specifically, this shortcoming is evident in "the lack of adequate services for Fetal Alcohol Syndrome and AIDS cases in the post-transfer scenario." Greater flexibility is needed, stressed Ms. Scott.

Non-insured health benefits were discussed next: "Also not available under the Health Program Transfer are the roughly $214 million being spent on non-insured health benefits (NIHBs) annually." NIHBs cover such things as prescription drugs, prosthetic devices, dental care, eye glasses and medical transportation. Ms. Scott recommended that the "administrative responsibility for NIHB...be transferred to Indigenous health authorities."

Another area of concern to Ms. Scott was the funding policies of the Social Development Branch of Indian and Northern Affairs. Absent from these budgets are community development and work activity projects. As well, within the new funding policy known as the Management Regime, there is no provision for "the establishment or operation of services for communities with fewer than 251 children." Ms. Scott acknowledged the reality of present "fiscal restraint," but felt "ethically obligated to highlight that this represents the substantive portion of isolated communities where children are at greatest risk." Aren't these children entitled to protection, too? she asked.

Deficits, Foundation and Aspirations Signal Need for Restructuring

William Mussell is a researcher, author and member of the Skwah Band, from the Sto:lo culture. He began his presentation by expressing concern over what he perceived as a lack of interaction among the participants at the Round Table. "I hope there is an opportunity for more discussion later in the day," he said.

Mr. Mussell made reference to "the two dimensions of the big picture, past and present." "We must know where we came from," he stressed, "before we know where we are going." It is from the elders that this knowledge will come, he said. Terms such as past, present and future are arbitrary, he continued, when you consider that time is more of a continuum than one static place or moment. But the history of First Nations peoples – their continuum – has been broken.

Extended family units can be thought of as an agent and client dynamic, said Mr. Mussel, with each person fulfilling a role and meeting their responsibilities within that role. Recent years have seen a tremendous breakdown of family roles – a separation of the agent from the client. Decisions that belong within the family have been made by outsiders. It is very important, said Mr. Mussell, that we bring together once again the client and the agent.

The issue of self-government will also create a client/agent dynamic, said Mr. Mussell, in that a "reciprocal interaction" will be required from First Nations peoples. At the moment, he is "very concerned that our own organizations are engaged in a one-way exchange of information," even at events such as this Round Table. No increased knowledge is derived from these exchanges, he concluded.

"There must be an opportunity for questions and the exchange of feelings," said Mr. Mussell. In regard to age, he said, different aged peoples have different needs. Care must be taken to meet the needs of all. It is with care and honest communication that the real change will occur.

If we are serious about solutions, said Mr. Mussell, everyone must respect and value each other's life experience. Our relations with people on the outside of our communities have affected the relations within our community as well, he said, creating feelings of unease and secrecy. We must model change within ourselves, and stimulate feelings of empathy. Any new strategy must focus on sharing.

Mr. Mussell discussed the "Information Wheel", which he said has subjected Aboriginal peoples to an outsider's perspective of themselves. We need to develop a new curriculum, he said, and "we should also produce research that will stir an appreciation of our history. We are taught in the school systems the reactions of Europeans to Aboriginal people but how did our forefathers react to them?"

Balance, between the heart, the mind and the spirit, is essential to the well-being of First Nations people, said Mr. Mussell. This means growth in the holistic realm.

On the subject of the teaching/learning model, Mr. Mussell said that the life experiences we know best, are the things that we can understand fully and share easily with others. And we create our own knowledge, he said. Learning how to learn is more important than memorizing information.

"We haven't lost our culture or history," affirmed Mr. Mussell, "because culture is a dynamic, living creation – we are always moving forward." The confusion comes from the outside, from people who do not understand the abstract nature of culture. "We have an opportunity to enrich our culture as we pass it on to the next generation," said Mr. Mussell. "We must listen to our internal environment."

Reciprocal interaction holds the key to the promotion of health within Aboriginal communities, Mr. Mussell concluded.

Treaty Right to Health

Alma Favel-King is the Executive Director for the Health and Social Development portfolio of the Federation of Saskatchewan Indian Nations. She began her presentation by acknowledging Chief Scott of the Kinistin Band, for whom she has great respect.

"I am not an expert in the area of treaty rights," said Ms. Favel-King, "but I can address some points on this subject." She referred to three questions posed in the discussion paper:

- How will the federal government transfer process enabling community control of health services and the recognition of treaty rights to health impact on the future of First Nations people?
- Will this process facilitate a holistic approach to health maintenance and how will this be achieved?
- How will the role of provincial and federal health agencies change?

The treaty right to health is not practised by the federal and provincial governments, said Ms. Favel-King. "We were told by the elders that our forefathers entered into a treaty process to ensure the survival of future generations," she said. There was confusion on this issue, however, because the word "health" did not even exist in some Aboriginal languages (e.g., in Cree, there is a phrase for well-being, but no single word denoting the western concept of health.) Regardless of these confusions, the elders acted in good faith and viewed the promise of a "medicine chest" as "access and availability of a wide-range of primary, secondary and tertiary health services."

Until the 1940s, the Department of Indian Affairs "maintained responsibility for all aspects of programs and services to Indian people," said Ms. Favel-King. After this time, the responsibilities were transferred to Health and Welfare, Medical Services Branch (MSB). Indian Affairs retained some services, but the two departments did not operate efficiently in combination: "The working relationship between these two departments has not always been geared toward meeting the needs of First Nations but rather that of carrying out the department's mandate as directed by the legislators of the day."

The MSB adopted a western European definition of health, said Ms. Favel-King. In regard to action on behalf on First Nations, the MSB and Indian Affairs used a ping-pong approach, she said. Furthermore, there "has been no documented case where the two departments have ever agreed to a joint process to address the treaty right to health issue."

Ms. Favel-King outlined four requirements for change:

- the recognition of the right of self-government;
- although the *Constitution Act, 1982* declared the re-affirmation of treaty and Aboriginal rights, the federal government has not provided the leadership necessary to put into practice what is contained in this legislation. Steps have to be taken to ensure that treaty understandings become the basis of any programs, policies, procedures adopted by the federal government;
- a reorganization of the federal government with respect to the responsibility of all programs and services for First Nations would be required;

- that an office of a federal treaty commissioner or treaty ombudsman be established. This office would monitor and be a watchdog over how the federal government meets its treaty obligations to First Nations governments.

A short question and answer period followed the conclusion of Ms. Favel-King's presentation. Bill Mussell added thoughts on "self-management," which is his favoured expression for self-government. He referred to "co-reliance", where families can rely on one another and survive and grow. The growth will be achieved by sharing, he said, by both giving and receiving. "Passive dependence" will diminish, he concluded, as we learn to share our feelings.

Dr. Harriet Kuhnlein directed several questions to the three speakers on the relationship of First Nations peoples with the land (traditional food systems). Bill Mussell replied that the "identity of the people is anchored in the land," even to the extent that their names often reflect the geography of their homeland.

Round Table 2: Policies to Facilitate Aboriginal Control of Health

Round Table moderator Alwyn Morris welcomed the participants.

David Newhouse is a professor of Native Studies at Trent University and Chair of the Joint National Committee on Aboriginal AIDS Education and Prevention.

Richard Jock, a member of the Mohawks of Akwesasne, is Director of the First Nations Health Commission.

Lou Demerais is Executive Director of the Vancouver Native Health Society.

Ron George is National President of the Native Council of Canada, and a Hereditary Chief of the Wet'suwet'en Nation.

Patrick Johnston is Executive Director of the Canadian Council on Social Development in Ottawa.

Jane Gottfriedson represented the Aboriginal Women's Council.

Dr. Catherine Cook has been a fly-in physician in nursing stations in Northern Manitoba for four years.

Dr. Marlyn Cox is a fly-in physician and a member of the Native Physicians' Association of Canada.

Sheila Genaille is Research Director for the Metis Nation of Alberta in Edmonton and advisor with the Constitutional Reform Committee.

Judy Moses is Director of Aboriginal Services for the B.C. Ministry of Health.

Michael Sims is Director General, Program Policy Branch, Indian Affairs.

Marie Fortier is Acting Assistant Deputy Minister, Medical Services Branch, Health and Welfare Canada.

Stephen Chase is responsible for federal, provincial, and Aboriginal policy matters for health and social services, government of New Brunswick.

Huguette Sauvageau represented the Ministry of Health and Social Services, government of Quebec.

Mr. Morris opened the discussion by restating the fundamental question:

> Aboriginal communities and individuals are assuming greater responsibility for health. What policies can facilitate that process? What are the recommendations for implementing a holistic strategy?

Jane Gottfriedson presented an overview of the work of the Aboriginal Women's Council, an organization representing many groups whose members work on a daily basis to improve the lives of people in the community. All the groups were established and are controlled by the grassroots, she said.

The groups have been active in many areas. Projects include establishing healing circles; preparing a lay counsellor's handbook to stimulate community participation in dealing with alcohol and drug abuse, family violence, HIV/AIDS and other issues; a literacy program; and Urban Images of Aboriginal Peoples, training for severely disadvantaged community members. The goal of these initiatives is to empower individuals to help themselves and their family and friends. The focus remains on individual and community involvement partly because there is a lack of resources for other kinds of initiatives. "The challenges we face are very grave," said Ms. Gottfriedson. "To lead the world in the number of suicides is an unacceptable situation."

She made a number of recommendations to the Royal Commission, including the following:

- Lasting solutions need adequate resources, under the control of Aboriginal people. Aboriginal people must have input at the highest decision-making levels.
- Health care systems must incorporate Aboriginal philosophy and ensure a holistic approach to the issues.
- Comprehensive land claims must be adequately funded, and the funds should not simply be redirected from other programs.
- The databases used for budget projections must be based on the real demographics of Aboriginal populations.

Ron George explained that the Native Council of Canada is looking at how to move toward a framework for health legislation that supports all Aboriginal peoples. He proposed an "Authorities Regulation Act" that would "cover up the cracks in the policies that our members fall between."

Mr. George said that the Community Futures Program's allocation of $170 million is used strictly for Aboriginal children living on reserves, even though the allocation was calculated with all Aboriginal children in mind. "The 1991 census showed that two-thirds of Aboriginal people live off-reserve," he added.

He lamented the failure of the Charlottetown Accord, which would have ensured equal access to resources for all Aboriginal peoples. There needs to be constitutional recognition of off-reserve people, he said, and self-government would mean that off-reserve people would design their own health services. He added that there are already enough people working on behalf of on-reserve populations.

Mr. George said that the movement toward increased control over health care must involve women, youth and elders in active roles. He criticized the 60 per cent cut in off-reserve housing, noting that "we have no land base and we need to upgrade our standard of living." The lack of housing for his members has reached a critical point, he added. Off-reserve people must have access to adequate resources. "There is nothing that off-reserve groups can access except on an ad hoc basis. The federal and provincial governments are using us as political footballs." He stressed the need to untangle the jurisdictional conflicts between levels of government.

His final comment concerned treaty rights. One of his organization's biggest problems is that the federal government treats treaty rights as status, he said. "They like to say that status equals treaty, but there's no connection whatsoever." He noted that many treaties were written before the Indian Act was introduced, and he urged participants to be clear about the distinction between treaty rights and status rights.

Patrick Johnston said he had "taken in a lot over the past few days" and he could only give back one observation. He recalled his involvement about 10 years previously in meetings about problems facing Aboriginal communities. At that time, one of the biggest problems was the removal of children from the communities by government social service agencies. Mr. Johnston noted that during the previous days, he had heard nothing about this issue; for him, it was a positive development. "Aboriginal communities are reclaiming responsibility" and there are now many community-controlled family and children's services organizations.

Mr. Johnston said the reason for the increase in community control was that "Aboriginal people took action themselves. They said, 'enough is enough, we're going to do it ourselves'." In some cases, bands instituted their own by-laws, not waiting for government policy to change. He suggested that Aboriginal people shouldn't always wait for policies to change, because that may never happen.

"The solution starts with us."

David Newhouse didn't know if more money would solve the problem of lack of adequate health care for Aboriginal people. "We have to stop giving responsibility away to other people," he said. "When we give away responsibility, we give away our lives. The solution starts with us. We are responsible for our health." New policies and structures that support service delivery to Aboriginal peoples must be developed.

Mr. Newhouse was optimistic about the ability of Aboriginal people to take on the task. He noted that in 1972, there were 600 Indian students in Canadian colleges and universities; in 1992, the number was 23,000. (The figures are based on the federal funding for Indian post-secondary students.) "There have been tremendous advances in education," he said, and the challenge is to find ways to bring the graduates back to the communities where they can help work toward solutions for community problems.

"This Royal Commission is the first in the history of royal commissions where most of the work is done by Aboriginal peoples," he continued, noting the wide range of expertise in the room. "We have the human capital to do the job."

There is a need for community guidance mechanisms to direct the programs, Mr. Newhouse said. He sees the federal government serving as a tax base for communities "telling us how to spend the money. We need to find ways to break the link with the federal government." Aboriginal people should begin to define accountability to themselves, not to the federal government.

Improving health will be a long-term process, and it must encompass improving standards of housing and economic development. "When we talk of health, we need to increase people's incomes," he said.

Lou Demerais works in what he said was the poorest riding in Canada, Vancouver's Downtown Eastside. His organization, the Vancouver Native Health Society, is "trying to put something in place to improve" that situation. In order for real change to happen, several factors must be addressed, including the following:

- Aboriginal people must have their own health service institutions and control over spending.
- Governments must recognize the need for traditional healing.
- Adequate funds need to be allocated to health services.

His organization has set up a healing centre where traditional healers work alongside western doctors. He is ambivalent about having the government more involved in traditional healing methods. "Anytime you get government recognition of something, you also get government regulation," he said. "That would be the death knell of traditional healing." If traditional healing is to work in clinical settings, "it needs to be self-regulated, not government-regulated."

"Both levels of government are responsible for funding Aboriginal health," Mr. Demerais continued, because both governments are responsible for "screwing up" the lives of Aboriginal people. As well, churches should be contributing their own funds to Aboriginal health care initiatives, by "handing over money to us." In general, "we need less bureaucratic interference in the process," he said. He predicted that governments would resist giving up control, but said that the response should be "we'll make a few mistakes but we can't do any worse than you're doing now."

Mr. Demerais related a recent problem faced by his organization involving an investigation of alleged mismanagement of funds, instigated, he said, by rumour-mongers within the government. He told the story to illustrate "the things we have to go through just to provide services."

Dr. Marlyn Cox was "frustrated" by some of the presentations made at the event so far. "We've heard about a lot of pain and anger in communities," she said. Dr. Cox provides primary care to a community of more than 4,000 people. She and the other staff see more than 100 people each day. There are not enough resources, and "what we ask for to provide quality care is not being listened to."

"It's frustrating to deal with Medical Services Branch (MSB)," said Dr. Cox. "Some days, it's just easier to ignore them." She suggested the reason that no Aboriginal doctors from MSB were at the table was because they have information on how the money is spent, and "their lips are sealed."

"We have to find a way to do away with MSB," Dr. Cox continued, suggesting that the Branch develop a policy working toward its own demise by 1997.

"We have heard our people pleading to give us responsibility and power to take care of our people," she said. She noted that "First Nations people are big business in health." In one community, more than $2 million was spent sending children to treatment centres outside the community, while the community itself has been asking in vain for their own treatment centre.

Dr. Cox concluded that she "never gets a response when she phones MSB," partly because many of the officials are only "acting" officials who will not commit themselves. She asked Marie Fortier to respond to her concerns.

Ms. Fortier agreed that the long-term objective of MSB should be to disappear, but said "we need to work together through a long process" toward that end. Responding to Dr. Cox's comment about the lack of MSB doctors at the table, Ms. Fortier said the reason for the absence was that the subject of discussion was policy, not service delivery. She added that there were indeed many "acting" officials in MSB, and it was a situation she hoped to improve within the next few months.

Turning her comments to the transfer initiative, Ms. Fortier said that the "current transfer initiative is the first generation of transfer initiatives" and its limits are "very real," operating within the current legislative framework. Now, after almost 70 communities have entered into transfer initiatives, there has been opportunity to evaluate the program.

"We need to work at a community level to bring better co-ordination of efforts" at improving health care, she said, citing the Innuulitsivik Hospital midwifery program in Quebec as one example of a positive outcome of collaboration between MSB and the community.

Responding to David Newhouse's comments, Ms. Fortier said that "if the impression still exists that transfer communities still report to the federal government, that is not the intent." Of course, she added, there must always be financial accountability – "you'll never get rid of it" – but authority for health care in transfer communities rests with the communities themselves.

Mr. Newhouse challenged her statement, saying that the federal government transfers funds to the provinces for health care "with no questions asked." Ms. Fortier responded that "you're talking government-to-government transfers, and that's another level," adding that there was accountability, even at that level.

Richard Jock commented that "We're not going to talk about how to work with the status quo. I hope there will be fundamental changes" to the relationship between the government and communities for control of health care. He cautioned against "getting sucked in" to debates about sectoral boundaries.

Mr. Jock said the reason why First Nations are funded through contribution agreements is that "legally, First Nations don't exist", and policy was created to deal with the situation. But a relationship between the government and a body with no legal basis is not a good relationship, he said. "This must change." He criticized the government for refusing to deal with treaty rights. "Treaty rights must be affirmed, recognized and implemented," he stressed.

"Empowerment" usually refers to the individual, Mr. Jock continued, but treaty rights provide the same kind of empowerment. The federal government should not be let off the hook from their responsibility for treaty rights to health care, he said. In the United States, there are many examples of the U.S. government dealing fairly with Indians through treaty rights, he added.

"Move from a 'welfare' approach to a 'rights' approach."

The solution is to move from a welfare approach to health care to a rights approach. The economics of the situation need to be examined, he said, referring to earlier presentations about the danger of Aboriginal people being marginalized if health care priorities are shifted.

Judy Moses stressed that governments need to understand the importance of a holistic approach to health care. "Jurisdictional debates are an excuse for inaction," she said. The B.C. Ministry of Health is moving toward decentralization and regionalization. Ms. Moses believed that the presence of an NDP government in the province represented a window of opportunity for change.

Ms. Moses said that structural change must involve the active participation of people working within the system, Aboriginal people who remain accountable to their people. She explained that she and her colleagues have worked very hard to get $5 million in funding for treatment programs out to Aboriginal control. The funds have been transferred to regional boards which have in turn funded more than 200 projects this past year alone. The transfer arrangements are "not perfect", because the spending parameters are narrow and not holistic, she said, but it could serve as a model for policy change in other areas of the country.

Michael Sims said that western society has focused on an individual, not collective, approach to health care, and "we have no precedents, no lessons to give you [Aboriginal people]. We're groping just like you are." A key question, he said, was "how can you teach what you learn to others?"

Mr. Sims said that forums like the Round Table were good venues for sharing information about health care initiatives, and suggested that an important component of moving toward more Aboriginal control of health care was "finding ways to systematically share information."

The moderator challenged Mr. Sims's statement, saying that information sharing wasn't enough if "you're still caught in the framework" of a traditional approach. Mr. Sims responded that none of the health care programs for Aboriginal people were legislated; all are policies, with general authority coming from the *Indian Act*. "The general framework can all be changed," he added, urging Aboriginal people to take action on their own initiatives. "Just do it," he said.

"Métis people are a political football"

Sheila Genaille interjected that "not all Aboriginal people in the country come under the *Indian Act*." When Métis people approach the provincial and territorial governments for health care, they are told to go to the federal government. Echoing Ron George's comment, she said that Métis people are "a political football." Sorting out the jurisdictional conflicts is key to the solution of Aboriginal control of health care, she said.

The practice of categorizing issues as 'Aboriginal' is a "game that masks the desperate state of affairs in Métis communities," Ms. Genaille said. She asked Round Table participants and authors of the position papers to be clear about the use of terms such as Aboriginal or Indigenous because "when we use these terms without clarification, we perpetuate a Canadian tragedy."

"The Métis ask that you not generate status-blind data, papers, presentations and recommendations," she continued. "If you mean Indian or Inuit, then say so....Collectively, we share the same problems," but the Métis social and health problems are amplified because of the jurisdictional dilemma of the Métis.

Ms. Genaille said that before change in health care occurs, politicians and bureaucrats must "change their attitudes toward Métis." Funding must be made more equitable to Métis people. When speaking of traditional healing, the question must always be asked: "Whose tradition?" Approaches to spirituality and healing cannot be generalized. She concluded by urging the Royal Commission to increase the participation of Métis people.

Stephen Chase said "the sheer scope and complexity of the problem is intimidating", but policy makers have begun to recognize that there are ways to approach the problem and deal with it on a piece-by-piece basis. Change is possible within the existing framework, he said.

Mr. Chase believed that provinces had much to offer Aboriginal communities working toward more control of health care. "Provinces have a broad-based experienced with health, social services, mental health and addictions," he said, and this experience can be used by communities as they develop programs and services.

He added that in addition to a holistic approach to health, a socio-economic approach is also important; if the goal is community self-sufficiency, improving the economic situation of a community is "every bit as important" as improving its health. He said that strategies for working toward self-sufficiency should include the following components:

- political willpower
- effective partnerships
- holistic and socio-economic strategies
- a well co-ordinated, multi-disciplinary approach to service delivery
- established goals and measurement of results

Huguette Sauvageau made the suggestion that the communities under the James Bay Agreement negotiated by the federal government, the government of Quebec, Hydro Quebec, the Inuit and the Cree, might serve as a model for other communities working toward more autonomy.

In his closing comments, moderator Alwyn Morris noted that Aboriginal people are a minority in this country for political reasons, but given the minority situation, "we have to make sure that we find a way to have an impact."

Plenary Session

The first speaker at the plenary session, Carrie Hayword, Aboriginal health co-ordinator for the Ontario Ministry of Health, told the gathering of an initiative under way in her province that "so far, seems to be succeeding." The family violence initiative was a collective effort of five organizations representing First Nations' interests, 11 provincial ministries, and two federal departments in an ex officio capacity. The ongoing challenges of the program include communication, especially reaching agreement on the definition of common terms; addressing the history of mutual distrust among the three major players; co-ordinating all the participants; and harnessing and directing the resources more holistically into community-based systems.

Jean Aquash, an Anishnawbekwee elder from Walpole Island in Ontario, said she was confused about how the word holistic had been used at the Round Table. She recalled "the old people" teaching that holistic meant a combination of mind, body, spirit and emotions, and a holistic approach would therefore be characterized by kindness, unconditional love, truth and honesty. However, the word holistic had been "used flippantly during the last few days," said Ms. Aquash. "What does holistic funding mean?" she asked – does it mean money handed over in kindness and unconditional love?

Dr. Catherine Cook said she has been confused about her role at the Round Table and "unclear as to what was expected of me"; she suggested that it would have been helpful to have a clearly defined idea of "who or what we're attempting to provide services for." She added that solutions to improving the health of Aboriginal people should not separate health and education, because "as education improves, so shall health; as health improves, so shall education."

Dr. Cook said that the transfer process needs continual re-evaluation. There should be long-term planning of funding. She concluded with comments about non-insured health benefits, which are "a mystery" to her. She wondered how much of the $450 million in the program is directly benefiting communities, and how much ends up paying for service providers.

Dr. Michael Monture, from the Six Nations Grand River Territory and a medical officer with MSB, said the solutions to the problem will differ, depending on "who we are trying to address," and it is important to recognize the similarities and differences between Aboriginal groups. Other issues to explore include whether rights should be linked to geography (land base), entrenched in the Constitution or contained within the Indian Act. He said rights should apply to all Aboriginal peoples, regardless of identification, but acknowledged that this approach will be limited by funding realities. Dr. Monture suggested that "using holistic and health in the same sentence is redundant, because the two are the same."

Tuma Young, co-ordinator of the Mi'Kmaq AIDS Task Force in Nova Scotia, said that "we should just go ahead and *do* it. Go ahead, don't wait for the federal government, the provincial government." He said that if his group had waited for funding from Health and Welfare, the program would never have begun. Among the group's success stories is convincing all the First Nations in the Atlantic region to pass resolutions to incorporate HIV/AIDS awareness into everything they do.

Day 3

Panel Presentation of Discussion Papers

Health Care Improvements for Labrador Inuit

Iris Allen, Executive Director of the Labrador Inuit Health Commission (LIHC), noted that the health conditions of Labrador Inuit are considerably worse than those of the average Canadian. The reasons include low income, unemployment or under-employment, inadequate education, sub-standard housing, alcohol abuse, tobacco use, poor water and sewer infrastructure, and family violence. "Even as our communities are pulling together and developing plans," she said, "we feel helpless" to improve the situation.

Created in 1985 as an affiliate of the Labrador Inuit Association (LIA), the goals of the LIHC include improving housing, employment, and other living conditions that affect the health of the Labrador Inuit.

Core programs of the LIHC include a Community Health Representative Program, with CHRs providing health education in five communities, and required in two more; a Health Liaison Program to assist Labrador Inuit in navigating the health care system and providing interpretation; a Non-Insured Health Benefits program, which is one of only two Aboriginal-administered programs of its kind in the country; and a seven-month-old Dental Therapy Program, which is already having success in improving the oral health of school-age children. In addition, LIHC has recently hired a family violence co-ordinator, a mental health co-ordinator, and a suicide intervention field worker.

In the future, said Ms. Allen, the LIHC hopes to be instrumental in developing a comprehensive training package for community health and services workers in all pertinent areas of mental health; facilitating the creation of community crisis response teams, community counselling, and crisis lines; and obtaining the services of a psychologist to provide staff training in counselling skills, conduct workshops, and provide one-to-one counselling.

The LIHC uses existing resources to promote health careers through individual counselling, tours of health facilities and educational settings, and advocacy. The LIHC and LIA have been instrumental in getting the Nursing Access Program at Labrador College off the ground, and take pride in the several Labrador Inuit currently enrolled in nursing studies in Labrador and Newfoundland. LIHC has also taken a proactive role in monitoring all the health research taking place in Labrador.

Members of the LIA and LIHC recently completed a series of community consultations with the aim of developing a five-year plan for the amalgamation of all health programs for the Labrador Inuit under a Community Health Department of the LIA. This plan, said Ms. Allen, will involve constant and ongoing staff education; trained staff will pass on their knowledge to the membership of the LIA. The LIHC is developing a Community Health Plan which would deal with the specifics of this ambitious undertaking.

Ms. Allen identified several barriers to the continued forward movement of Labrador Inuit health care. Jurisdictional issues regarding program eligibility pose a time-consuming impediment. There are four groups defining health policy for the Labrador Inuit: the federal Medical Services Branch, the provincial Department of Health, Grenfell Regional Health Services, and the LIA through membership in the LIHC. These groups have different understandings of the needs of Labrador Inuit and how they should be met and, despite efforts on everyone's part, the groups do not work well together.

The CHR program has not reached its full potential because of lack of ongoing training, inadequate supervision and co-ordination, and lack of recognition of CHRs as full, participating members of the health care team by health professionals.

The isolation of the Labrador Inuit as the only Inuit group in the Atlantic region provides little opportunity to network with other Inuit groups. This makes it difficult to address the lack of understanding in outside groups of the inherent differences between Inuit and other Aboriginal people, as well as the hardships posed by geographic isolation, a harsh climate, limited economic opportunities and obstacles to transportation.

Another barrier cited by Ms. Allen was the severely limited availability of services for Inuit with disabilities. Limited wheelchair accessibility in homes and public buildings, lack of training programs and employment opportunities, limited or non-existent home support programs, inadequate or inappropriate methods of transportation, and poor knowledge of services that are available – all impede the full participation of Inuit with disabilities in their communities. Other barriers are inadequate staffing of nursing stations and the need for Inuit to travel outside their communities for specialist services.

Recommendations for improving the health of Labrador Inuit include the following:

- The federal and provincial governments together should make interim decisions on the eligibility of Labrador Inuit for health and social programs while awaiting the results of the land claims process.
- The MSB should commit funds to provide ongoing training programs to CHRs, NNADAP and mental health workers.
- All levels of government delivering health care must work together.
- Financial and professional assistance to Labrador Inuit communities should be increased.
- Labrador Inuit must have the authority to establish health boards and committees to plan, implement and control community health services.
- Services must be brought to the people rather than people having to travel to the services.
- Health care careers must be promoted among Inuit youth.
- Working water and sewer systems, adequate housing and meaningful employment in isolated communities are imperative.
- Well developed and easily mobilized resources must be made available to communities in crisis.
- Inuit with disabilities need accessibility to new and existing public buildings and private homes; opportunities for meaningful employment and involvement in community activities; and ongoing home care and respite programs.

Health and Social Issues of Aboriginal People with Disabilities

Brenda Sinclair of the Alberta Health Care Commission Office said she felt humbled because "I am not an expert on disability. The words in this paper are the words of the people, who are the real experts." The paper addressed 11 areas of concern, said Ms. Sinclair, posing three questions in each area: What problems are people with disabilities facing? What would people with disabilities like done about them? Who do people with disabilities feel is responsible for implementing solutions?

The people spoke extensively about their need for housing, health care, access to traditional healing, and additional home care opportunities. Ms. Sinclair found that educational needs expressed by able-bodied Aboriginal people were a non-issue among Aboriginal people with disabilities because opportunities to attend college "fade before the daily struggle of putting food on the table and adding wood to the stove."

Isolation is a significant problem for Aboriginal people with disabilities, said Ms. Sinclair. Not only are they suffering physical isolation because of a lack of transportation and accessible buildings, but also community isolation because no one at the community level has the mandate to care for their needs. Even where services are available, she said, information about them is not getting through the bureaucratic maze to those who need it and those, like the CHRs, who could help them gain access to it.

At a conference last year of Aboriginal people with disabilities, some participants stated: "We are no longer willing to be forgotten. We are not asking people to do our work for us. We can do our own work. We ask only that our presence in the community be recognized and our participation in the community be supported physically, emotionally, mentally and spiritually."

Ms. Sinclair asked who has the mandate to give voice to the needs of all Aboriginal people with disabilities. She expressed her hope that provincial organizations for Aboriginal people with disabilities would represent all Aboriginal people with disabilities, whether Métis, status or non-status, living on or off reserves.

At the local level, there is a need for support groups for people with disabilities and their caregivers. In addition to providing social and emotional support, these groups should give people with disabilities a voice to ensure that community members and leaders become accountable for the needs of all members of the community.

Ms. Sinclair's paper addressed several broad areas in which she proposed recommendations. These areas included empowerment of people with disabilities; review and re-visioning of access to western health care and traditional healing opportunities; personal supports for people with disabilities; accessibility at home and in the community; and the need for transportation.

It is important to note that the same issues being discussed today, said Ms. Sinclair, were discussed at a think tank on Aboriginal people with disabilities held in 1988. "Today the recommendations of that think tank are only words in a book on someone's shelf," she said, emphasizing the need to ensure that recommendations made at this time be acted upon.

The issues, she said, involve respect, honour, caring and sharing. "How do we as a people treat each other?" she asked. "In our quest for healthy communities, we must push to the forefront the well-being of our brothers and sisters living with the burden of disability."

Ms. Sinclair concluded by saying that the English translation of her Cree name means 'Eagle Woman Who Stands Strong for the People'. "I hope I have brought honour to the people by living up to that name here today."

Beyond the Caregivers: Health and Social Services Policy for the '90s

Sharon Helin acknowledged the presence of so many people in the room who were able and qualified to address the issue of culturally appropriate care. Ms. Helin stressed that she did not speak on behalf of all First Nations people, but from her own experience and the experiences of those with whom she shares her life. "I am not an expert," she said. "While we sit in a comfortable hotel we must not forget that someone in Fort Simpson may at this moment be sitting at a loading dock waiting for a plane to take them to medical care." They are the real experts, she said.

"We are living in a world of shifting paradigms," she said. Hospital beds are closing, user fees are being charged, the province of British Columbia is reorganizing its health care system, and there will be a federal election this year; Aboriginal needs for health representation must be placed in this context, she said. "From Nuu-chah-nulth to Kahnawake, we must build on the successes already achieved by First Nations people."

In speaking of culturally appropriate health care, Ms. Helin chose to focus on care of the elderly as a result of her experiences with her 92-year-old grandmother. "I once heard a prayer offered to the Great Spirit to be with our elders and stretch the length of their days," she said; Western medicine sees old people in the past tense, describing the full lives they've lived before they die. The important thing, she said, is to focus on helping old people continue to have good lives.

Ms. Helin described a recent situation in which her grandmother fell and was injured. A series of western health care professionals failed to discover anything to explain the pain she was experiencing. Five days after her initial examination and X-ray, she was almost unconscious from the pain. It was finally discovered that she had five compression fractures in her spine. The most frightening element of this story, said Ms. Helin, is that "she has me to speak for her, but many of our elders have no one to speak for them."

"We need to humanize our discussions about health care jurisdictions instead of always being guided by cost," she said. "We need institutional change guided by caregivers. We need a commitment from caregivers to examine decision-making processes and provide access for First Nations people to the closed boardrooms where those decisions are made."

Getting just one Aboriginal person on a hospital board is not enough, she said. One person alone will face little success in conveying a First Nations view of health to 11 people who support the views of the dominant culture. Ideally, institutions should not be making decisions on behalf of Aboriginal people. "Yet institutions will be around for a long time so we must learn to live with them."

Speaking of transfer initiatives, Ms. Helin said "government policy has increased the gaps between the haves and have-nots in Indian country." Transfer policies are creating a situation in which only large bands are economically healthy enough to fit program criteria, but "all First Nations people need access to better health care."

In the midst of the shifting models, First Nations people have experienced one constant approach to health care that has been successful for years: traditional healing.

Ms. Helin highlighted the following needs: for self-government; for the federal government not to treat Aboriginal people differently than non-Aboriginal people regarding transfer payments for health care; for Aboriginal people in communities to have employment opportunities in the "big business" of health care; for Aboriginal input into development and implementation of policy; for improved Aboriginal access to health care programs; and for culturally appropriate health programs.

"We always hear talk of a mythical 'they'," she concluded. "But there is no 'they', there is only us. If we want change, we must take the responsibility to make it happen."

Pathways to a Dream: Professional Education in the Health Sciences

Lynn Chabot presented this paper on behalf of its author, Dianne Longboat, who was unable to attend. Ms. Longboat works at the Office of Aboriginal Student Services and Programs at the University of Toronto, and Ms. Chabot, previously Recruitment Officer for the Aboriginal Health Professionals Program at the University of Toronto, has returned to her community, Kitigan Zibi Anishnabeg, to work on economic development.

Ms. Longboat's paper, based on the work of the Aboriginal Health Professionals Program, looked at overcoming the barriers facing Aboriginal people entering and completing professional health careers. The paper identified academic barriers to university entrance, as well as institutional, financial, geographic, personal and social barriers. The most fundamental of these, said Ms. Chabot, revolves around a lack of interest among young people in studying maths and sciences. Even those with an interest in these areas at the elementary level tend to lose interest by the time they reach high school. But without high school fundamentals, students are barred from most careers in the health sciences before they reach university.

The University of Toronto has two programs designed to maintain interest in maths and science: the First Nations Summer Science Program, and the Aboriginal Science and Mathematics Pilot Project. Other university programs have been implemented to support Aboriginal students once they arrive.

Academic and personal counselling programs are available, and increasing efforts are going into culturally appropriate curriculum redesign.

"While it is important for our young people to have up-to-date knowledge on current medical issues and practices, this must not happen at the expense of their cultural knowledge," she said. Through a slow process of co-operation between First Nations people and the university administration, knowledge of traditional practices is being incorporated into course content.

"Although we have found solutions in many areas," said Ms. Chabot, "we are always stymied by lack of funds." Most funding bodies are interested in funding pilot projects which last, at best, a few years. Ongoing programs are needed, but many careers in health care require training that extends beyond the period for which financial assistance is available, leaving students with few alternatives once the money runs out, she said. Until the need for ongoing funding of health care students and culturally appropriate programming is addressed, First Nations people will continue to have difficulty fulfilling dreams of greater numbers of Aboriginal health care professionals.

Defining Disability

In response to a question posed after the presentations were made, Ms. Sinclair defined disability as any impairment of hearing, speech, sight or mobility, but said she also included people with literacy problems, diabetes, and other chronic diseases. The participant who asked the question said he agreed with her definition but warned of difficulties she would have in convincing government officials of her position.

Ms. Chabot identified a lack of role models as the biggest single problem in encouraging young people to believe they can pursue careers in health care. She noted a mentoring or job-shadowing program at the University of Toronto and she said a similar program in areas distant from the city should be helpful in making youth believe, "Yes, I can do this."

Peter Ernerk, Executive Director of the Inuit Cultural Institute, said that the biggest problem facing health care workers in the Northwest Territories is service delivery. Too many people must travel to southern Canada for health care. He praised the efforts of ministers of the government of the Northwest Territories, the majority of whom are Inuit, to improve health conditions for northern peoples. In addition to promoting the importance of preventive health practices, it is vital to give people a knowledge of their rights as patients.

Mr. Ernerk praised the hard work of nurses in the N.W.T. but bemoaned the presence of only one physician to serve the region of Keewatin. He stressed the need to treat people's emotional as well as physical pain, pointing out the dire need for Inuit professionals able to speak with unilingual patients in their own language to understand and treat that pain. He emphasized that in the

Northwest Territories, as elsewhere, improvement of health care conditions for Aboriginal people is a federal responsibility.

Dr. Ed Connors, a Kahnawake band member and psychologist, asked why we have been unable to apply a holistic model of health in our communities. "Perhaps it is because we haven't been thinking holistically." He said that Aboriginal people base their understanding of health and holistic health on definitions created by the outside world, and said that as long as we continue to do this "we will miss the mark." Professionals in western health all have different labels and mandates for care. They often work at odds with each other, leaving clients and families confused. By the time a suicidal person has passed through several professionals who all think someone else is better mandated to help, the person might be dead, he said. "We must dialogue to develop our own definition," he said, suggesting as a starting point the Ojibwa term for health which means "good life".

Brenda Sinclair responded by talking about the different ways in which western and traditional healers look at the same problem. As an example, she talked of a schizophrenic patient who agreed with his doctor and his pharmacist that his was a mental illness. His community, however, perceived his illness as spiritual. This difference between western and traditional perceptions, she said, requires a shift in the type of healing used.

Elder Glen Douglas responded to Dr. Connors by saying that First Nations people already do have a definition of holistic health, and to learn it one must only go to the elders and ask. He said many elders are frustrated by the number of times people have not listened to them, but they remain the holders of knowledge, wisdom, skills and patience. He expressed his own concern at the absence of elders at this Royal Commission, and wondered if it would affect the Commission's credibility with the elders at his home. He also expressed frustration that the traditional gift of tobacco made to an elder in exchange for his wisdom was not offered to him at these meetings. In closing his remarks, and the discussion of the papers presented, he challenged participants to think of the two words used repeatedly by him in his prayers of the past two days, which define Aboriginal rights.

Round Table 3: Overcoming Barriers to Health Care

Moderator Dr. Jay Wortman reminded the participants that the Round Table was "not a forum for prepared speeches," but rather a place for the exchange of ideas and information by experts in the field of Aboriginal health care. He reviewed the three questions that the thirteen speakers would be addressing:

> What are the roles and responsibilities of the health care partners in ensuring that non-Aboriginal institutions are responsible to Aboriginal health needs? In particular, the specific needs of

Aboriginal people living in remote and northern areas and Aboriginal people with disabilities? What are the obstacles that need to be overcome?

Dr. Wortman expressed hope that the alternative of "health promotion" would soon replace the current model of paternalistic health care.

James Smokey Tomkins, President of the National Aboriginal Network on Disability, stated that disability is a social and economic issue. He was disappointed at the lack of discussion on Aboriginal people with disabilities. "You have to include all the people [in the communities], or your circle is incomplete," he said. He concluded by cautioning Commissioners not to omit the issues of people with disabilities when it came time to consider new policies and programs.

Dr. Isaac Sobol, a medical health officer and family physician with the Nisga'a Valley Health Board, spoke about the biases against First Nations people shown by non-Aboriginal people in institutional settings. Choosing workers with a different orientation toward Aboriginal people, as well as placing health services within Aboriginal communities, would eliminate this type of prejudice, he said. Health care workers need to have an appropriate historical perspective of Aboriginal people, he emphasized.

Dr. Roland Chrisjohn, a member of the Oneida First Nation and a registered clinical psychologist, has worked in community-based research projects at the Blood Reserve in Alberta and at Williams Lake, B.C. "I call for revolutionary change in institutional health care and practices," he said. "How relevant is the western style of medicine – including the practice of psychology, which has no consideration of the spirit – when applied to the health care of Aboriginal peoples?" he queried.

A non-Aboriginal health professional, Dr. Chris Derocher told a story about his time in the Yukon. "In the decade I worked in the Yukon," he explained, "I had never attended a Potlatch, because I had never been invited to one. After 10 years, when I mentioned this to a Native woman in the community, she told me that I didn't need an invitation, all I needed was to care about the people who were at the Potlatch and just come." Imagine taking a decade to discover this cultural difference, said Dr. Derocher. "It taught me never to assume I knew all the differences between Native and non-Native worlds," he said. He also applied this realization in his work as a doctor.

Carrie Hayward is the Aboriginal Health Co-ordinator for the Ontario Ministry of Health. Her current priority is the development of an Aboriginal Health Policy in partnership with Aboriginal organizations. "I am an advocate," said Ms. Hayward, "I work for Aboriginal people." As an advocate, Ms. Hayward recognizes the tremendous distances that separate Aboriginal health care from the care that other Canadians receive. She works hard, she said, to obtain monies from bureaucracies and apply them to the areas of greatest need.

A professor of Anthropology at the University of Alberta, and the Director of the Centre for the Cross-Cultural Study of Health and Healing, Dr. David Young has worked with traditional Aboriginal healers in northern Canada. "Who are the experts in health care?" he asked and then supplied the answer: the healers. Healers do not always receive the respect they deserve from young people, he said. To remedy this, he suggested the medical community re-empower northern traditional medicine by putting it on a legal footing. This has been done successfully in China, he said, and could be established in Canada, as well. By conferring a legal status on traditional healing practices, the status of the profession would rise, and would draw into its sphere the younger generation. At the same time, it would protect healers from prosecution and interference from the larger medical community. Dr. Young also recommended that funding be available to help young people in the North study traditional medicine.

Helene Sioui Trudel, a representative from the National Indian Inuit CHR Organization, spoke about biases held by young Aboriginal people and how it is easy to go from one extreme to another, neither extreme representing an accurate picture of Aboriginal peoples. She referred to current attitudes toward western medical practices; at the moment, she said, health practitioners are much more oriented toward the treatment of disease than to disease prevention. She called Aboriginal elders "resources in the community" and emphasized the importance of listening to the older generation. As for herself, she is "fighting all the time" to improve health care services for First Nations people.

A Fundamental Principle of Safety

"We should adopt a fundamental principle of safety for Native people," said Clare McNab, a Cree Métis woman from the prairies. This means mental, emotional and spiritual safety, she said. The context of health care practices is also important to consider. Once an Aboriginal health care professional has been trained in a large urban centre, he or she often returns to a small community, where they have to re-learn who they are and reacquaint themselves with the people they are treating.

Conrad Saulis is the Director of the Native Council of Canada. The desire within Aboriginal communities to take responsibility for their own health and to reinstate traditional medicine practices is strong, said Mr. Saulis. Non-Aboriginal people must acknowledge the expertise of Aboriginal healers and understand that traditional health care is the best way to heal Aboriginal peoples. Because Aboriginal people feel comfortable and secure seeking advice from elders regarding health issues, the non-Aboriginal institutions should strive to be partners with us, he said, and accept the fact that we are equal. This recognition is imperative, he stated. Echoing the opening remarks of Dr. Wortman, Mr. Saulis said that paternalism needs to die out. Even when research on health is done, he said, the work should benefit the Aboriginal community and not be undertaken to provide an academic with material for another article.

"I am very pleased to hear about the successful reinstatement of traditional health practices in China," said Jean Goodwill, the past president of the Aboriginal Nurses Association of Canada. "Let us hope this success will be repeated in Canada," she said. When traditional practices are coupled with the high level of skill displayed by Aboriginal nurses, she continued, the end result will be a vastly improved and relevant system of health for First Nations people.

Dr. Michael Monture, from the Upper Mohawk Nation, works with the Medical Services Branch of Health and Welfare Canada. He spoke about the importance of effective communication, comparing language to a basic building block from which the attainment of goals can be achieved. He also referred to the difficulty of overcoming colonial attitudes and how these attitudes continue negatively to affect the lives of First Nations peoples.

It is crucial to promote health careers among Aboriginal peoples, said Marilyn Sark, President of the Aboriginal Nurses Association of Canada. Not only does the Association do this, she said, it also acts as an agent to promote better health care for Aboriginal people. "We are a collaborative body," said Sark, because we work with the government and the Aboriginal community. "In our capacity as role models for young Native people, we do our best to convey the satisfactions and challenges of a career in health care," she concluded.

During a discussion of traditional Aboriginal healers, Dr. David Young said that "Native healers refer people to western-trained doctors, but these doctors do not in turn refer cases to Native healers, even though the latter's success in such areas as the treatment of chronic stress diseases is very high." James Smokey Tomkins added that "there are two types of healing in traditional practices – the use of herbs and the emphasis on the spirit. Why can't we insist on the acceptance of traditional healing? What are the objections of western-trained doctors?"

Marilyn Sark asked the other participants if they were concerned that some traditional healers might abuse traditional medicine.

In response, Dr. David Young said that "we need some kind of self-regulation process. Beyond that, the local grapevine is effective – word goes out about who is good – or bad." James Smokey Tomkins agreed.

Dr. Michael Monture said that "there is no difference between good or inadequate doctors who are western-trained or who practise traditional medicine. People soon discover who they can trust." Jean Goodwill added that "the general population is very sceptical about spiritual aspects of traditional healing. This is one obstacle to overcome."

Helene Sioui Trudel said that "it is the recognition of our own people [in the area of traditional medicine] that we need to develop. We can trust our own healers and take the time to define health – nutrition, exercise and the spirit – in our own way."

Moderator Dr. Jay Wortman said he now has "a much deeper appreciation of traditional medicine. I do not hesitate to recommend it. It doesn't matter to me that the western scientific community cannot validate traditional medicine to their own satisfaction. I know that it works."

Conrad Saulis wished that Aboriginal youth "were more involved with this process of discussion. We have to respect all groups within the community – they should be here in greater numbers. Also, where are the friendship centres?" He added that "there should always be a representative from one of the people with disabilities' associations at these conferences. Their needs must not be overlooked."

The last speaker was Dr. Vince T. Tookenay, a member of the Native Physicians of Canada. After reviewing a brief history of his organization, Dr. Tookenay made a more general comment on First Nations peoples in Canada: "We haven't defined our own paradigm. We hear elements from other people, but this isn't enough."

Dr. Tookenay recommended the formation of a National Native Institute of Health, where all First Nations peoples can participate in the formation of a vital and relevant program of health care.

Dr. Tookenay reminded participants that before self-government is achieved, Aboriginal peoples need to be fully in control of a health care system that meets the needs of all its users.

Dr. Wortman opened the discussion to other participants. Woodrow Morrison, a Haida with degrees in economics and law, said that before discussing the problems, it was necessary to look at the symptoms. He said the world is suffering from a "global melanoma" caused by British imperialists who "destroyed the environment and people wherever they went." He recommended, to audience applause, that future Round Tables adopt the format of the traditional talking circle, so nobody can dominate the discussion.

Elder Jean Aquash said that "we are the healers, and we need to be heard."

Report from the Rapporteur

Professor John O'Neil was asked by the Royal Commission to synthesize and analyze the presentations and interventions made over the course of the Round Table.

Mr. O'Neil began by briefly reviewing his experiences, since 1975, studying Aboriginal health care systems, suggesting these experiences might have helped his reflections on the Round Table, but he added that his academic background also might have made him somewhat over-analytical about the material. "How many PhDs does it take to screw in a light bulb?" he asked. "None – they just sit in the dark and contemplate different paradigms."

Noting the frustration expressed by several participants about the lack of time for discussion, he suggested that future Round Tables adopt a small discussion format, to give participants more time to express their views.

Many solutions were proposed to the issues at hand, he said. Noting that the Commission was anxious to find long-term solutions to problems facing Aboriginal peoples, solutions that might mean a basic restructuring of Canadian society, Mr. O'Neil stressed that "health is central to these issues."

"We don't deliver health," he said. Health is something interwoven with daily living, and self-government is clearly one long-term policy solution to improving the daily lives of Aboriginal peoples. Mr. O'Neil speculated briefly about what self-government would look like. "It's not just about power," but also about economics and resources. Self-government should address the issues facing children, people with disabilities, and all people who suffer in Aboriginal communities, and "self-government has to reflect all the issues we've talked about in the last few days," he said.

Some of the community initiatives discussed during the Round Table "are examples of what self-government should look like," Mr. O'Neil continued, adding that he was amazed by some of the initiatives presented. Self-government is a long-term solution, but there must be immediate action to address the daily suffering in communities. "I've heard a clock ticking through the meeting – people are dying while we sit here talking." He added that the struggles of community members from Davis Inlet to Vancouver's Downtown Eastside were "practically identical" – there are the same kinds of distress and the same lack of access to resources.

From his perspective as a political economist, Mr. O'Neil believes that the responsibility of those working for social change is to "level the playing field," to create a structural environment were healthy individuals and communities are possible. Some of that responsibility lies with the communities, and he repeated the advice given by several participants: "Just do it."

He added that levelling the playing field is the responsibility of the Royal Commission, in its recommendations to the government at the end of the process.

Referring to Robert Evans's presentation on health economics – in which Mr. Evans said that "something happened in the last 10 years" to the economy that resulted in the deterioration of the health care system – Mr. O'Neil said that the fiscal policies of the conservative governments of Mulroney, Reagan and Thatcher must surely have been responsible for the deterioration, and replacing those governments with ones determined to improve the situation must surely be part of the solution. "Political will starts in the prime minister's office," he said, echoing a comment made by a participant.

Dr. Vince Tookenay had suggested to Mr. Evans that an Institute of Aboriginal Health be established, and Mr. Evans agreed. "It should be established in the very near future," he said, adding his belief that large institutions would be willing to contribute financially to the project.

Mr. Evans recalled visiting Australia shortly after one of the state governments adopted a policy of spending 10 per cent of its health care budgets on Aboriginal health, after a study determined that 10 per cent of the state population were Aboriginal people. Mr. Evans suggested that a similar study in Canada tied to a policy review might result in a "considerably larger" allocation of funds for Aboriginal health in this country. Some of this money could go toward funding the proposed Institute.

The Institute could have regional branches and would be based on the principle of Aboriginal rights – in the broadest sense possible, to extend access to health care to all Aboriginal people across the country.

Part of the Institute could be a National Aboriginal Health Research program, under Aboriginal control. Funding for the initiative would be drawn from many sources, and Mr. O'Neil predicted that post-secondary institutions would be very interested in aligning themselves with the program, resulting in spin-off benefits such as training programs for Aboriginal students.

Also associated with the Institute could be a National Council of Elders and Traditional Healers, a self-regulating body that could serve many purposes, including assisting people who don't have access to traditional healers.

These initiatives would be associated with the various associations for Aboriginal health care workers (such as the Indian and Inuit Nurses of Canada, the Native Physicians' Association of Canada, etc.) Association with the Institute would allow "cross-fertilization among the health care professionals," said Mr. O'Neil.

He suggested the formation of Community Healing Centres in communities that were willing to take on the task of running health care institutions. "New hospitals aren't easy to establish," he noted. The centres would be rooted in human values and could encompass many kinds of healing, including treatment centres.

Another idea is a Healthy Options Program that would direct health care funds into improving recreational facilities and programs in communities.

Mr. O'Neil remarked that the room was filled with "a group of extraordinary people" and that the human resources available to provide health care services for Aboriginal communities were "stretched extremely thin". He noted the potential for burnout.

He added that he is aware of the many silent voices in Aboriginal communities, especially isolated communities: people who are not able to communicate their needs to health care workers and not able to advocate on their own behalf. He also noted that there are many unsung heros across the country – Aboriginal people who have pioneered initiatives in health care – who need to be more recognized for their efforts.

Round Table Chairman Louis T. Montour thanked Mr. O'Neil for an "incredibly insightful and powerful report." He thanked Commissioners and the behind-the-scenes staff of the Royal Commission who worked hard on the event. Commissioner Allan Blakeney thanked the many people who contributed to the Round Table, the presenters and everyone who asked questions from the floor. He gave a special thanks to elders Jean Aquash and Glen Douglas and Chairman Dr. Louis T. Montour.

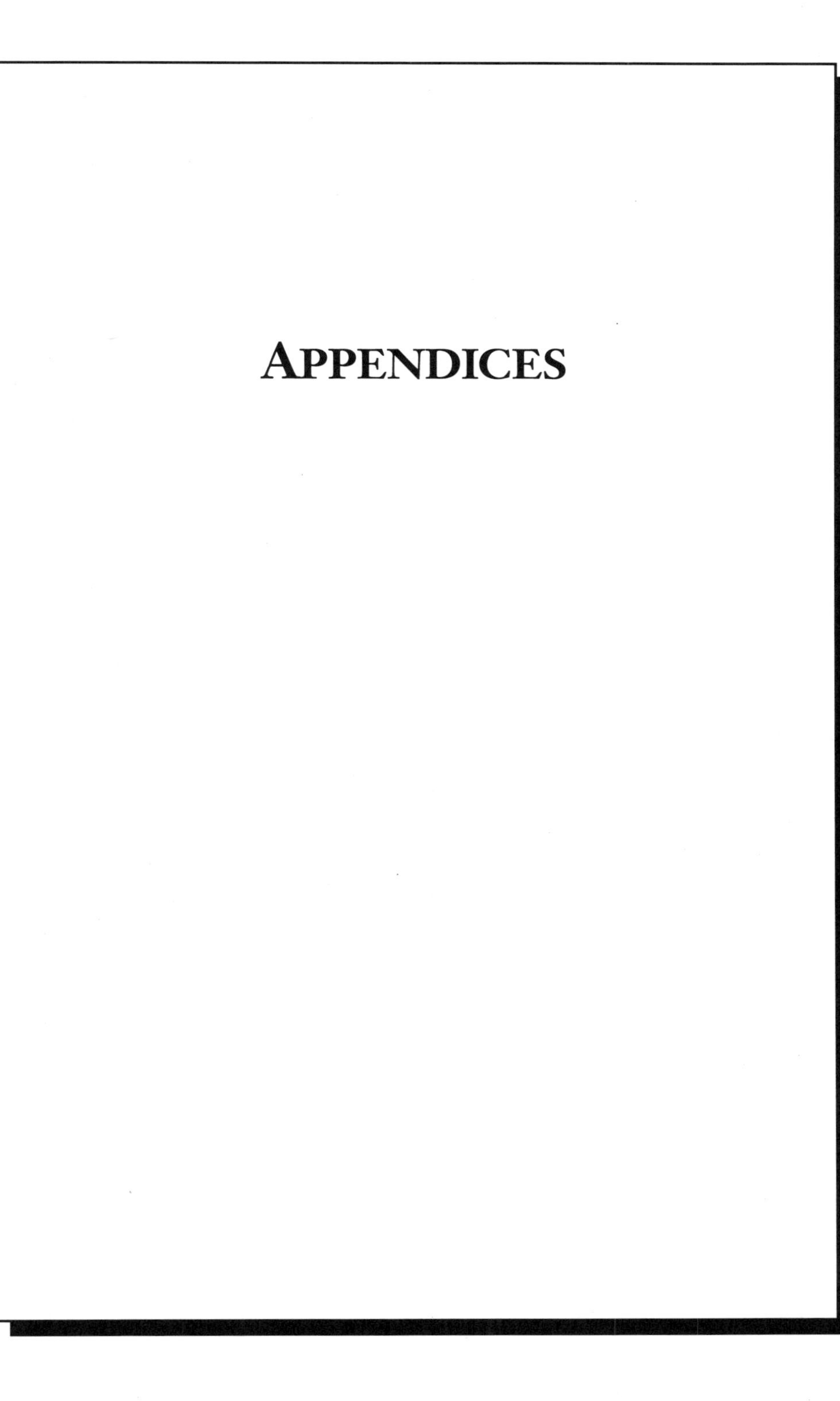

APPENDICES

Round Table Program

Introduction

The past few decades have seen numerous studies on the health and well-being of Aboriginal people, including:

- *Indian Conditions: A Survey*, Department of Indian Affairs, 1981
- *Urban Research Project*, National Association of Friendship Centres, 1985
- *National Native Child Care Study*, Assembly of First Nations, 1989
- *The Circle of Care*, Native Council of Canada, 1990
- *Métis Families*, co-written by the Métis Nation of Alberta and Métis Child and Family Services, 1990

These studies paint a grim picture of the state of well-being in Aboriginal communities, but few of their recommendations have been implemented. As a result, little improvement has been apparent in the past three decades or more; health and social services remain inadequate, inaccessible or culturally inappropriate for the communities they serve, and Aboriginal people remain at substantially greater risk than the general population with respect to virtually all physical ills, including respiratory, circulatory, gastro-intestinal and infectious diseases, parasitic infectious, accidental injuries and poisoning.

Health and well-being in Aboriginal communities are closely related to poor environmental and economic conditions, inadequate housing and sanitary facilities, and the social dislocation occasioned by the disruption of support networks such as the extended family through divorce and separation, the birth of children in single-parent families, child wardship, and the adoption of Aboriginal children outside their cultural milieu. Poor diet and lack of exercise or recreational opportunities for Aboriginal youth are contributing factors to the increasing statistics on early obesity, heart attacks and diabetes.

Of particular concern are the situations of Aboriginal women, youth and elders and issues such as family violence, youth suicide, and drug and alcohol addiction.

Recent initiatives transferring administrative responsibility to Indian/Inuit communities reflect growing federal recognition that health services must be designed and delivered by Aboriginal people. These arrangements do not satisfy all concerns, however; the needs of Aboriginal people in urban centres remain to be addressed, for example, as do issues of jurisdiction and control.

The Round Table will bring together federal and provincial policy developers, representatives of national health and social development organizations, and others with expertise in health and community development to analyze where change is needed and why progress in implementing recommendations has been so slow.

Over the three days of the Round Table, participants will be able to consider several fundamental questions about Aboriginal concepts of health and how these can be reflected in services delivered in their communities, in remote and northern areas, and by non-Aboriginal institutions. The issues will be elaborated through presentation of discussion papers and examples/models of health-related initiatives in several Aboriginal communities. Participants will be asked to consider what changes in policy and practice are necessary, to identify obstacles to change in communities, institutions and governments, and to suggest concrete measures to remove these roadblocks in moving toward health for all.

Goal of the Round Table

The Round Table will facilitate discussion on changes to health care and maintenance which are more holistic. All stakeholders in achieving health for Aboriginal Peoples will be challenged to overcome barriers to substantive change. The Round Table is founded upon the analysis and recommendations of previous inquiries and will provide an opportunity to consolidate valuable information that may be used in the formulation of practical solutions.

A report will be produced to synthesize and analyze discussion at the Round Table and develop a series of questions to help guide future direction in health. Daily summaries of the discussion will also be available to participants. The results of Round Table discussions will contribute to the development of the Royal Commission's final recommendations.

Round Table Advisers

Jean Goodwill, Saskatchewan Indian Federated Colleges (Saskatchewan) and President, Canadian Society for Circumpolar Health

Patrick Johnston, Executive Director, Canadian Council on Social Development (Ottawa)

Dr. Louis T. Montour, Medical Director, Kateri Memorial Hospital (Kahnawake, Quebec)

William Mussell, Sal'I'Shan Institute (British Columbia)

Round Table Participants

Round Table participants were invited to attend based on the following criteria:

1. Participants, from both the Aboriginal and non-Aboriginal communities, who are expert and knowledgable in the area of health and social issues.
2. Those who have experience in the creation and implementation of systems of health and social issues for Aboriginal people.
3. A balance of gender, age and Aboriginal identification was sought.

Fundamental Questions

Question 1

What are the traditional/spiritual understandings of health and healing held by Aboriginal peoples?

Question 2

What is preventing the application of holistic community health strategies in critical situations such as youth suicide, family violence, addictions and other serious ills?

Question 3

What are some of the successful models for Aboriginal communities to take responsibility for the design and delivery of health and social services? What other approaches besides the administrative transfer model could be considered? What are the advantages and disadvantages of various models?

Question 4

How will community control and the recognition of treaty rights to health affect health care and maintenance?

Question 5

How can law, policy and funding arrangements be changed to respond better to holistic health programming for Aboriginal peoples?

Question 6

How can health care be improved for Aboriginal people living in remote and northern areas? For Aboriginal persons with disabilities? Where are the obstacles?

Question 7

Where Aboriginal health services continue to be delivered by non-Aboriginal institutions, what adjustments need to be made in service delivery? What policies should be implemented by governments to ensure that hospitals, health centres, social services, etc. make the required changes? How can training institutes assist in recognizing the value of traditional approaches to health?

Question 8

How can the supply of Aboriginal health care and social service workers be increased? What are the barriers to entry of Aboriginal people into these careers? How can the barriers be removed? What are the features of successful program initiatives and strategies in education for Aboriginal students? Who should take the needed steps?

National Round Table on Aboriginal Health and Social Issues

Program

TUESDAY, MARCH 9, 1993

19:00 - 21:00
Registration

DAY 1
WEDNESDAY, MARCH 10, 1993

7:30 - 8:30
Registration

8:30 - 8:50
Round Table Opening

Call to Order
Dr. Louis T. Montour, Round Table Chairman

Opening Prayer
Elder Glen Douglas

Welcoming Comments
Frank Rivers, Squamish Nation
Georges Erasmus and Judge René Dussault
Co-Chairs, Royal Commission

8:50 - 9:00
Outline of Day 1 Agenda and Objectives and Introduction of Panel

Dr. Louis T. Montour, Round Table Chairman

DAY 1
WEDNESDAY, MARCH 10, 1993

9:00 - 10:00
Panel Presentation Of Discussion Papers

Discussion Paper A
Background paper on current trends in Aboriginal health as well as a consolidation of recommendations in previous reports and the extent of their implementation.
John O'Neil

Discussion Paper B
The maintenance of health, emphasizing the shift from medical/treatment model to more promotion and prevention and the need to find an acceptable balance.
Rosemary Proctor (presented by Karen Ginsberg)

Discussion Period

Moderator: Dr. Jay Wortman

10:00 - 10:15
Break

10:15 - 12:00
Panel of Elders

Traditional understandings of Indian, Métis, Inuit health and healing held by Aboriginal peoples with a discussion of holistic community health approaches.
Questions and Answers

Moderator: Marlene Brant Castellano

12:00 - 13:30
Luncheon Keynote Speaker, Dr. Harriet Kuhnlein

Global Nutrition and the Holistic Environment of Indigenous Peoples

---

13:30 - 14:30
Panel Presentation Of Discussion Papers

Discussion Paper C
What are the root causes and precipitating factors in suicide? What is blocking the action required to deal with youth suicide in Aboriginal communities? How can we remove those barriers?
Dr. Clare Brant

Discussion Paper D
What is blocking the action required to deal with violence, specifically family violence, in Aboriginal communities? How can we remove those barriers?
Professor Emma LaRocque (presented by Jo-Ann Daniels)

Discussion Period

Moderator: Peter Ernerk

14:30 - 14:45
Break

DAY 1
WEDNESDAY, MARCH 10, 1993

14:45 - 16:45

Round Table I - Discussion of Fundamental Questions

What is preventing the application of holistic community health strategies to deal with critical situations such as youth suicide, family violence, addiction and other serious ills? How can we support holistic community health strategies to deal with critical situations? Why has this not been done? Who should take these steps?

Questions and Answers
Moderator: Dr. Jay Wortman

16:45 - 17:15

Plenary Session

Dr. Louis T. Montour, Round Table Chairman

17:15

Closing Prayer

Elder Glen Douglas

18:00 - 20:00

Reception

DAY 2
THURSDAY, MARCH 11, 1993

8:30

Day 2 Opening

Call to Order
Dr. Louis T. Montour, Round Table Chairman
Opening Prayer
Elder Glen Douglas
Outline of Day 2 Agenda and Objectives
Dr. Louis T. Montour, Round Table Chairman

DAY 2
THURSDAY, MARCH 11, 1993

8:45 - 10:15

Panel Presentation Of Four Community Social Initiatives

1. *Grand Lac Victoria Community*

An Algonquin project to restore the community's social/spiritual/physical and cultural health.

Presenter: **Richard Kistabish, Health Program Co-ordinator, Grand Lac Victoria Band Council**

2. *Métis Child and Family Services, Alberta*

An urban-based social service organization culturally sensitive to Métis.

Presenter: **Carolyn Pettifer, President and Founding Executive Director**

3. *Alkali Lake, British Columbia*

A dramatic reversal from widespread addictions to almost total sobriety.

Presenters: **Carol Howarth, Director of Social Services, and Fred Johnson/Joyce Johnson, Band Counsellor, Drug and Alcohol Programs**

4. *Atikamekw Health and Social Services Project*

Took control, developed, and implemented an integrated approach to health and social services for three Atikamekw communities, despite difficulty with provincial regulations and jurisdiction.

Presenter: **Louis Hanrahan, Former Director of Health and Social Services for the Conseil de la Nation Atikamekw**

Questions and Answers

Moderator: **Alwyn Morris**

10:15 - 10:30

Break

10:30 - 12:00

Panel Presentation Of Four Community Medical Initiatives

1. *Innuulitsivik Hospital and Social Services Centre, Midwifery, Povungnituk, Quebec*

The only Aboriginal midwifery program in Quebec. Initiated by and for the women from six Inuit communities.

Presenter: **Aani Tuluguk**

2. *Anishnabe Health, Toronto*

An urban-based health centre serving the Aboriginal population.

Presenters: **Priscilla George, President, and Barbara Nahwegahbow, Executive Director**

3. *Kateri Hospital, Kahnawake, Quebec*

A community-based hospital with emergency, chronic care and physiotherapeutic services.

Presenter: **Keith Leclaire, Director of Administration**

4. *Nuu Chah Nulth, British Columbia*

A tribal council's experience with the Medical Services Branch Transfer Initiative.

Presenter: **Richard Watts, Chairman**

Questions and Answers

Moderator: **Peter Ernerk**

DAY 2
THURSDAY, MARCH 11, 1993

12:00 - 13:30

Luncheon Keynote Speaker, Professor Robert Evans on Health Economics

---

13:30 - 14:45

Panel Presentation Of Discussion Papers

Discussion Paper E

How can programs, policies and funding arrangements be changed to respond better to holistic health challenges and health promotion?

Kim Scott

Discussion Paper F

What are some of the workable models that allow Aboriginal individuals/communities to take responsibility for health?

Bill Mussell

Discussion Paper G

How will community control of services and the recognition of treaty rights to health affect holistic strategies to maintain and restore health?

Alma Favel-King

Discussion Period

Moderator: Dr. Jay Wortman

14:45 - 16:45

Round Table II - Discussion of Fundamental Questions

Aboriginal communities and individuals are assuming greater responsibility for health. What policies can facilitate that process? What are the recommendations for implementing a holistic strategy?

Moderator: Alwyn Morris

16:45 - 17:45

Plenary Session

Chairman: Dr. Louis T. Montour, Round Table Chairman

17:30

Closing Prayer

Elder Glen Douglas

DAY 3
FRIDAY, MARCH 12, 1993

8:30

Day 3 Opening

Call to Order
Dr. Louis T. Montour

Opening Prayer
Elder Glen Douglas

Outline of Day 3 Agenda and Objectives
Dr. Louis T. Montour, Round Table Chairman

8:45 - 10:15

Panel Presentation of Discussion Papers

Discussion Paper H
How can health care be improved for Aboriginal people living in remote and northern areas?
Iris Allen and William Anderson

Discussion Paper I
How can health care be improved for Aboriginal people living with disabilities?
Brenda Sinclair

Discussion Paper J
Where Aboriginal health services continue to be delivered by non-Aboriginal institutions, what adjustments need to be made in service delivery to make it more culturally appropriate? What policies should be implemented by governments to ensure that hospitals, health centres, social services, etc. make the required changes? What changes would this imply in the way practitioners deliver Aboriginal health care? How can training institutions and professional bodies assist in recognizing the value of Aboriginal approaches to health?
Sharon Helin

Discussion Paper K
How do we increase the number of Aboriginal health care practitioners? What are the features of successful health care education programs? What prevents ongoing support for successful education strategies? What changes are required to ensure ongoing support of successful strategies?
Dianne Longboat (presented by Lynn Chabot)

Discussion Period

Moderator: Alwyn Morris

10:15 - 12:15

Round Table III – Discussion of Fundamental Questions

What are the roles and responsibilities of the health care partners in ensuring that non-Aboriginal institutions are responsive to Aboriginal health needs? In particular the specific needs of Aboriginal people living in remote and northern areas and Aboriginal people with disabilities? What are the obstacles that need to be overcome?

Questions and Answers

Moderator: Dr. Jay Wortman

DAY 3
FRIDAY, MARCH 12, 1993

12:15 - 12:45
Report from Rapporteur
Professor John O'Neil

12:45 - 13:00
Closing Prayer
Elder Glen Douglas

Round Table Participants and Observers

Elders

Jean Aquash, Onoway, Alberta

Norman Chartrand, Camperville, Manitoba

Glen Douglas, Keremeos, British Columbia

Daisy Watt, Kuujjuaq, Quebec

Chairman

Dr. Louis T. Montour, Medical Director, Kateri Memorial Hospital, Kahnawake, Quebec

Advisers

Jean Goodwill, SIFC, Fort Qu'Appelle, Saskatchewan

Patrick Johnston, Executive Director, Canadian Council on Social Development

Dr. Louis T. Montour, Medical Director, Kateri Memorial Hospital, Kahnawake, Quebec

William Mussell, Sal'I'Shan Institute

Rapporteur

Professor John O'Neil, Department of Community Health Sciences, University of Manitoba

Keynote Speakers

Dr. Harriet Kuhnlein, Director, Centre for Nutrition and the Environment of Indigenous Peoples, McGill University

Professor Robert Evans, Department of Economics, University of British Columbia

Moderators

Peter Ernerk, Executive Director, Inuit Cultural Institute

Alwyn Morris, Policy Adviser, Federal/Provincial Relations Office, government of Canada

Dr. Jay Wortman, AIDS and STDs, Health and Welfare Canada

Community – Social

Louis Hanrahan, Former Director, Health and Social Services, Conseil de la Nation Atikamekw

Richard Kistabish, Aide-Conseil à la Coordination, Val d'Or, Quebec

Carolyn Pettifer, President and Founding Executive Director, Métis Child and Family Services

Community – Health

Priscilla George, President, Anishnawbe Health Toronto/ Barbra A. Nahwegahbow, Executive Director

Keith Leclaire, Director of Auxiliary Services, Kateri Memorial Hospital, Kahnawake, Quebec

Aani P. Tulugak, Innuulitsivik Hospital and Social Services Centre, Povungnituk, Quebec

Richard Watts, Chairman, Nuu-chah-nulth Tribal Council, Port Alberni, British Columbia

Authors

Iris Allen, Labrador Inuit Health Commission, North West River, Labrador

Dr. Clare Brant, Shannonville, Ontario

Sharon Helin, Sharon Helin & Associates

Alma Favel King, Director of Health, Federation of Saskatchewan Indian Nations

Dianne Longboat, Aboriginal Student Services, University of Toronto

William Mussell, Sal'I'Shan Institute

Kim Scott, Senior Policy Analyst, Royal Commission on Aboriginal Peoples

Brenda Joy Sinclair, Alberta Indian Health Care Commission

Professor John O'Neil, Department of Community Health Sciences, University of Manitoba

Rosemary Proctor, Deputy Minister, Ministry of Community and Social Services, Ontario

Professor Emma LaRocque, Department of Native Studies, University of Manitoba

Aboriginal Organizations

Marianne Demmer, Inuit Tapirisat of Canada

Sheila D. Genaille, President, Métis National Council of Women

Ron George, President, Native Council of Canada

Roda Grey, Health Coordinator, Pauktuutit, Inuit Women's Association

Mark Gryba, Métis National Council

Richard Jock, Director of First Nations Health Commission, Assembly of First Nations

Martha Montour, National Coordinator, Native Women's Association of Canada

Conrad Saulis, Director, Health and Social, Native Council of Canada

Federal Government Representatives

Mike Sims, Director General, Program Policy, Indian Affairs, Department of Indian Affairs and Northern Development

Marie Fortier, Acting Assistant Deputy Minister, Medical Services Branch, Health and Welfare Canada

Provincial/Territorial Government Representatives

Nova Scotia/New Brunswick
Stephen Chase, Director, Federal-Provincial Relations, Department of Health and Community Services

Newfoundland
Primrose Bishop, Assistant Deputy Minister, Department of Health

Quebec
Huguette Sauvageau, Chargée de programmes, Ministère de la santé et des services sociaux

Ontario
Carrie Hayward, Aboriginal Health Coordinator, Ontario Ministry of Health

Manitoba
Pete Sarsfield, Director, Health and Wellness Branch, Department of Health

Saskatchewan
Lynn Minja, Special Projects Officer, Department of Health

Alberta
Dr. Lynn Hewitt, Director, Research and Planning, Alberta Health and Welfare

British Columbia
Marnie Dobell, Acting Director of Policy, Ministry of Health

Northwest Territories
Elaine Berthelet, Assistant Deputy Minister, Department of Health

Other Participants

Dr. Yvon Allard, St. Boniface, Manitoba

Dr. Irwin Antone, South West Middlesex Health Centre

Dr. Judy Bartlett, Medical Services Branch, Health and Welfare Canada

Charlene Belleau, Canim Lake Band

Lea Bill, Siksika Lodge Treatment Centre

Professor Carol Brown, Native Access Program

Lynn Chabot, Community Projects Assistant, Kitigan Zibi Anishnabeg

Dr. Roland Chrisjohn, Professor, Department of Psychology, University of Guelph

Dr. Ed Connors, Sacred Circle, Ojibway Tribal Family Services

Catherine Cook, Associate Director, J.A. Hildes Northern Medical Unit, University of Manitoba

Dr. Marlyn Cox, Native Physicians Association of Canada

Jo-Ann Daniels, Executive Trustee of Otpemisiwak

Lou H. Demerais, Executive Director, Vancouver Native Health Society

Dr. Chris Derocher, Canadian Medical Association

Madeleine Dion Stout, Director, Aboriginal Education Research and Culture, Carleton University

Norman Evans, President, Pacific Métis Federation

Dr. Margo S. George, Research and Project Coordinator, Canadian Medical Association

Jane Gottfriedson, President, Aboriginal Women's Council

Eric Gourdeau, Comité de santé mentale du Québec

Wayne C. Helgason, Executive Director, Ma Mawi Wi Chi Itata Centre Inc.

H. Philip Hepworth, Director, Information Training Cost Shared Program, Health and Welfare Canada

Maggie Hodgson, Executive Director, Nechi Institute on Alcohol and Drugs

Carol Howorth, Director of Social Services, Alkali Lake Indian Band

John Hucker, Secretary General, Canadian Human Rights Commission

Barbara Louis, Secretary/Treasurer, Alberta Indian Health Care Commission

Professor David Lynes, Lakehead University

Clare McNab, Assistant Coordinator of the National Native Access Program to Nursing, University of Saskatchewan

Dr. Michael Monture, Native Physicians Association of Canada

Joan Moore, Director Health and Social Services, Conseil de la Nation Atikamekw

Judy Moses, Director, Aboriginal Services, Ministry of Health, Province of British Columbia

David Newhouse, Associate Professor, Trent University

Norbert Prefontaine, Consultant, Canadian Society for International Health

Chief Katie Rich, Mushuau Innu Band Council, Davis Inlet

Marilyn Sark, President, Aboriginal Nurses Assoc. of Canada

Conrad Saulis, Native Council of Canada

Helene Sioui-Trudel, Coordinator, National Indian and Inuit Community Health Representative Organization

Isaac Sobol, Chairman, CPHA Rural Health Division, Canadian Public Health Association, Family Physician and Medical Officer of Health, Nisga's Valley Health Board

James "Smokey" Tomkins, President, National Aboriginal Network on Disability

Dr. Vincent F. Tookenay, President, Native Physicians Association

Russell J. Willier, High Prairie, Alberta

Darlene Yellow Old Woman, Director, Treaty 7 Zone, Medical Services Branch

Dr. David E. Young, Studies in Traditional Medicine, University of Alberta, Dept. of Anthropology

Thomas (Tuma) Young, Coordinator, Mi'Kmaq Aids Task Force

Observers

Pearl Alfred, Nimpkish Band, Alert Bay, British Columbia

Marie Anderson, Executive Director, Hey Way Noqu (Nlakapux Interior Salish)

Barbara Britton, Policy Analyst, Ministry of Aboriginal Affairs, Government of British Columbia

Harvey Brooks, Aboriginal Council of Surrey

Connie Campbell, Regional Director, Métis Child and Family Services

Dr. Roland Chamberland, Grand Lac Victoria

Donna Connors, Kenora, Ontario

Greg Coyes, Director, National Film Board — Studies I, Edmonton, Alberta

Diana Day, Employment Co-ordinator, AIMS Job Development/Urban Images

Linda Day, Executive Director, Healing our Spirit, B.C. First Nations AIDS Society

Kimberly-Ann Davey, Vancouver, British Columbia

Cynthia Desmeules-Bertolin, Lawyer, Métis National Council

Catherine M. Einarson, Vancouver, British Columbia

Bev Gabora, Program Policy Manager, Adult Care, Indian and Northern Affairs Canada

Ken Goodwill, Band Council Member, Standing Buffalo Reservation

Rosaline Heinel, N.W. Angle #33 Band, Surrey, British Columbia

Elaine Herbert, MSW Student, Shuswap, Vancouver, British Columbia

Rhea Joseph, Health Care Planning Consultant, Native Brotherhood of B.C.

Patricia E. Kelly, Vancouver, British Columbia

Paul Kyba, Assistant Regional Director, Operations-Indian Health Services, Medical Services Branch, Health and Welfare Canada

Gene Littlejohn, Dreamspeaker, AIMS Job Development

Walter Louyine, AIMS Job Development

Matthew McKay, AIMS Job Development

Tim Michel, Aboriginal Health Coordinator, U.R.B.A.N. Society

Harold Morin, Executive Director, Central Interior Native Health Society

Woodrow Morrison, Consultant (Haida), Kindaanq Saang Consulting

Wayne Negonabe,AIMS Job Development

Theresa Netsena, Coordinator, Aboriginal Women's Council

Gloria Nicolson, Executive Director, Professional Native Women's Association U.R.B.A.N. Society

Colleen Okeymou, Facilitator, Native Outreach Program

Earl Pelletier, Health Coordinator, Métis Society of Saskatchewan

Dwight Powless, Fort Coquitlam, British Columbia

Richard Powless, AFN Intervention Coordinator, Assembly of First Nations

Simon Read, Manager, Nuu-chah-nulth Health Board

Frank A. Rivers, Councillor, Squamish Nation Council

Peter Roberts, Grenfell Regional Health Services

Judith Ross, Chief, Policy Development, Health and Welfare Canada

Grace Sanchez, Communications Officer, Statistics Canada

Josephine Sandy, Chairman of the Board, Ojibway Tribal Family Services

Albert Scott, Vice-Chair, Health and Social Services, F.S.I.N. (Kinistin Band)

Seis'Lom, Life Skills Counsellor, Allied Indian and Metis Society Job Development Program

Anne Sheffield, Assistant Deputy Minister, Health, Yukon Territorial Government

Robert Simon, Board of Directors, Urban Images for Native Women

Angela Slaughter, Liaison Office, Department of Indian and Northern Affairs

Dan Smith, President, United Native Nations of B.C.

Michel Smith, Program Development Consultant, S.S.P.B. – Health and Welfare Canada

George Speck, Assistant Band Manager, Nimpkish Band

Debbie Tattrie, Policy Adviser, Medical Services Branch, Health and Welfare Canada

Viola Thomas, Publications Coordinator/Field Worker, Legal Services Native Programs

Gordon Tootoosis, Albion, British Columbia

Dino Trakostanec, Dream Speaker, AIMS Job Development

Marilyn Van Bibber, Private Consultant, Delta, British Columbia

Nancy Van Heest, Researcher, Aboriginal Women's Council

Ernie Voyageur, Mathematics Instructor, North Island College

Gina Whiteduck, Senior Adviser, Child Welfare, Assembly of First Nation

Daniel Whetung, Native Health Division, Ministry of Health, Government of British Columbia

Kim Williams, Administration Officer, Ministry of Aboriginal Affairs, Government of British Columbia

Connie Willier, NNADAP Counsellor

Yvonne Willer, Owner, Moostoos Arts and Crafts

Royal Commission Staff

Marie Bergeron
Jerome Berthelette
Myrtle Bush
Marlene Brant Castellano
Karen Collins
Jim Compton
Dara Culhane
Deborah Hanley
Karen Ginsberg
Mel Maracle
Hugh McCullum
Becky Printup

For further information:
Royal Commission on Aboriginal Peoples
P.O. Box 1993, Station B
Ottawa, Ontario
K1P 1B2

Telephone: (613) 943-2075
Facsimile: (613) 943-0304

Toll-free:
1-800-363-8235 (English, French, Chipewyan)
1-800-387-2148 (Cree, Inuktitut, Ojibwa)